Ultrasound-Guided Liver Surgery

Guido Torzilli
Editor

Ultrasound-Guided Liver Surgery

An Atlas

Springer

Editor
Guido Torzilli
Department of Hepatobiliary Surgery
Humanitas Research Hospital—IRCCS
University of Milan, School of Medicine
Rozzano, Milano
Italy

ISBN 978-88-470-5832-3 ISBN 978-88-470-5510-0 (eBook)
DOI 10.1007/978-88-470-5510-0
Springer Milan Heidelberg New York Dordrecht London

Softcover reprint of the hardcover 1st edition 2014

Printed on acid-free paper

Springer is part of Springer Science+Business Media (www.springer.com)

To my family, to my Masters, and to all the colleagues who feel a passion for what they do for the benefit of their patients

Foreword

Liver resection had been carried out since before World War II. However, Ichio Honjo and Lortat-Jacob's successful right liver resection by ways of controlled method after the war established the era of right liver resection, left liver resection and left lobe resection (S2 + S3 resection) from the 1950s to the 1970s.

Then came the end of the 1970s, and the introduction of intraoperative ultrasound had suddenly enabled detection of small tumors within the liver which until then was not possible to locate from the surface of the liver either palpatively or visually. Stereo visualization of the positional relationship of the vessels and the tumors, and identification of tumor thrombus in the vessels and intrahepatic metastases were realized. Radical resections of deeply situated tumors were made possible, segmentectomy/subsegmentectomy with the use of intraoperative ultrasound-guided puncture technique was introduced, and the liver can now be transected while exposing the main hepatic vein running between the segments within the liver. All these are the fruits brought about by the technological advancement of intraoperative ultrasound during 1980s up to 2010.

Doctor Guido Torzilli first came to visit me at the beginning of 1990s when I was holding a position of professorship at the Shinshu University. He had been an avid learner from the beginning, with a stern, uncompromising and reliable characteristic that I had no reservations in offering Dr. Torzilli the position of research assistant, when I moved to the University of Tokyo in 1994. At the end of his one-year study, he submitted a thesis and was awarded a doctorate from the University of Tokyo. He has always been a skillful surgeon and a prolific writer who does not hesitate to share his knowledge through publishing his works, and today, he is one of the few surgeons in Europe with reliable intraoperative ultrasound technique, whose surgical accomplishments are much acknowledged around the world. Dr. Torzilli is also respected for his dedication in organizing European School of Surgical Ultrasound meetings every year since 2006.

Doctor Torzilli's new book *Ultrasound-guided Liver Surgery* covers every issue about intraoperative ultrasound in hepatobiliary surgery, from basic information on ultrasound, guidance on liver scanning procedure, liver evaluation according to its anatomical characteristics, intraoperative diagnosis and staging, contrast-enhanced ultrasonography, planning up of the surgical strategy, liver transplantation, laparoscopic ultrasound, intraoperative radiofrequency ablation, to ultrasound guidance in robotic surgery. This book is worth being owned by surgeons who wish to newly acquire what has now become the essential technique for a successful hepatobiliary surgery, and by the veterans to update their knowledge.

Masatoshi Makuuchi, MD, PhD
Professor Emeritus of the University of Tokyo
President of the Japanese Red Cross Medical Center

Foreword

In 1988, ultrasound was already an established diagnostic tool for abdominal diseases and was *per se* anyway a revolutionary advancement for a medical community used to consider the liver, the spleen, the pancreas, and the pelvic organs as a sort of unexplored world, "*hic sunt leones*", like it was named in the ancient maps. Still nowadays I feel emotion when I put the probe on the abdomen of a patient often solving, by doing this, his diagnostic problem. However, it was at that time that new applications of ultrasound started to be established too, such as guided punctures of organs, tumors, and collections. That year in November, while I was running a course on interventional ultrasound, GuidoTorzilli, who was getting the MD degree, came to visit me and wished to join my course. Although I was initially skeptical, his passion and willingness convinced me to accept his application: it was well-founded trust. Once gotten the MD degree, in a span of a few months he developed enough skill to become consultant in ultrasound in my hospital.

For some years I had been investigating the possibility to treat small liver tumor with percutaneous ethanol injection (PEI) [1]. Indeed, if it was possible to disclose a lesion, puncture it, and sample the tissue in real time, why should it have been unfeasible to inject something able to induce toxicity in it? The field of investigation was fascinating and potentially enormous. Was that therapeutic efficacy equal for primary or metastastic liver tumors? Was an eventual different therapeutic efficacy depending on the origin of the primary tumor? How much necrosis would have been achievable? Which morbidity? Guido was passionate too in that clinical research, and we wrote together the first report about 3-year survival of cirrhotic patients with hepatocellular carcinoma (HCC) and treated with PEI [2]. Data were surprising, with survival after PEI similar to results obtained with surgery: with that contribution a debate started about the role of surgery and ablation for liver tumors, which is still open.

However, Guido, despite his great interest for these new applications, had a dream: becoming a surgeon and specifically a hepato-biliary surgeon. Although disappointed, anyway I supported his design and I asked Professor Makuuchi to accept him in his Department as a visiting doctor: by that, the interventional ultrasound community was losing a potentially valuable member. However, we got in touch, having the chance to follow his training.

Meanwhile, many studies on PEI were published and the comparison with surgery became a source of deep discussions in the international meetings. In the mid 1990s, PEI started to be progressively substituted by thermal ablation [3]. This new tool demonstrated the ability to destroy a tumor in a few minutes, hence justifying randomized trials versus surgery for early HCC, which showed long-term outcome as similar despite the lower invasivity, and the limited costs of ablation. Moreover, at least for the tumors in a very early stage, we were able to prove that ablation could be somehow "surgical," justifying its affirmation as the gold standard approach for these particular subsets of patients [4]. However, although proud of that, the doubt that surgical results were biased by an inadequate way of facing the problem, with too extensive and risky hepatectomies, started growing in my mind.

That idea found its confirmation some years ago, when I had the chance again to share working experience with Guido, at the Humanitas Research Hospital in Milan. Accurate patient selection, "radiological" knowledge of the preoperative imaging, the absolute mastery of intraoperative ultrasound resulting in targeted resection of the liver, with low morbidty and mortality, although often referred to patients presenting high complexities, convinced me that surgery could play still a great role. As the French are used to saying: "Chapeau!" We share now the knowledge that ablation should be limited to small lesions and surgery offered to patients with more complex diseases, provided that the surgical team offers adequate expertise—expertise in which ultrasound plays a fundamental role and for which the need for an adequate training has to be accounted. From this perspective, this book is certainly unique, and for the richness of images and details about new techniques, it seems to me, although I am not a surgeon, a must-have for those who wish to get into the world of a new and modern concept of liver surgery guided by ultrasound.

Tito Livraghi, MD
Member Emeritus of the Italian Society of Ultrasound
Member Emeritus of the Italian Society of Radiology
Former Director Department of Radiology
Hospital of Vimercate
Vimercate, Milan
Italy

References

1. Livraghi T, Festi D, Monti F et al (1986) US-guided percutaneous alcohol injection of small hepatic and abdominal tumors. Radiology 161(2):309–312
2. Livraghi T, Bolondi L, Lazzaroni S et al (1992) Percutaneous ethanol injection in the treatment of hepatocellular carcinoma in cirrhosis. A study on 207 patients. Cancer 69(4):925–929
3. Livraghi T, Goldberg SN, Lazzaroni S et al (1999) Small hepatocellular carcinoma: treatment with radio-frequency ablation versus ethanol injection. Radiology 210(3):655–661
4. Livraghi T, Meloni F, Di Stasi M et al (2008) Sustained complete response and complications rates after radiofrequency ablation of very early hepatocellular carcinoma in cirrhosis: Is resection still the treatment of choice? Hepatology 47(1): 82–89

Preface

Milan, Italy, in autumn of 1984: a young student in his 3rd year of the 6-year curriculum at the School of Medicine, University of Milan, I had just started an internship at the 1st Surgical Department, chaired by Giuseppe Pezzuoli, where I met Jannis Spiropoulos from Greece. He was doing his residency in surgery, and with the eagerness of a person who had migrated to find a better life he had already picked up a considerable knowledge of ultrasound and was running a service for the department. Jannis trusted me and I could learn the basics of ultrasound from him. He became my first Master – in fact, without him this book would never have been written.

Then, shortly before graduation, late in 1988, I had the privilege to meet Tito Livraghi, worldwide recognized pioneer of interventional ultrasound and of ablation techniques for liver tumors, the most cited radiologist in the medical literature within the last 60 years: he became my mentor and taught me interventional ultrasound and ultimately I had the honor of co-authoring some important papers with him. He is my second Master, and in fact, without him this book would never have been written.

Having proven my firm intention to complete my residency in surgery, rather than becoming a radiologist, Livraghi introduced me to Masatoshi Makuuchi. I was still a resident in surgery, when in the summer of 1992 I travelled to Matsumoto, Japan, and had the honor to meet Professor Makuuchi in person, the worldwide recognized pioneer of modern liver surgery, living donor liver transplantation, and of intraoperative ultrasound: this encounter should definitely change my life. Having attained his sympathy he arranged for me a prestigious fellowship of the Foundation for the Promotion of Cancer Research, and employed me as Assistant Professor – with patience and trust he taught me to carry out liver surgery and most of the things that I write about in this book. Masatoshi Makuuchi has been my third Master, and truly, without him this book would never have been written.

From the year 2000, back in Italy, it was Natale Olivari who gave me the opportunity to start my own program of liver surgery in his Surgical Department at Lodi, a small town nearby Milan, and in 2004, Marco Montorsi offered me to continue that program at the University of Milan. In the last 15 years – from Tokyo to Milan and Lodi – I have worked passionately and met other inspiring personalities in my field who supported my program within the national and international surgical communities. Jacques Belghiti, with whom I have had the honor of organizing meetings around the world, has been particularly supportive and I cherish his strong appreciation and continued support, and am particularly grateful of being his friend. Gennaro Nuzzo and Lorenzo Capussotti offered their warm and friendly consideration as I returned to Italy from Japan – their support has helped me to become accepted, respected, and now well established within the Italian surgical community. Henri Bismuth then asked me to coauthor two book chapters with him, which I consider a particular honor.

But this book is also inspired by the many great surgeons and colleagues who I've had the privilege of meeting, sharing time and exchanging ideas with, many of which are now good friends, some having made valuable contributions to this book. All, in their own way, have helped with their trust and efforts and expertise.

My strongest appreciation goes to my beloved mother and my late father: a poor family of workers who always trusted me and always unconditionally supported my studies. Most importantly, the most important person in my life, my wife Chiara, a doctor like me, and mother of our three wonderful children, has provided everything to make this possible: my professional life (the clinic, the many meetings, and ... this book!) has stolen from them and from myself quite many days and nights. To them, I wholeheartedly address my love and recognition.

This book, in the complexity of its contents, is the result of the efforts, talents, and passion of my fellows and of friends who accepted to contribute with their expertise. It is a book focused on a way of interpreting surgery, from the simple act to the more complex procedures, as ready sequence of sophisticated maneuvers aimed to treat a disease, respecting the organ and respecting the patients and their lives: an approach and attitude which has been endowed on me by my master Masatoshi Makuuchi. I see it as part of my responsibilty to transmit such wisdom to my fellows, and I hope you will sense this between the lines. The readers, especially the younger readers, may possibly feel initially discouraged by the apparent high degree of complexity of the techniques and maneuvers. For them, I have recalled my personal encounters, which profoundly changed my life, and which I hope will draw out the importance of trust and passion, which feature each of those prominent stages and encounters in my own life....trust, being passionate, and breathing the passion of your masters...if even a glimpse of this is conferred to you by this book, it will already be worth all the effort and a reason to be proud of.

Guido Torzilli, MD, Ph.D, FACS

Contents

Part I Introductory Aspects

1 **Technological Requirements for Ultrasound-Guided Liver Surgery** . . . 3
Guido Torzilli, Fabio Procopio and Daniele Del Fabbro

2 **Technical Tricks to Start Exploring the Liver with Ultrasound** . . . 15
Guido Torzilli, Daniele Del Fabbro and Matteo Cimino

3 **Exploring the Liver by Ultrasound Along its Anatomy** . . . 25
Guido Torzilli, Guido Costa and Florin Botea

Part II Diagnosis and Staging

4 **Diagnosis and Staging: Intraoperative Ultrasound** . . . 43
Guido Torzilli, Matteo Donadon and Matteo Cimino

5 **Diagnosis and Staging: Contrast-Enhanced Intraoperative Ultrasound (CEIOUS) Using Intravascular Contrast Agents** . . . 55
Guido Torzilli, Matteo Donadon and Guido Costa

6 **Contrast-Enhanced Intraoperative Ultrasound Using Liver-Specific Contrast Agents** . . . 67
Junichi Arita and Norihiro Kokudo

Part III Hepatobiliary Surgery

7 **Planning of the Surgical Strategy** . . . 75
Guido Torzilli, Fabio Procopio and Guido Costa

8 **Resection Guidance** . . . 117
Guido Torzilli, Fabio Procopio and Guido Costa

9 Intraoperative Cholangio Ultrasound in the Study of the Biliary Tree 169
Guido Torzilli, Fabio Procopio and Angela Palmisano

Part IV Liver Transplantation

10 Liver Transplantation from Deceased Donors 185
Matteo Cescon, Fabio Piscaglia, Alessandro Cucchetti and Antonio Daniele Pinna

11 Liver Transplantation from Living Donors 209
Kiyoshi Hasegawa, Yasuhiko Sugawara and Norihiro Kokudo

Part V Minimally Invasive Surgery and Interventional Procedures

12 Laparoscopic Ultrasound: Impact in Liver Surgery 217
Alessandro Ferrero, Luca Viganò, Roberto Lo Tesoriere and Lorenzo Capussotti

13 Ultrasound-Guided Intraoperative Ablation Therapies. . . . 231
Roberto Santambrogio, Matteo Barabino and Enrico Opocher

14 Robotic Ultrasound-Guided Liver Resections. 249
Alberto Patriti, Marco Carlani and Luciano Casciola

15 Trends and Future Prospects in the Use of Ultrasound in Liver Surgery. 267
Guido Torzilli, Matteo Donadon and Matteo Cimino

Index 277

Part I
Introductory Aspects

Technological Requirements for Ultrasound-Guided Liver Surgery

1

Guido Torzilli, Fabio Procopio, and Daniele Del Fabbro

1.1 Basic Principles of Ultrasound

Ultrasound imaging is based on the 'pulse-echo' principle: a short burst of ultrasound is emitted from a transducer, directed into a tissue, and as consequence, part of the echoes produced by the interaction of sound with tissue are reflected back to the transducer. They are converted to electrical signals and sent to the ultrasound machine for being elaborated as images. Ultrasound, in practice, measures the mechanical properties of the tissue: indeed, tissues feature different acoustic impedance, which is the product of tissue density and ultrasound speed in passing through the tissue.

The key component of the transducer, whose function is to convert electrical impulses into ultrasound waves and vice versa, are the piezoelectric crystals, which change their shape once electricity and echoes are applied.

Image resolution is determined by the frequency at which ultrasound is emitted. However, higher frequencies are associated with higher absorption of the sound energy, therefore their utility in exploring deep structures is limited.

Among the basic features of ultrasound, the one that is of particular relevance for the surgeon is knowledge of the probe, since the latter, as further elaborated throughout this textbook, has to allow for different applications from unusual kinds of exploration to true ultrasound-guided surgical maneuvers with demanding peculiarities which also need to be taken into account.

1.2 The Probe

Probes are preferred that can be sterilized and can then stay in direct contact with the targeted organ. This may reduce eventual artefacts created by imperfect adhesion between the probe and the sterile cover of the ultrasound, even if a sufficient amount of gel has been applied for the purpose of avoiding air bubbles and for facilitating signal transmission. Nowadays, efficient systems are available for sterilizing intraoperative ultrasound (IOUS) probes, as, for instance, the hydrogen peroxide gas plasma technology (Sterrad; ASP, Rome, Italy).

High-frequency echoprobes (7.5–10 MHz) are commonly recommended to perform intraoperative ultrasound (IOUS), since, as mentioned, they allow a higher spatial resolution than those working at lower frequencies (2.5–5 MHz). The latter, at least up to the recent past, have played a role during the initial exploration providing a better panoramicity, which compensates the lower spatial resolution

G. Torzilli (✉) · F. Procopio · D. Del Fabbro
Department of Hepatobiliary Surgery,
Humanitas Research Hospital-IRCCS,
University of Milan-School of Medicine,
Via A. Manzoni 56, 20089 Rozzano, MI, Italy
e-mail: guido.torzilli@humanitas.it;
guido.torzilli@unimi.it

G. Torzilli (ed.), *Ultrasound-Guided Liver Surgery*,
DOI: 10.1007/978-88-470-5510-0_1, © Springer-Verlag Italia 2014

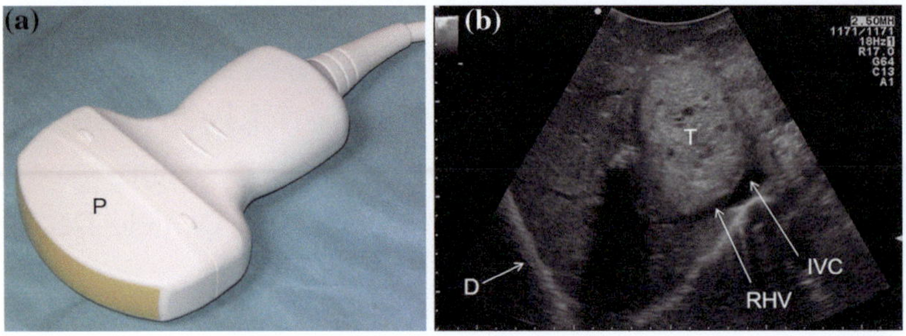

Fig. 1.1 **a** A convex probe for percutaneous exploration, used intraoperatively for an initial overview, and for cases where an improved panoramicity of the exploration is needed. Particular features: relatively low frequency, possibility to depict deep structures though loosing in spatial resolution; **b** A convex-probe scan: one scan reveals a tumor (*T*) in the liver, right hepatic vein (*RHV*), retrohepatic inferior vena cava (*IVC*), and diaphragm (*D*)

(Fig. 1.1a, b). However, it should be pointed out that a higher spatial resolution at the superficial portion of the liver would often be less important than the overall visibility of the deeper structures, since the most superficial portions are also palpable and can be inspected visually, both indeed still being fundamental steps of liver exploration [1]. In the latter situation, once a nodule is slightly visible at IOUS but is not palpable especially in a cirrhotic liver, a glove filled with deaerated sterile water can be positioned between the probe and the liver surface for better visualization of the lesion itself (Fig. 1.2): standoff pads are commercially available for the same purpose. Similarly, water can fill the resection area to check its status and moreover excluding the presence of the residual tumor (Fig. 1.3). Lower-frequency echoprobes, as described below, are also useful for allowing contrast-enhanced IOUS (CEIOUS). Therefore, having both lower- and higher-frequency probes would be the best solution: new probes with a wider range of frequencies (3–11 MHz) are now available (Fig. 1.4a–d).

A crucial point to be evaluated while selecting a probe is its shape and volume. Indeed, an optimal probe should represent the best compromise between the size, which should be small to allow its handling in deep and narrowed spaces, and the ultrasonographic scanning window, which should be large enough to provide a widest possible area of exploration in a single

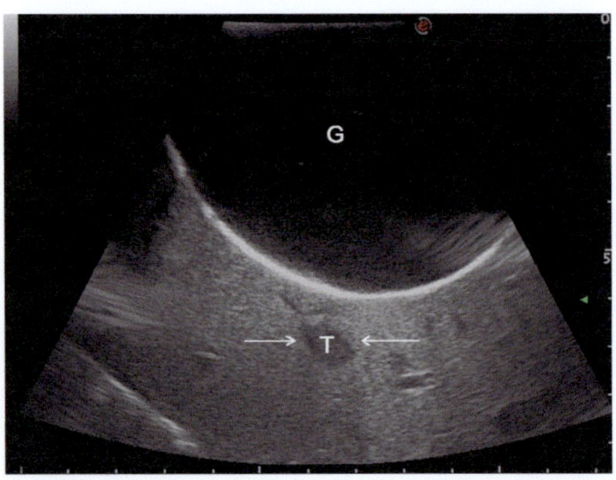

Fig. 1.2 For better exploration of the superficial structures, a glove filled with deaerated water (*G*) is positioned between the probe and the targeted surface; *arrows* indicate a small lesion (*T*)

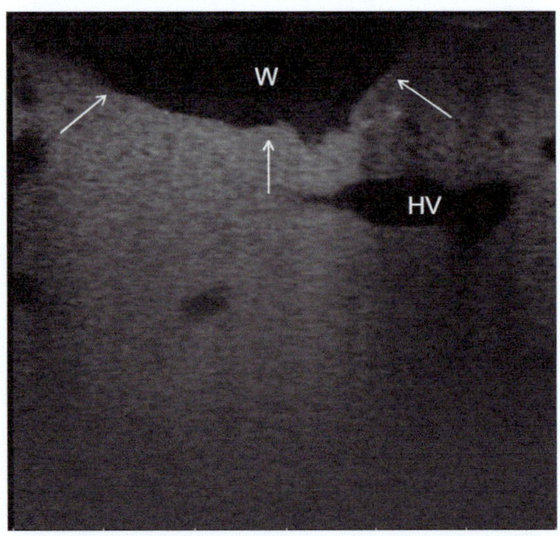

Fig. 1.3 The cut surface (*arrows*) can be explored by filling the cavity with deaerated water (*W*); hepatic vein (*HV*)

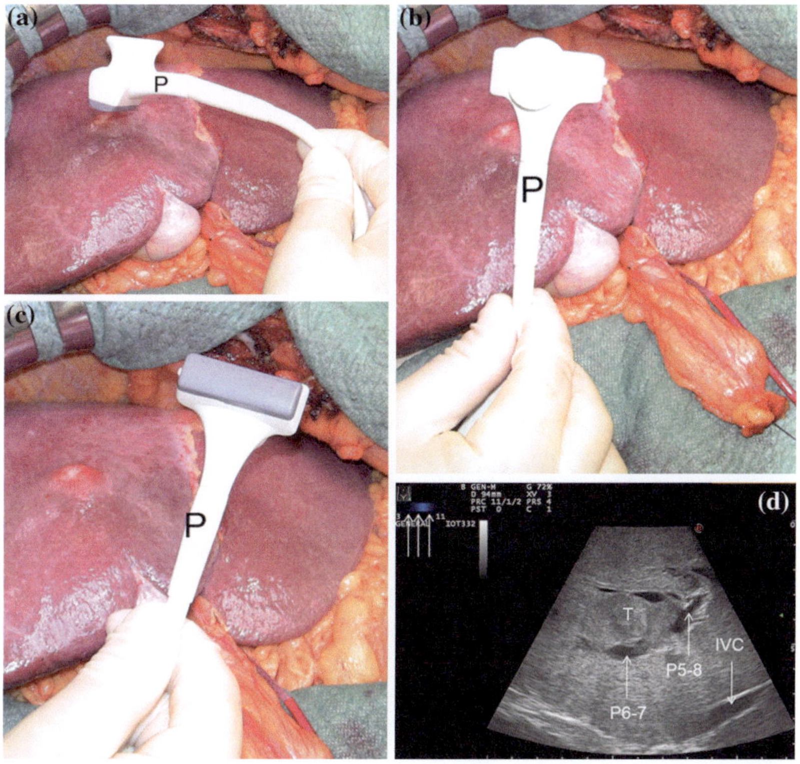

Fig. 1.4 Profile (**a**), dorsal (**b**), and scanning side (**c**) of a micro-T-shaped linear echoprobe (Esaote SpA, Genova, Italy) designed for surgical maneuvers, featuring a trapezoid scanning window and a wide (3–11 MHz) range of frequencies (*arrows*) (**d**); tumor (*T*); portal branch to segments 5 and 8 (*P5-8*); portal branch to segments 6 and 7 (*P6-7*); inferior vena cava (*IVC*)

view; the adherence to the surface of the target organ should be high enough for enabling an adequate stability along its handling and for avoiding gas interposition, reducing the number of possible artefacts in organ exploration. The most frequently used probes are T-shaped with linear (Fig. 1.5a, b) or convex scanning head (Fig. 1.6a, b), interdigital (Fig. 1.7a, b), and microconvex (Fig. 1.8a, b). The microconvex probe provides the best solution regarding the aforementioned desirable criteria. Indeed, the T-shaped probe, while remaining more stable and being associated with higher image resolution, has a lower ratio between lateral length and ultrasonographic scanning window than the microconvex one. Linear transducers, with enlarged scanning windows, have more recently become available (trapezoid scanning window): these combine the stability of the linear probes and their higher image resolution with larger scanning windows and a limited volume (Figs. 1.4a–d, 1.9a, b). Another aspect to be considered in evaluating a probe is whether it can be used for surgical maneuvers as those described in Chap. 8 for which the echoprobe is acting as a kind of surgical instrument (see Fig. 1.10a–c).

Another important feature of probes to be considered is whether they allow to survey eventual interventional maneuvers, such as puncturing targets within the liver, e.g., vessels, nodules, and areas which are to be reached along the dissection. Adapters can be coupled to the probe (Fig. 1.11), or the probes themselves can be designed for that purpose on an intraoperative setting. For instance, there are biplanar probes which combine two scanning surfaces working on different axes which can be useful to help

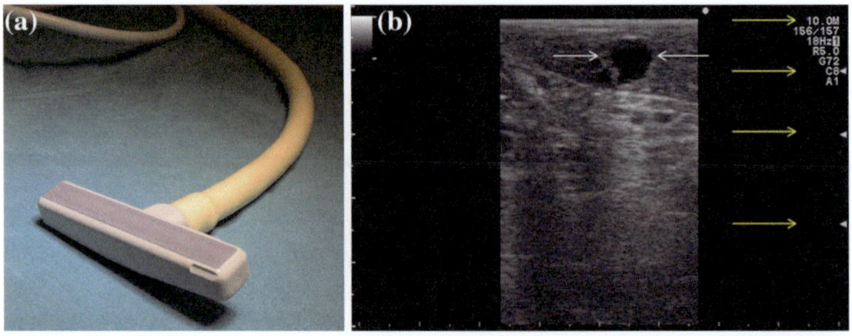

Fig. 1.5 **a** The scanning side of a T-shaped linear echoprobe (Hitachi-Aloka Medical; Tokyo, Japan); **b** the scanning area is also disclosed and a small lesion (cyst) is shown: this high-frequency echoprobe (5–10 MHz) is featured by a high resolution but a low power of ultrasound penetration, which means relatively limited panoramicity. The *yellow arrows* indicate from top to bottom the frequency at which it is working in that precise moment (10 MHz) and the three focal levels

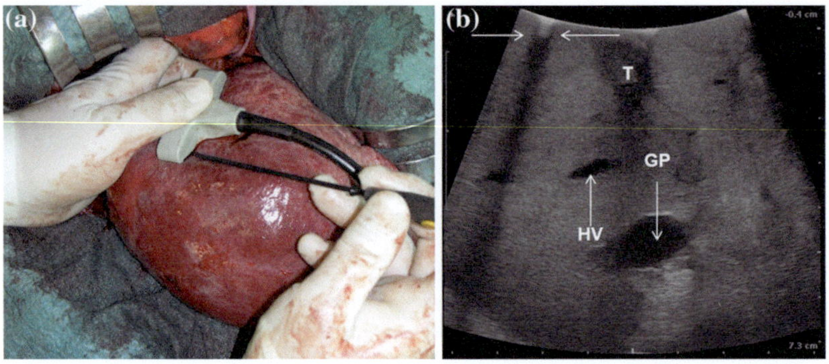

Fig. 1.6 **a** The scanning side of a T-shaped convex echoprobe (BK Medical APS, Peabody MA, USA) with an electrocautery positioned between the liver and the probe; **b** the scanning area is also disclosed and a small lesion (*T*) is shown together with the posterior echo (*arrows*) generated by the tip of the electrocautery; glissonian pedicle (*GP*); hepatic vein (*HV*)

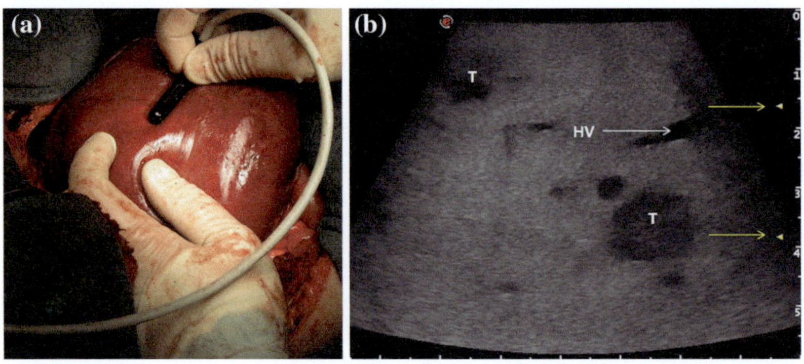

Fig. 1.7 **a** A interdigital linear echoprobe (Esaote SpA, Genova, Italy); **b** the trapezoid scanning area is also disclosed and two lesions (*T*) are shown. *Yellow arrows* indicate the two focal levels; hepatic vein (*HV*)

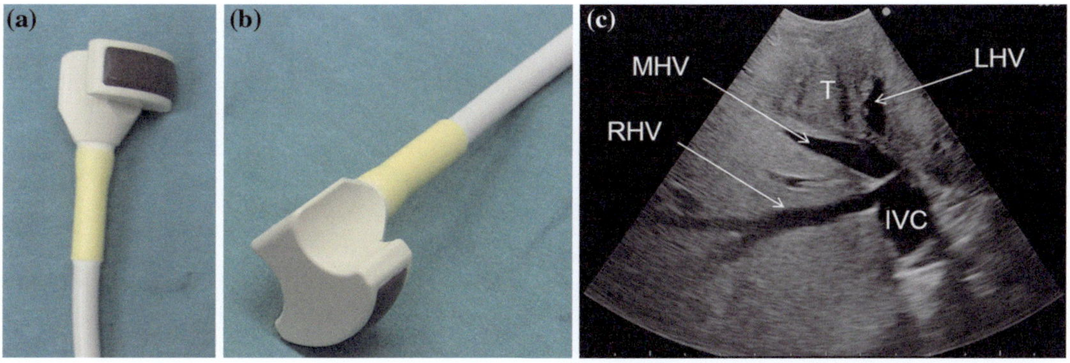

Fig. 1.8 The scanning side (**a**) and opposite side (**b**) of a microconvex echoprobe (Hitachi-Aloka Medical; Tokyo, Japan). The scanning area is also disclosed (**c**) the wide-frequency-range echoprobe (2–7 MHz) in one scan shows the liver with a tumor (*T*)—right (*RHV*), middle (*MHV*), and left (*LHV*) hepatic veins are recognizable; inferior vena cava (*IVC*)

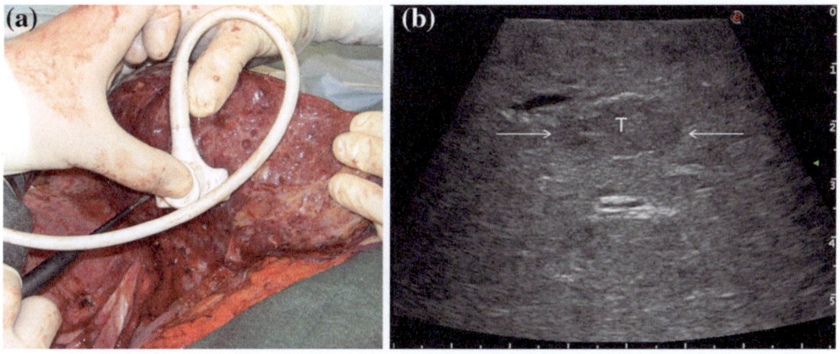

Fig. 1.9 An intraoperative micro-T-shaped linear probe (Esaote SpA, Genova, Italy) (**a**). Featuring a trapezoidal scanning window (**b**). This probe combines the stability of a linear transducer and the wideness of the scanning window of a convex probe. It was designed also for allowing ultrasound-guided compressions maneuvers (see Chap. 8); tumor (*T*)

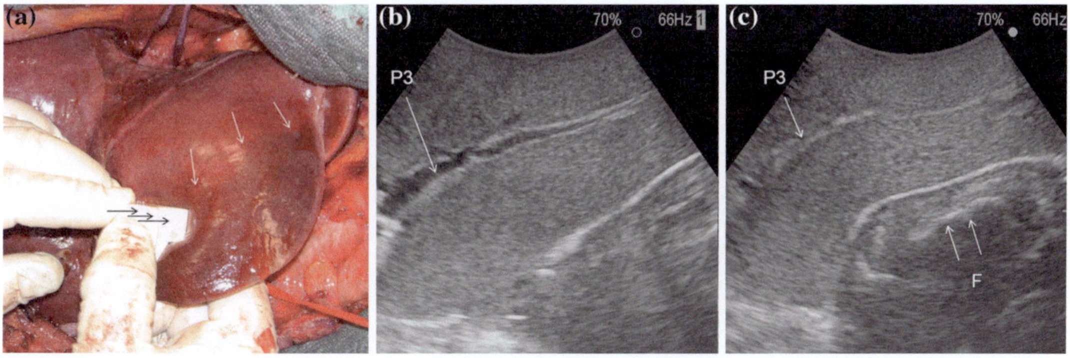

Fig. 1.10 **a** The simultaneous compression of the liver by the surgeon's fingertip and the probe for generating segmental transient ischemia and consequent change of color of that part; **b** this is obtained by selecting with IOUS the feeding glissonean pedicle (*P3*, in this case, since it is feeding segment 3); **c** once selected, the compression as shown in (**a**) is applied simultaneously using probe and fingertip (*F*)

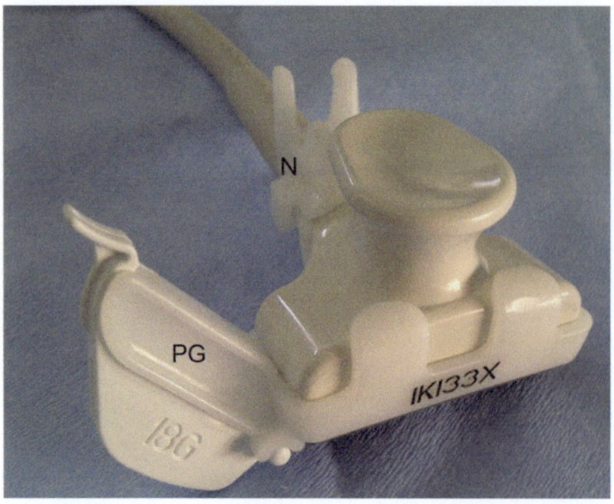

Fig. 1.11 A probe allocating the device for puncture guidance (*PG*) and for the navigation system (*N*) (see Chap. 15)

drive the needle to the target following its trajectory on two planes (Fig. 1.12).

1.3 Laparoscopic and Robotic Probes

Peculiar aspects of ultrasound probes used in laparoscopic exploration of the liver are to be separately addressed here.

Currently, laparoscopic transducers are available in several configurations that can fit through the 10-mm laparoscopic port. The simplest transducer configuration is the rigid, linear array. This transducer has a light-weight 10-mm-diameter shaft in which the distal 4 cm contain a linear-array transducer with a field of view of up to 90°. Such probes usually operate in the frequency range of 5–10 MHz and provide both excellent near-field visualization and resolution to a depth of 10 cm. The main advantage of such transducers is the large blunt shape that allows to substantially lift and manipulate the tissues and works best for organs with large flat surfaces, such as the liver. With these probes the liver can be explored in vertical direction (Fig. 1.13a), and also laterally by tilting the probes on their main axis (Fig. 1.13b). However, having a rigid shaft, they need to be placed in different laparoscopic sites for varying their scanning areas laterally, and moreover they cannot follow the curvature of the organ in its upper segments, which drastically limits their field of exploration.

In the newer configuration, the laparoscopic transducer is incorporated into a flexible tip with hidden cables controlled by knobs provided at

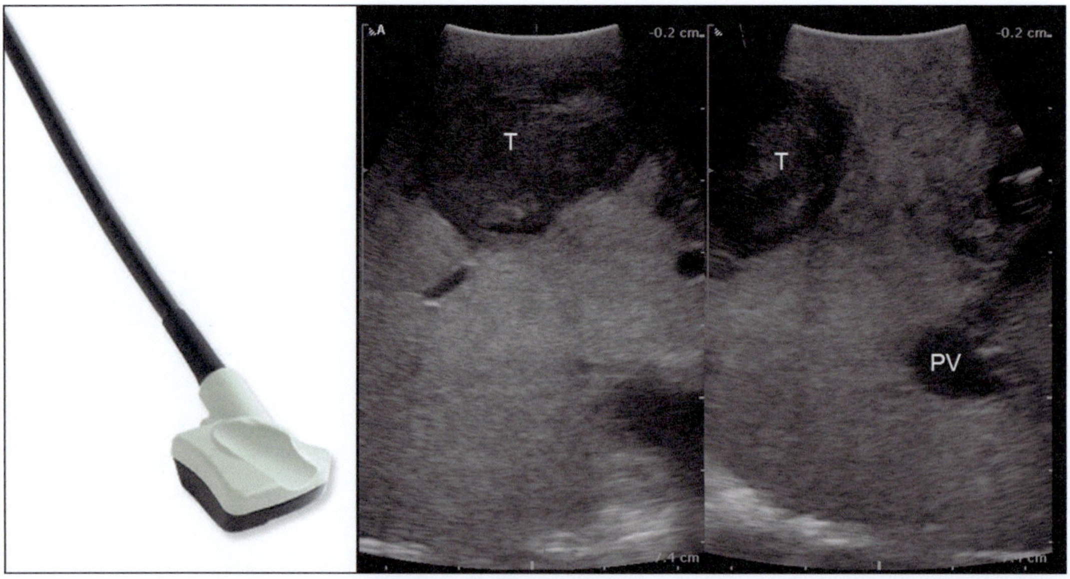

Fig. 1.12 (*left*) a biplanar probe (BK Medical APS, Peabody MA, USA); (*right*) the related images demonstrating a tumor observed in two different planes; tumor (*T*); portal vein (*PV*)

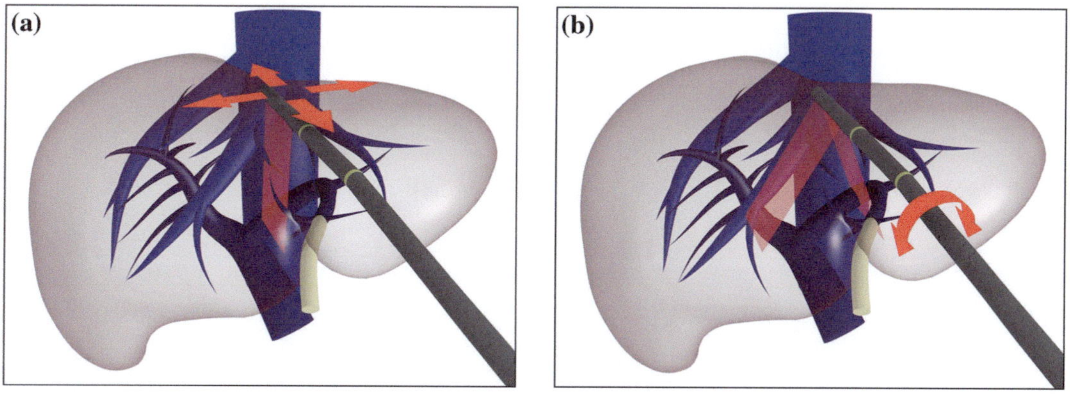

Fig. 1.13 The movement modalities of a rigid laparoscopic probe keeping a perpendicular (**a**) and an oblique (**b**) scanning

the proximal end of the shaft (Fig. 1.14a–c). The transducer can be flexed in one or two axes allowing the examination of a given structure in transverse and longitudinal views without need to be moved in different trocars. Furthermore, these probes can follow the curvature of the liver making feasible its exploration also for the upper segments (Fig. 1.15). Such laparoscopic ultrasound (LUS) probes operate at frequencies of 5–10 MHz and can be equipped with linear or convex arrays (Fig. 1.16a, b). As for the open exploration, this latter provides a wider field of view and works best for organs with curved surfaces where only a limited surface contact is possible, being more stable than the similar IOUS probe but conveying, as for any laparoscopic probe, the drawback of less adherence to the surface of the targeted organ than the one used for IOUS. The flexible probe ranges from 35 to 50 mm in length and 10 mm in diameter, which facilitates its insertion through the standard laparoscopic trocar.

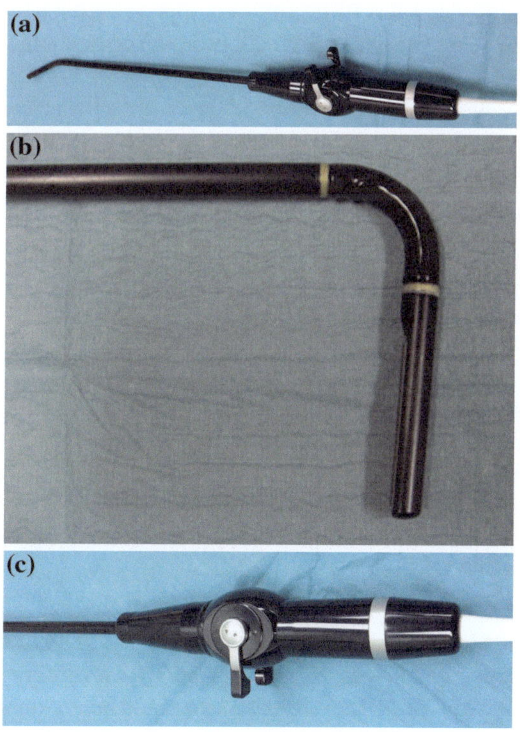

Fig. 1.14 **a** A flexible laparoscopic probe (Hitachi-Aloka Medical; Tokyo, Japan); **b** details of the flexible tip and **c** knobs

The newer LUS probes are also equipped to provide color-Doppler and power-Doppler functions and also enabling laparoscopic use of contrast agents.

More recently, robotic liver surgery probes (see Chap. 12) dedicated to this use have become available. They feature a cable as probe for open IOUS (indeed usable with this approach), and a particular grip to allow coupling with the forceps used in the robotic setting (Fig. 1.17).

1.4 The Ultrasound System

Ultrasound systems in a surgical environment should be easy to handle, i.e., movable, with articulated connections allowing independent

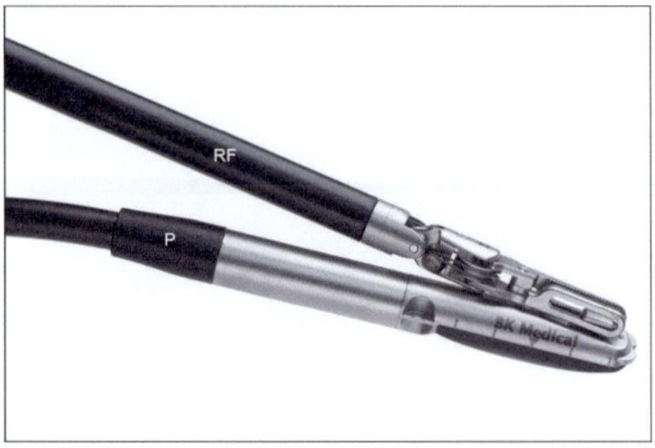

Fig. 1.17 A convex probe (BK Medical APS, Peabody MA, USA) (*P*) for robotic approach having a grip for handling by forceps designed for robotic use (*RF*)

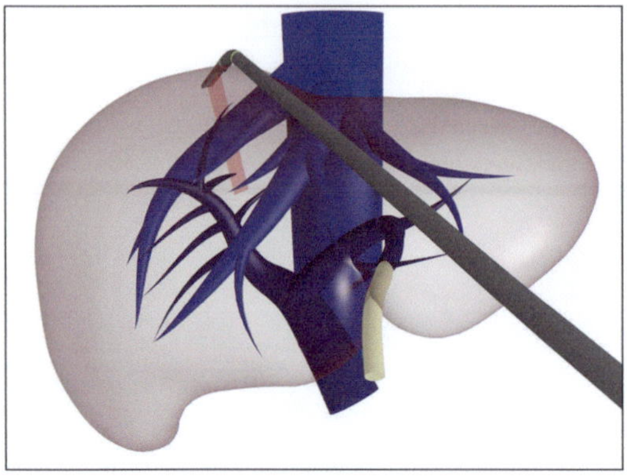

Fig. 1.15 The scanning modality of a flexible laparoscopic probe

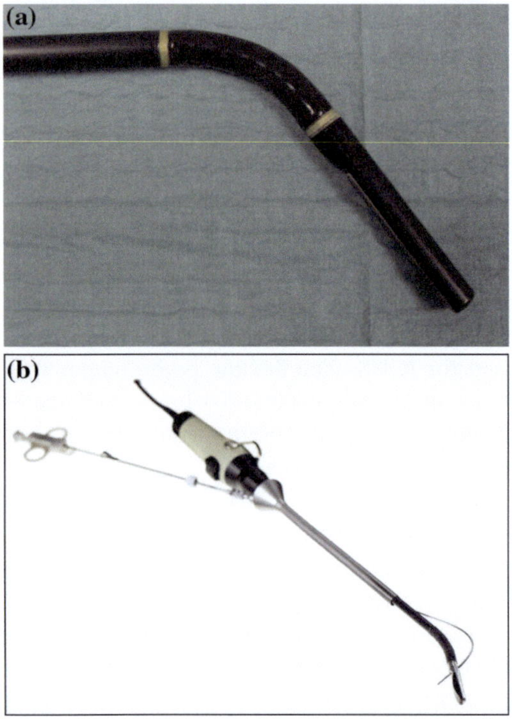

Fig. 1.16 The flexible tip of two laparoscopic probes respectively (**a**) linear (Hitachi-Aloka Medical; Tokyo, Japan) and (**b**) convex (BK Medical APS, Peabody MA, USA); the latter is also equipped with an operating channel for interventional procedures

movement of the screen, keyboard, and main hardware. The size should be compatible with the restrictions of the environment. Prompt management of each device and rapid manipulation of each instrument should be guaranteed (Fig. 1.18a). The keyboard should have a simple and easy to use layout, and the monitor screen, usuallly located on the other side of the patient, should be large enough for clear visibility by the surgeon (see Chap. 2, Fig. 1.18b, c). All these needs should not in any way impair the technological features of the system which has to be fully equipped not only for basic ultrasound examination but also for sophisticated analyses, as referred to again in the following chapters.

The system should be able to host several probes at the same time (Fig. 1.18d). Color-Doppler facilities (Fig. 1.19), and particularly new and more sensitive color flow modes (CFIOUS) (Fig. 1.20) should be considered for intraoperatively studying the in-and-outflow anatomy of the liver, and the modifications induce by the surgical maneuvers: this information, as further described in Chaps. 7 and 8, represents crucial data for possible surgical strategies that are otherwise unfeasible. As shown in Fig. 1.19, the color represents the direction of blood flow in relation to the probe's surface: red, the flow moving towards the probe; and blue, the flow away from the probe.

Compression maneuvers , as e.g., of an hepatic vein (see Chaps. 7 and 8), can modify the flow direction; so, based on color inversion it is possible to precisely confirm the flow direction (Fig. 1.21). CEIOUS is a latest advancement in intraoperative application of US. Here,

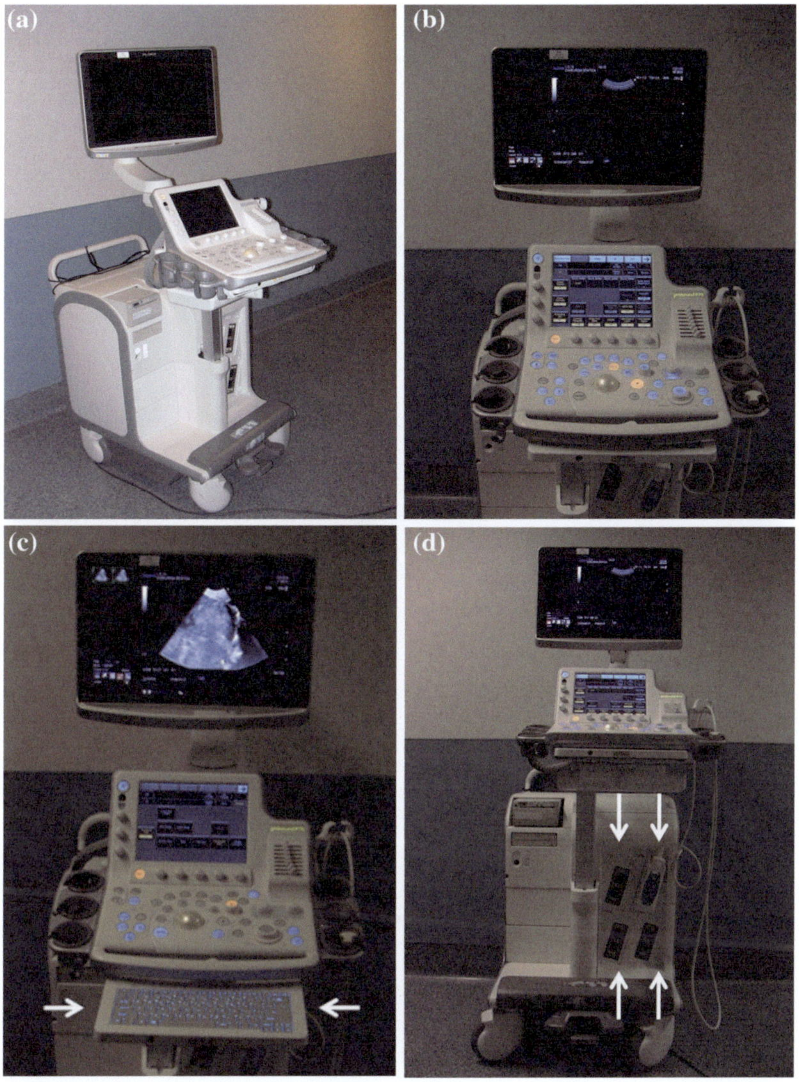

Fig. 1.18 **a** An ultrasound system designed also for intraoperative use; **b** keyboard and screen; **c** keyboard which can be expanded (*arrows*); **d** multiple allocation for probes (*arrows*)

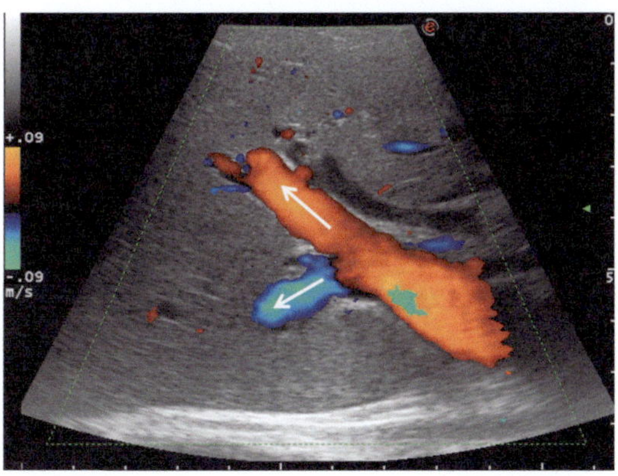

Fig. 1.19 Color-Doppler image with *arrows* indicating the flow directions

the vibration of gas-filled microbubbles contained in the injected contrast agents produces the visible contrast enhancement (Fig. 1.22) enabling a real-time continuous enhanced ultrasonic imaging.

The contrast agent used in most European countries consists of sulfur hexafluoride microbubbles stabilized by a phospholipid shell (SonoVue, Bracco Imaging, Milan, Italy). The anesthesiologist injects intravenously 2.4–4.8 ml of SonoVue per exploration through a peripheral vein: the amount of contrast is established according to the preference of the operator, generally half-sample (2.4 ml), if well prepared,

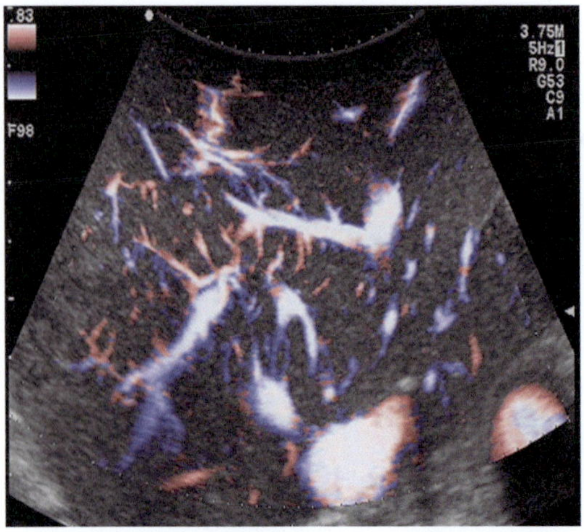

Fig. 1.20 Liver under color-flow imaging (CFIOUS)—analyzing blood flow independently from the angle of scanning (eflow; Hitachi-Aloka Medical; Tokyo, Japan), as opposed to the case of color-Doppler mode. This increases the sensitivity allows precise mapping also of slow motion flow (tiny vessels are clearly depicted here), higher detectability of small vessels, as compared to the case in Fig. 1.19 all of that keeping a directional flow pattern: *red*, flow moving towards the probe; *blue*, moving away from the probe

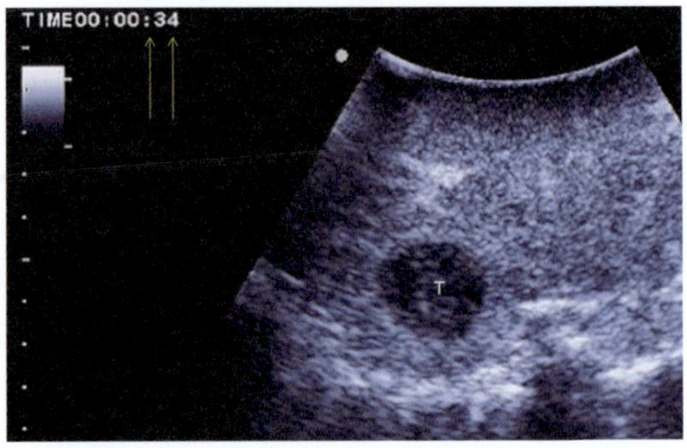

Fig. 1.22 Contrast-enhanced intraoperative ultrasound (CEIOUS) in which a lesion is shown (*T*) after 34 s from contrast agent injection (*yellow arrows*)

is sufficient. The purpose of contrast enhancement is to evaluate lesion vascularity, aiding in the characterization of those lesions eventually found intraoperatively at IOUS, and to detect new ones profitting from the enhanced brightness of the liver parenchyma especially along the delayed phases (Fig. 1.23).

A new hepatospecific contrast agent (Sonazoid, perfluorobutane, GE Healthcare, Oslo, Norway) will soon become commercially

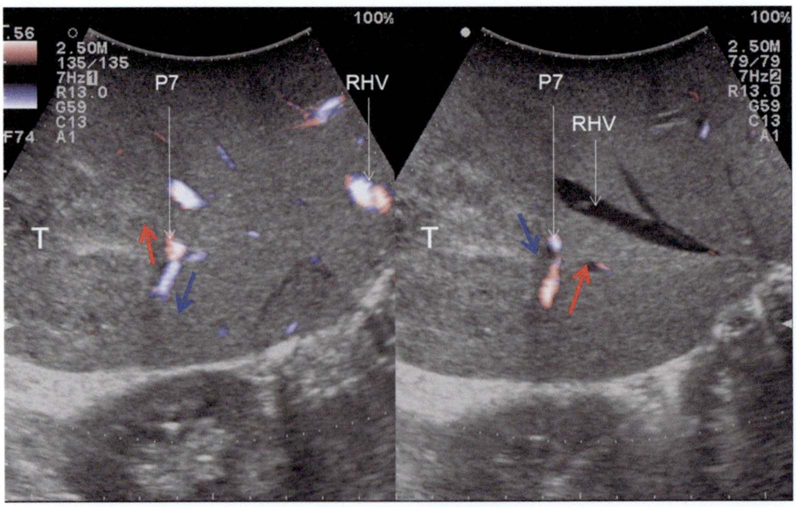

Fig. 1.21 Flow inversion in color-flow image (*colored arrows*); (*left*) right hepatic vein (*RHV*) not compressed and flow direction in segment 7 portal branch (*P7*) is hepatopetal; (*right*) once *RHV* is compressed, flow in *P7* becomes hepatofugal; tumor (*T*)

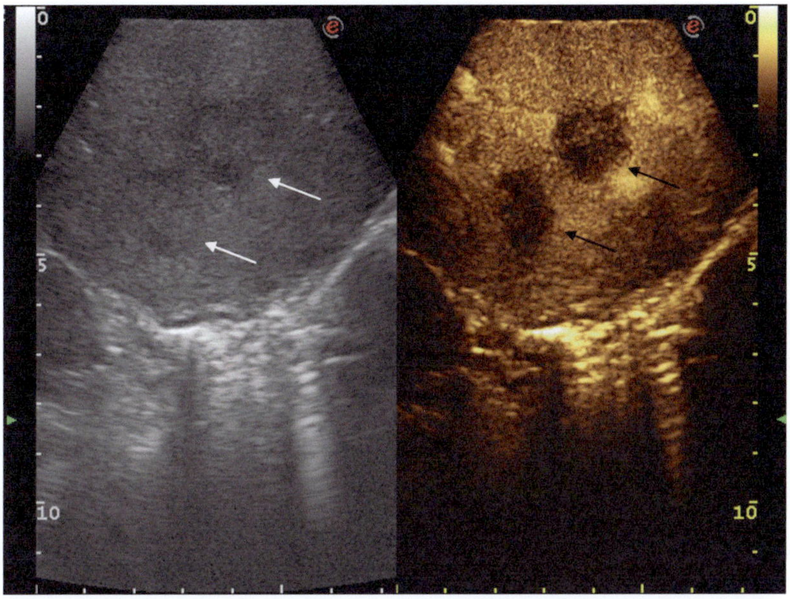

Fig. 1.23 (*right*) Contrast-enhanced intraoperative ultrasound (CEIOUS) revealing more lesions (*black arrows on the right-hand side*); (*left*) B-mode scanning is also possible that the same lesions appear, but are less clearly visible (*white arrows*)

available for clinical use: at the present time, it is clinically used only in Japan. This contrast agent, which functions not only as a vascular contrast agent (as SonoVue), but also as an hepatospecific contrast medium used in magnetic resonance, could provide new options for nodule analysis [2] and detection [3]. Chapter 6 focuses on this new contrast agent.

Images and video clips from the ultrasound systems are to be electronically stored, and can be linked the hospital networks via cable or wi-fi for viewing in real time in other locations.

References

1. Hata S, Imamura H, Aoki T et al (2011) Value of visual inspection, bimanual palpation, and intraoperative ultrasonography during hepatic resection for liver metastases of colorectal carcinoma. World J Surg 35:2779–2787
2. Kudo M (2007) New sonographic techniques for the diagnosis and treatment of hepatocellular carcinoma. Hepatol Res 37(Suppl 2):S193–S199
3. Nakano H, Ishida Y, Hatakeyama T et al (2008) Contrast-enhanced intraoperative ultrasonography equipped with late Kupffer-phase image obtained by sonazoid in patients with colorectal liver metastases. World J Gastroenterol 14:3207–3211

Technical Tricks to Start Exploring the Liver with Ultrasound

2

Guido Torzilli, Daniele Del Fabbro, and Matteo Cimino

The IOUS should always be carried out personally by the surgeon in charge of the surgical procedure, rather than by an assistant, radiologist, or technician. Optimally, ultrasound and operation are done by the same person. Only the surgeon has the required skills and background in interpreting ultrasound images in a surgical perspective, and will be able to judge possible surgical maneuvers by personally guiding the echoprobe. As mentioned in Chap. 1, the ultrasound system has to be positioned opposite the chief operator who should be facing the screen (Fig. 2.1). The screen has to be large enough for allowing optimal visibility at that distance and lights should be positioned with caution not to obscure the surgeon's visibility of the ultrasound screen. An unscrubbed team member should be at hand to manipulate the keyboard or a transparent and sterile keyboard pad may allow a scrubbed assistant to handle the keyboard directly (Fig. 2.2).

After entering the abdominal cavity and preceding IOUS exploration, the liver should be mobilized dividing the round and falciform ligaments (Fig. 2.3a) and eventual adhesions should be dissected to free the anterosuperior and inferior surfaces of the liver (Fig. 2.3b). Of course, adhesions with other organs or structures should not be severed as to possible tumor infiltration. In that case, IOUS can be helpful in ruling out or confirming the tumor invasion and allow for changing the surgical strategy accordingly. Palpation of the organ needs to precede the exploration with IOUS; indeed, as recently demonstrated [1], inspection and palpation of the liver are still of paramount importance.

By pulling the round ligament, the liver surface is widely exposed and following the portal branches and the hepatic veins, the liver can be entirely studied (Fig. 2.4). The probe should be managed using a pressure sufficient to ensure a good contact with the liver surface but not to compress the intrahepatic vascular structures and in particular the hepatic veins. Generally, at the onset one should not move the probe extensively over the liver surface but identify a vascular landmark which is generally represented by the main portal bifurcation. Then, once identified (see Chap. 3), just a minimal shifting of the probe on the liver surface would allow following all the portal pedicles, and exploring all liver segments by IOUS (Fig. 2.5a, b).

The hard and irregular surface of cirrhotic liver (Fig. 2.6), scars due to previous resection or strong adhesions in reoperated patients (Fig. 2.3b), or simply a heterogeneous ultrasound pattern make it somewhat difficult to detect small nodes both by palpation and IOUS exploration. Under such circumstances, searching a scanning window opposite the site of an

G. Torzilli (✉) · D. Del Fabbro · M. Cimino
Department of Hepatobiliary Surgery,
Humanitas Research Hospital-IRCCS,
University of Milan-School of Medicine,
Via A. Manzoni 56, 20089 Rozzano, MI, Italy
e-mail: guido.torzilli@humanitas.it;
guido.torzilli@unimi.it

G. Torzilli (ed.), *Ultrasound-Guided Liver Surgery*,
DOI: 10.1007/978-88-470-5510-0_2, © Springer-Verlag Italia 2014

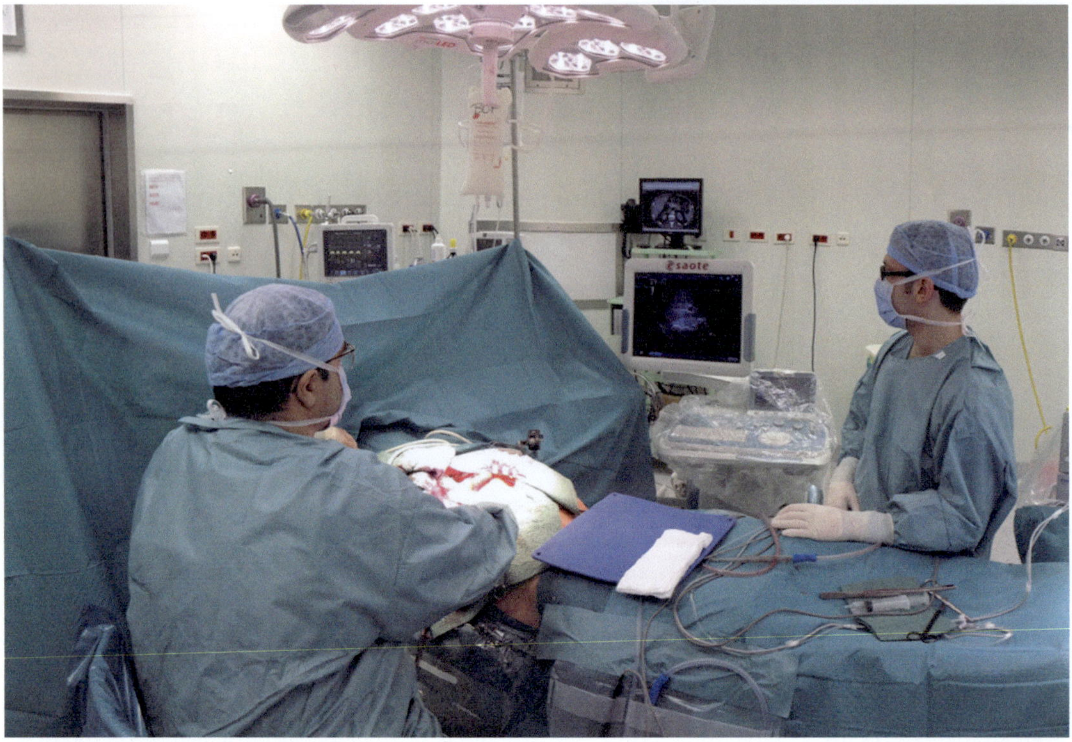

Fig. 2.1 Positioning of the ultrasound system in the operative theater: the operator faces the screen, which can be managed by the second or third assistant

unsuitable exploration to provide a deeper access than the initial superficial one would be essential to increase the chance to detect these lesions by IOUS (Fig. 2.7a, b). This maneuver can be further improved by keeping the fingertip on the liver surface opposed to that in contact with the probe, paying attention to match the fingertip plane with that of the scanning window (Fig. 2.7c, d).

The above example illustrates that the rationale of liver exploration with IOUS needs to follow each step of a surgical procedure, and should be repeated using different probes (Fig. 2.8a). If initially a mid-low-frequency probe (3.5–5 MHz) has been used to explore the deep structures prior to liver mobilization (Fig. 2.8a, b), a more detailed study of those areas of the organ initially not exposed could subsequently be achieved by a high-frequency probe (5–10 MHz). This is done by directly applying the probe on the liver surface once this is exposed after mobilization (Fig. 2.8a, c, d). In case of a rough surface (cirrhotic liver, scars from previous surgery, or strong adhesions) for which exploration should be carried out on the opposite side, a mid-low frequency would be preferred (Fig. 2.9a–d). Structures as the caval confluence which initially should be explored prior to full exposure (Fig. 2.10a), would best be explored again upon full exposure of the organ in spite of the artifacts generated by surgical dissection. Here, small probes should be used which are able to detail particular anatomical aspects (Fig. 2.10b) which may be useful for further refinement of the surgical strategy. This is specifically useful in the event of lesions at the caval confluence, which may generate artifacts that could mask the pattern of the confluence of the hepatic veins at initial exploration.

As described in detail in the next chapter, the liver should be explored using as landmarks the glissonian pedicles (inflow) or the hepatic veins

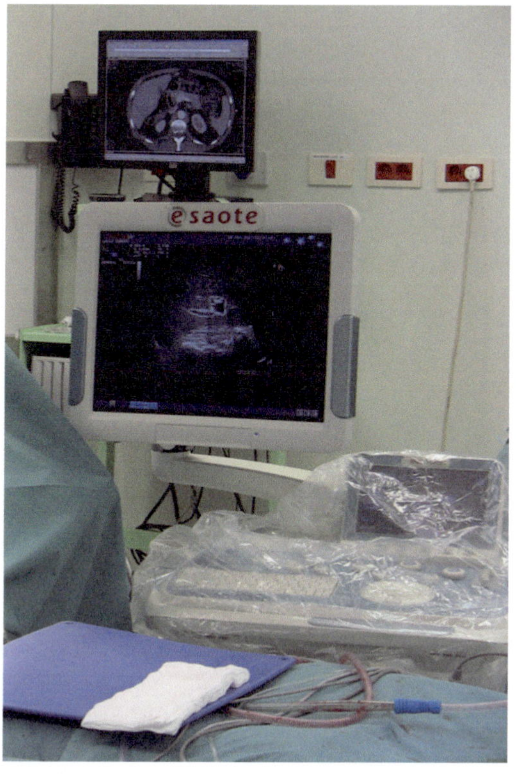

Fig. 2.2 An ultrasound system with a sterile pad covering the keyboard to allow its management by the surgical team directly

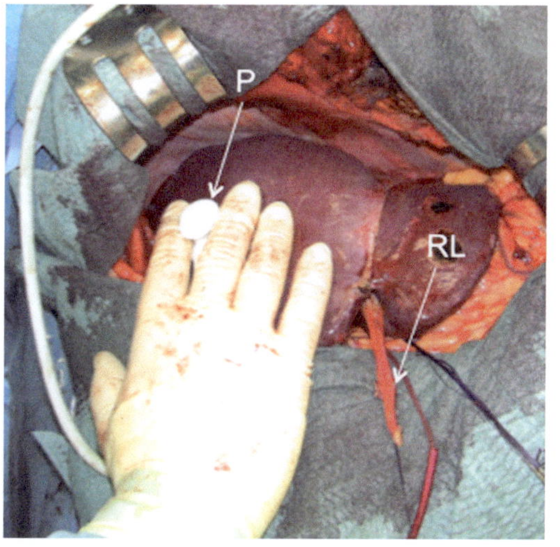

Fig. 2.4 A surgeon handling a probe and initially exploring the liver; round ligament (*RL*)

(outflow). To avoid ambiguity, in the following we use the *Brisbane terminology* for liver anatomy [2]. Prerequisite to the study of liver anatomy by IOUS (Chap. 3) one needs to acquire full knowledge of ultrasound semiology for distinguishing glissonean pedicles from hepatic veins. Glisson's capsule effects that the portal

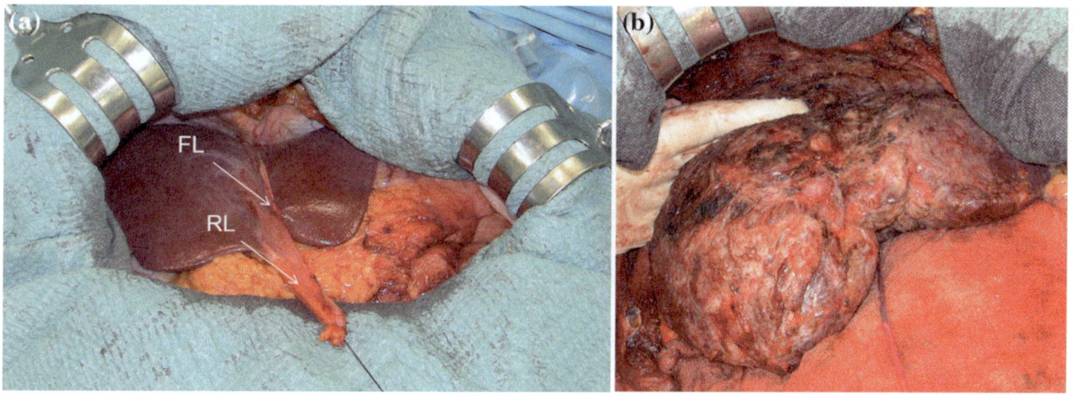

Fig. 2.3 **a** The liver is exposed for initial exploration once the falciform ligament (*FL*) has been cut and the caval confluence has not been exposed yet for avoiding artifacts upon IOUS; **b** liver exposed after extensive adhesions have been removed; round ligament (*RL*)

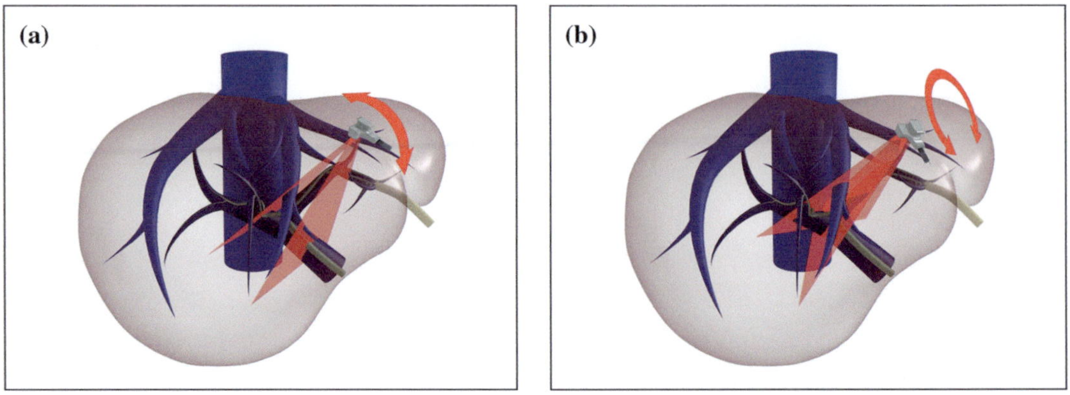

Fig. 2.5 Moving the probe while exploring the liver. This consists in minimal upward and downward tilting (**a**) or rotation (**b**) of the probe, avoiding its extensive shifting on the liver surface

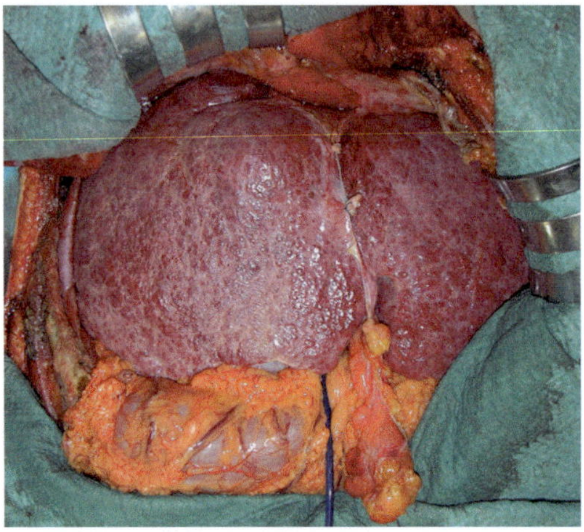

Fig. 2.6 Cirrhotic liver after initial exposure

pedicles, which run together with the arteries and the bile ducts, have thicker vessel walls than hepatic veins and for this reason they appear in IOUS as echo-free zones surrounded by a thicker hyperechogenic layer (Fig. 2.11a, b). Furthermore, other parallel, thinner vascular structures are visible, being the artery and the bile duct of the glissonian triad (Fig. 2.11c). The new sensitive color-flow modalities allow for differentiation of arterial, portal, and biliary elements also within thin glissonean sheets (Fig. 2.12). Hepatic veins appear as echo-free zones inside the liver parenchyma with the vessel wall appearing as a thin hyperechogenic line (Fig. 2.11a–c): hepatic vein wall can be thicker in cirrhotic liver and its lumen thinner due to stiffness of the organ (Fig. 2.13a, b). However, in principle distinction between hepatic veins and portal branches should be based not only on their appearance but mainly on their anatomy.

Bile duct appearance in IOUS is particular: normally they present as thin echo-free zones in the glissonian triad (Figs. 2.11c, 2.12, and 2.14); once dilated though, they appear as more evident echo-free zones with a serpiginous path (Fig. 2.15).

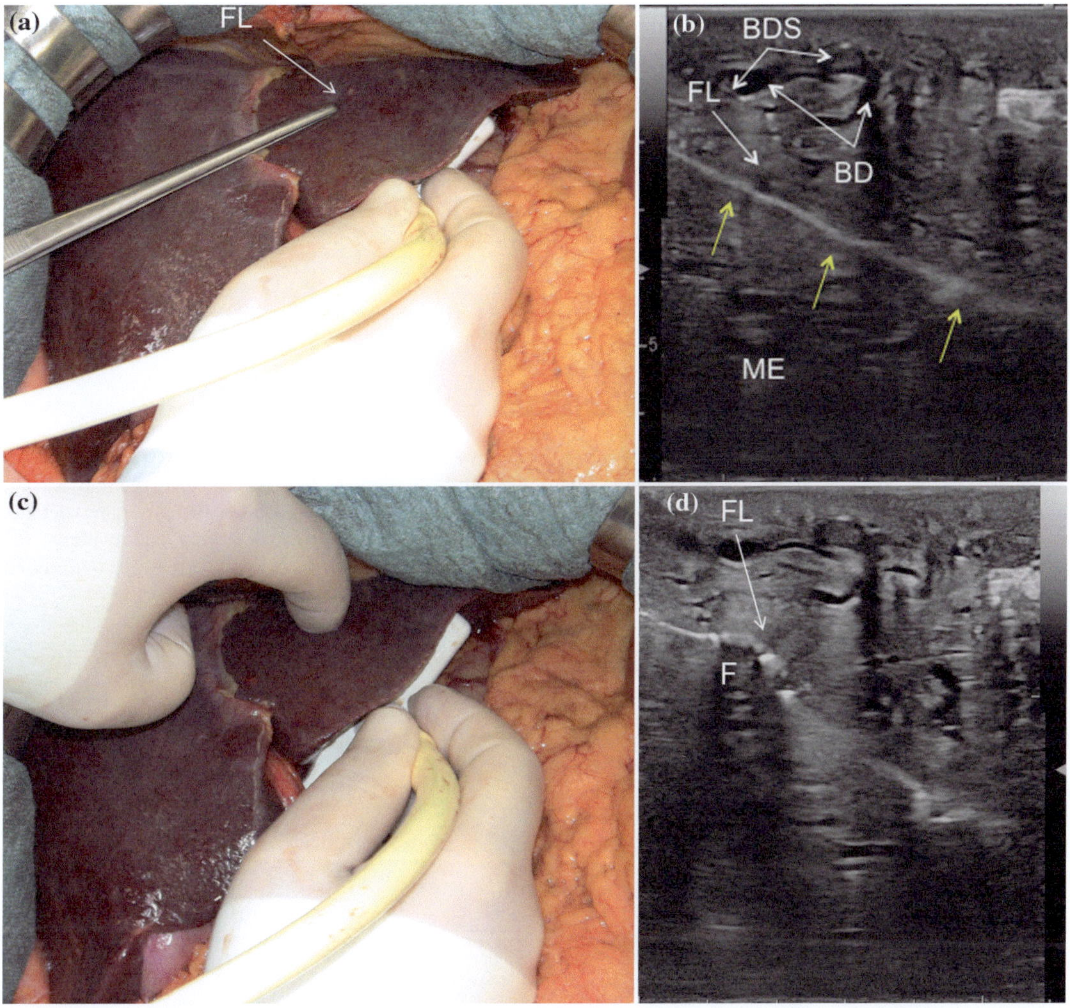

Fig. 2.7 Procedure of scanning superficial lesions without adopting water-filled gloves (see also Chaps. 1 and 4). The lesion visible at inspection (*FL*), indicated by the forceps, is searched for ultrasound confirmation having the probe scanning at the opposite side (**a**). In this case, the lesion could not be confirmed with certainty due to inhomogeneous liver bile duct dilation (*BD*) and the presence of biliary sludge (*BDS*) (**b**). For this reason a simultaneous finger palpation of the lesion (**c**), concurrently with IOUS, enables to precisely put in relation the suspected lesions at IOUS with the surgeon's fingertip (*F*) then confirming its existence and ultrasound appearance (**d**), which in this case is compatible with a fore site of a perihilar bile duct cancer; mirror effect (*ME*) (see Chap. 4); *yellow arrows* indicate the interface between the liver surface and the adjacent structures

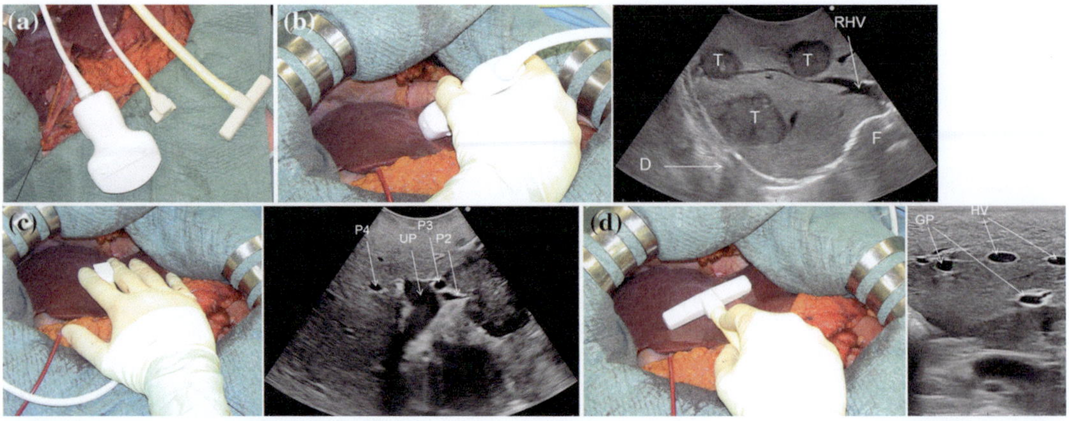

Fig. 2.8 Various probes (**a**) can be used for exploration taking advantage of their respective working frequencies, occasionally with improved panoramicity or more details. Indeed, a convex probe for percutaneous exploration can advantageously be used even intraoperatively (*left*) for enhanced panoramicity (*right*) of the scan (**b**). A microconvex probe (*left*) providing a wide scanning window when working at mid-frequencies also may enable sufficient panoramicity (*right*) (**c**). Conversely, a T-shaped linear array (*left*), generally working at higher frequencies and having a high density of crystals, is superior for providing detailed scans (right), though with reduced panoramicity (**d**); diaphragm (*D*); finger (*F*); glissonian pedicle (*GP*); hepatic vein (*HV*); portal pedicle to segment 2 (*P*2); portal pedicle to segment 3 (*P*3); portal pedicle to segment 4 (*P*4); right hepatic vein (*RHV*); tumor (*T*); umbilical portion (*UP*)

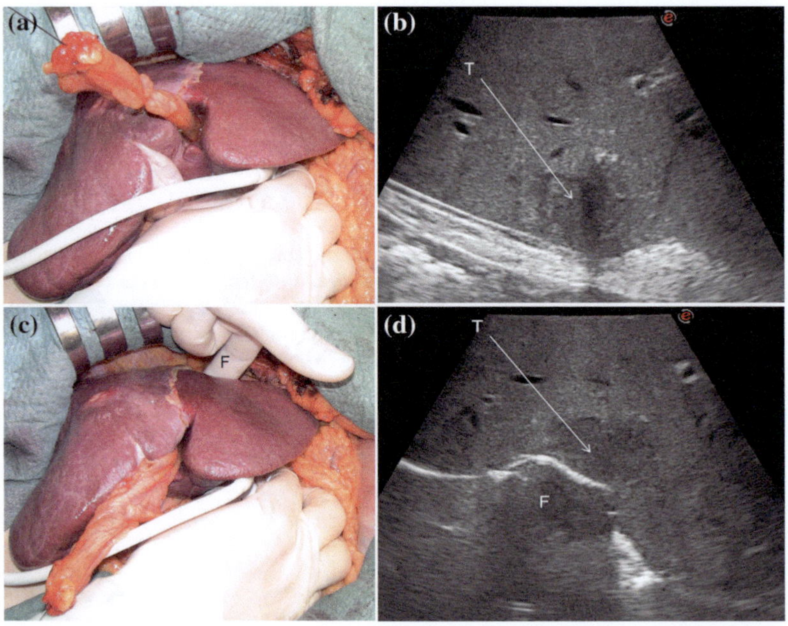

Fig. 2.9 Scanning of superficial lesions without adopting water-filled gloves, as in Fig. 2.7 (see also Chaps. 1 and 4). Lesion not visible, but superficial and palpable, is searched with the probe scanning at the opposite side (**a**), and is well depicted in IOUS (*T*), without (**b**), or with aid of fingertip palpation (**c**, **d**); surgeon's fingertip (*F*)

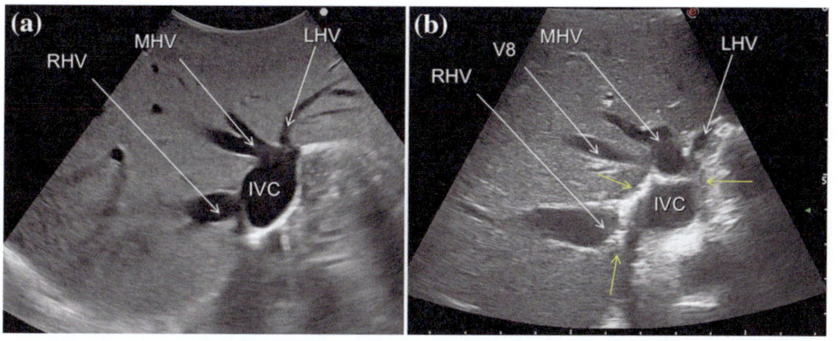

Fig. 2.10 **a** The caval confluence before onset of dissection; **b** upon exposure, artifacts due to air bubbles (*yellow arrows*) may affect the exploration during IOUS, though this does not generally compromise the disclosure of peculiar aspects as a thick vein draining segment 8 (*V8*) and flowing into the middle hepatic vein (*MHV*) close to its confluence or the existence of a left hepatic vein (*LHV*) which is flowing into the inferior vena cava (*IVC*) very laterally; right hepatic vein (*RHV*)

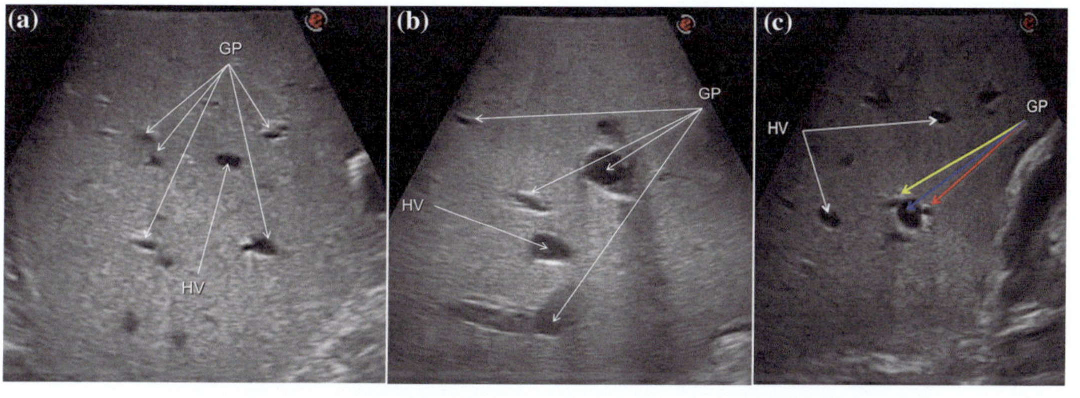

Fig. 2.11 **a** Tiny branches of the hepatic vein (*HV*) and glissonean pedicles (*GP*): despite the small diameters, they can be discerned by the different thickness of the hyperechogenic layer surrounding the anechoic area of the vessel lumen; **b** similar to the previous, here the different thickness of the hyperechogenic layer surrounding the vessel lumen in the case of GP and HV also is clearly seen; **c** triad composing a GP is disclosed by *blue arrows* for the portal branch, *red* for the artery, and *yellow* for the bile duct: a close look reveals the mickey-mouse pattern of the GP

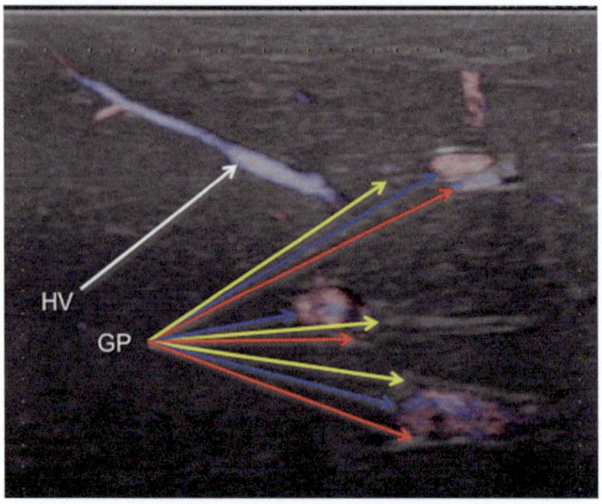

Fig. 2.12 Triple composition of the glissonian pedicle (*GP*) disclosed in color-flow IOUS, *colored arrows* indicating the various elements. The *color filling* the vessel lumen indicates the flow direction rather than the type of vessel; portal veins (*blue arrows*), arteries (*red arrows*), bile ducts (*yellow arrows*); hepatic vein (*HV*)

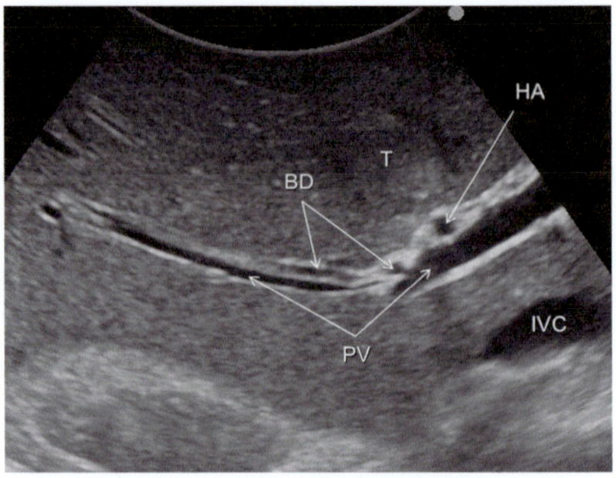

Fig. 2.14 A normal bile duct (*BD*) running straight and parallel to the other elements of the glissonean pedicle, despite adjacency to the tumor (*T*)—portal vein (*PV*); hepatic artery (*HA*); inferior vena cava (*IVC*)

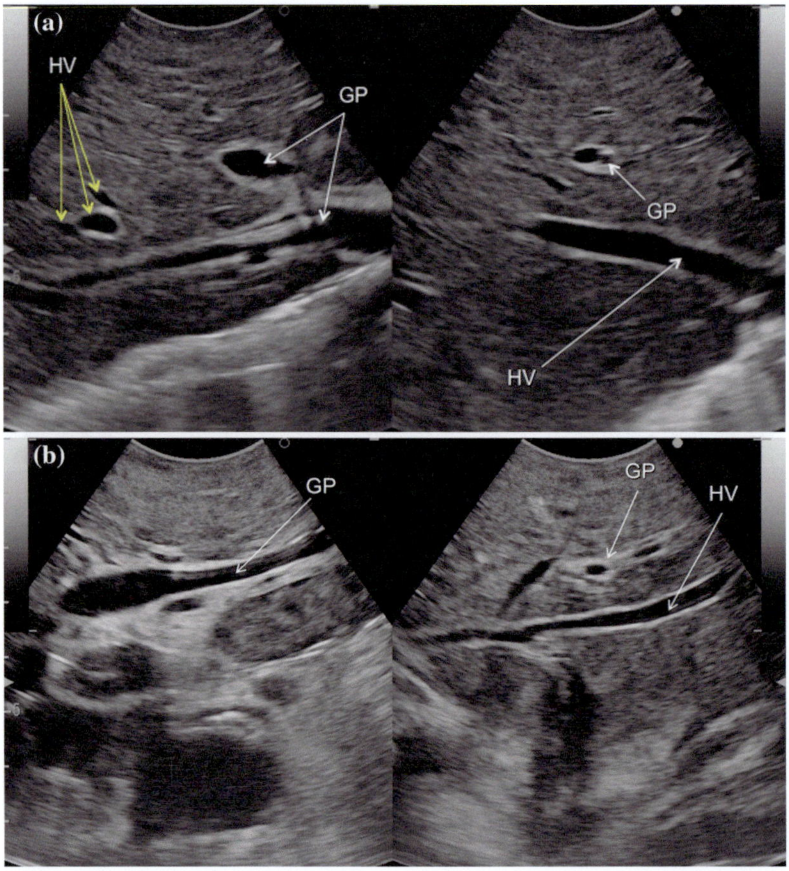

Fig. 2.13 Sometimes, particularly in fibrotic liver, as in cirrhotics, vessel wall thickness can be misleading (**a**, **b**), and even the triad could lead to a wrong interpretation. Indeed, sometimes an hepatic vein (*HV*), once the scan catches the confluence of multiple branches, could mimic a glissonean pedicle (*GP*), even mimicking the mickey-mouse pattern (to the left of the *yellow arrows* in **a**)

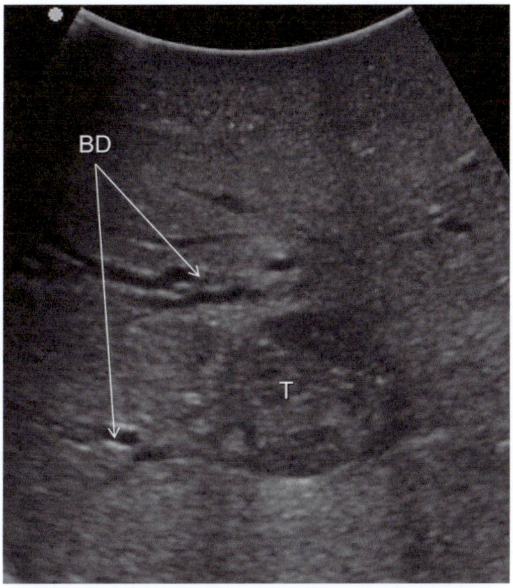

Fig. 2.15 Slightly dilated bile ducts (*BD*) due to the presence of a tumor (*T*), eventually compressing or infiltrating their confluence: the ducts become more evident in IOUS and assume a serpiginous trajectory

References

1. Hata S, Imamura H, Aoki T et al (2011) Value of visual inspection, bimanual palpation, and intraoperative ultrasonography during hepatic resection for liver metastases of colorectal carcinoma. World J Surg 35:2779–2787
2. Belghiti J, Clavien PA, Gadzijev et al. (2000) The Brisbane 2000 terminology of liver anatomy and resections. HPB 2:333–339

3 Exploring the Liver by Ultrasound Along its Anatomy

Guido Torzilli, Guido Costa, and Florin Botea

Adequate knowledge of liver anatomy, by surgical and ultrasound, is a requirement for performing IOUS: its vascular skeleton composed of the glissonian skeleton with its portal, arterial, and biliary elements and the hepatic veins are landmarks for liver exploration (Fig. 3.1). The *Brisbane terminology* for liver surgical anatomy is applied here [1].

The authors recommend liver explorations to start from the portal branches for the following reasons:

1. The portal bifurcation is generally the first structure encountered by positioning the probe on the liver's surface since it is located relatively in the center, and can be visualized by positioning the probe in a relatively wide area of the liver surface which can be located along an ideal midline dividing the liver into an upper and lower portion, grossly passing through the edge between the segments 5 and 8 and 4 superior and inferior (Fig. 3.2a, b).
2. Following the portal branches from their hilar origin to the periphery it is possible to explore all the segments without extensive movements but just titling the probe on the liver surface as recommended in Chap. 2 (Fig. 3.3a, b).
3. Tilting the probe and following the portal branches from the central part to the periphery of the organ it is possible to identify and explore systematically all the sectional branches (Figs. 3.4a, b, 3.5a, b), and all the segmental and subsegmental portions of the liver (Figs. 3.6, 3.7, 3.8, 3.9, 3.10, 3.11, 3.12, 3.13, 3.14). One is then capable to locate any eventual lesion in relation to those branches and to recognize any eventual anomalous branching patterns (Figs. 3.15a, b, 3.16).
4. Once all segmental glissonean pedicles have been explored between the portal branches feeding segment 2 and 3 the left hepatic vein (LHV) appears (Fig. 3.17) and the probe is tilted upward to see the hepatocaval confluence (Fig. 3.18a, b). This way it is also possible to identify the various patterns of hepatic vein confluence (Figs. 3.19, 3.20, 3.21, 3.22, 3.23, 3.24). From this scan, bending the probe downward one can entirely explore the paracaval portion of the liver appearing as covered by a virtual roof outlined by the three hepatic veins (Fig. 3.25). Proceeding to scan downward, one may find in some patients a thick accessory vein, such as a middle inferior right hepatic vein (MIRHV) (Fig. 3.26a, b) or an inferior right hepatic vein (IRHV) , the latter which typically runs behind the right sided portal branches (Figs. 3.26b, c, 3.27).

G. Torzilli (✉) · G. Costa · F. Botea
Department of Hepatobiliary Surgery,
Humanitas Research Hospital-IRCCS,
University of Milan-School of Medicine,
Via A. Manzoni 56, 20089 Rozzano, MI, Italy
e-mail: guido.torzilli@humanitas.it;
guido.torzilli@unimi.it

G. Torzilli (ed.), *Ultrasound-Guided Liver Surgery*,
DOI: 10.1007/978-88-470-5510-0_3, © Springer-Verlag Italia 2014

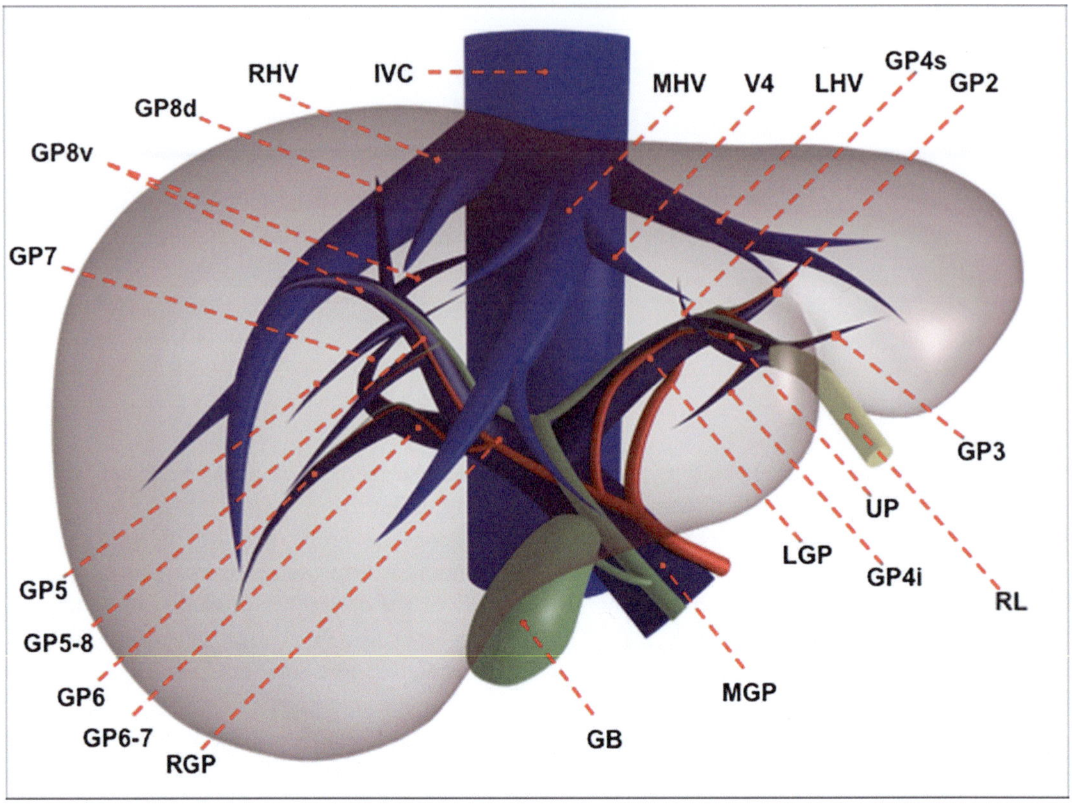

Fig. 3.1 The liver with its vasculobiliary skeleton; portal and hepatic veins (*blue*); hepatic arteries (*red*); bile ducts (*green*); gallbladder (*GB*); glissonian pedicle to segment 2 (*GP2*); glissonian pedicle to segment 3 (*GP3*); glissonian pedicle to segment 4 inferior (*GP4i*); glissonian pedicle to segment 4 superior (*GP4s*); glissonian pedicle to segment 5 (*GP5*); glissonian pedicle to segment 6 (*GP6*); glissonian pedicle to segment 7 (GP7); glissonian pedicle to segment 8 dorsal (*GP8d*); glissonian pedicle to segment 8 ventral (GP8v); glissonian pedicle to segments 5 and 8 (right anterior section) (*GP5-8*); glissonian pedicle to segments 6 and 7 (right posterior section) (*GP6-7*); inferior vena cava (*IVC*); left hepatic vein (*LHV*); middle hepatic vein (*MHV*); left glissonian pedicle (*LGP*); main glissonian pedicle (*MGP*); right glissonian pedicle (*RGP*); right hepatic vein (*RHV*); round ligament (*RL*); umbilical portion (*UP*)

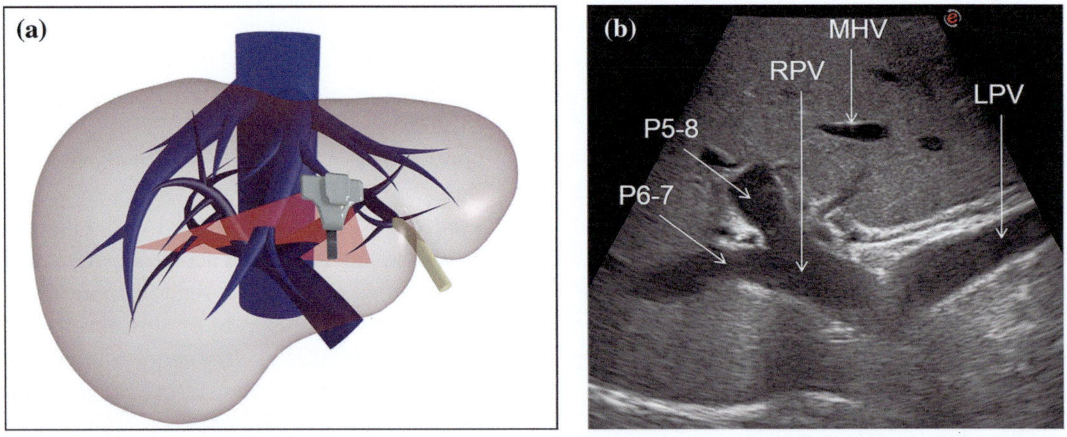

Fig. 3.2 *Left* (**a**) scan disclosing the main portal bifurcation and *right* (**b**) IOUS image; left portal vein (*LPV*); middle hepatic vein (*MHV*); right portal vein (*RPV*); portal branch to segments 5 and 8 (*P5-8*) (right anterior section); portal branch to segments 6 and 7 (*P6-7*) (right posterior section)

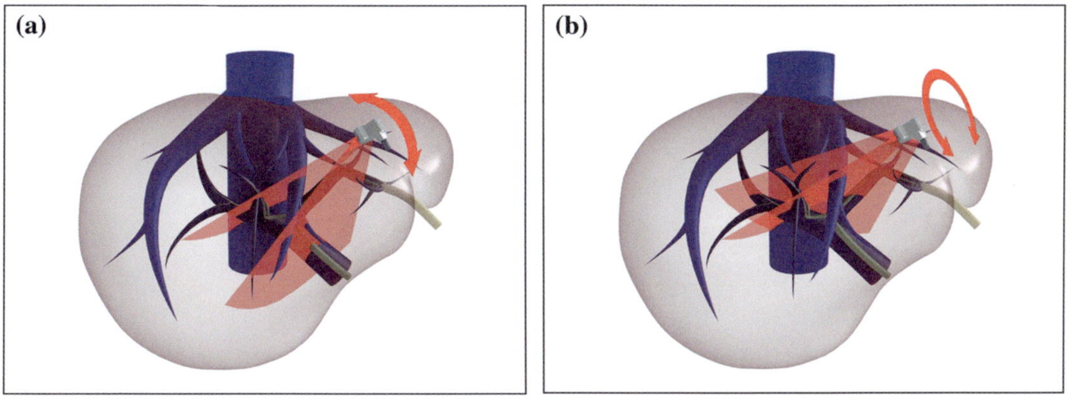

Fig. 3.3 Useful movements for liver exploration (as also shown in Chap. 2), involving up- and downward tilting (**a**) and axial rotation (**b**)

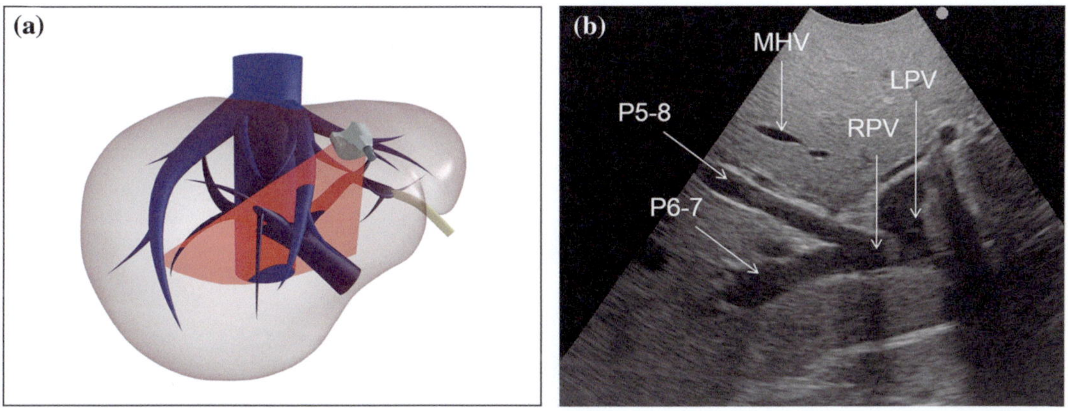

Fig. 3.4 *Left* (**a**) scan, *right* (**b**) IOUS image; left portal vein (*LPV*); middle hepatic vein (*MHV*); right portal vein (*RPV*); portal branch to segments 5 and 8 (right anterior section) (*P5-8*); portal branch to segments 6 and 7 (right posterior section) (*P6-7*)

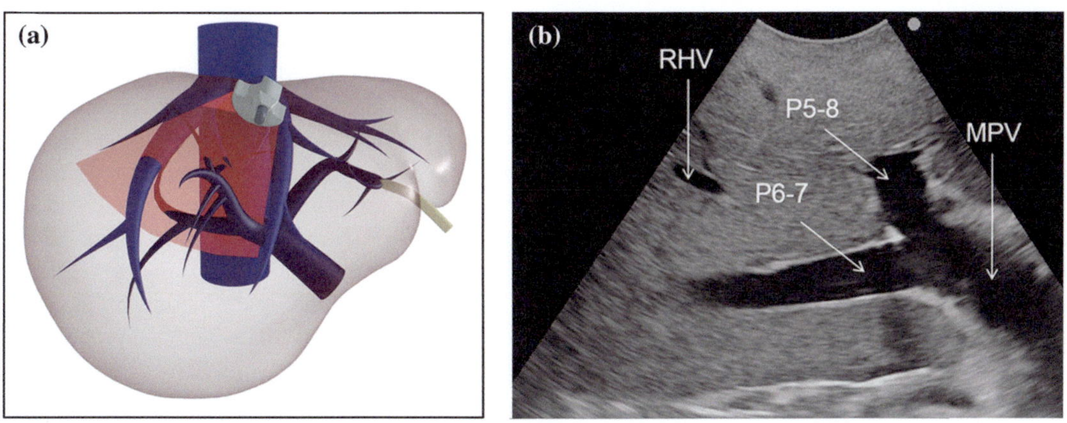

Fig. 3.5 *Left* (**a**) scan; *right* (**b**) IOUS image; right hepatic vein (*RHV*); portal branch to segments 5 and 8 (right anterior section) (P5-8); portal branch to segments 6 and 7 (right posterior section) (*P6-7*)

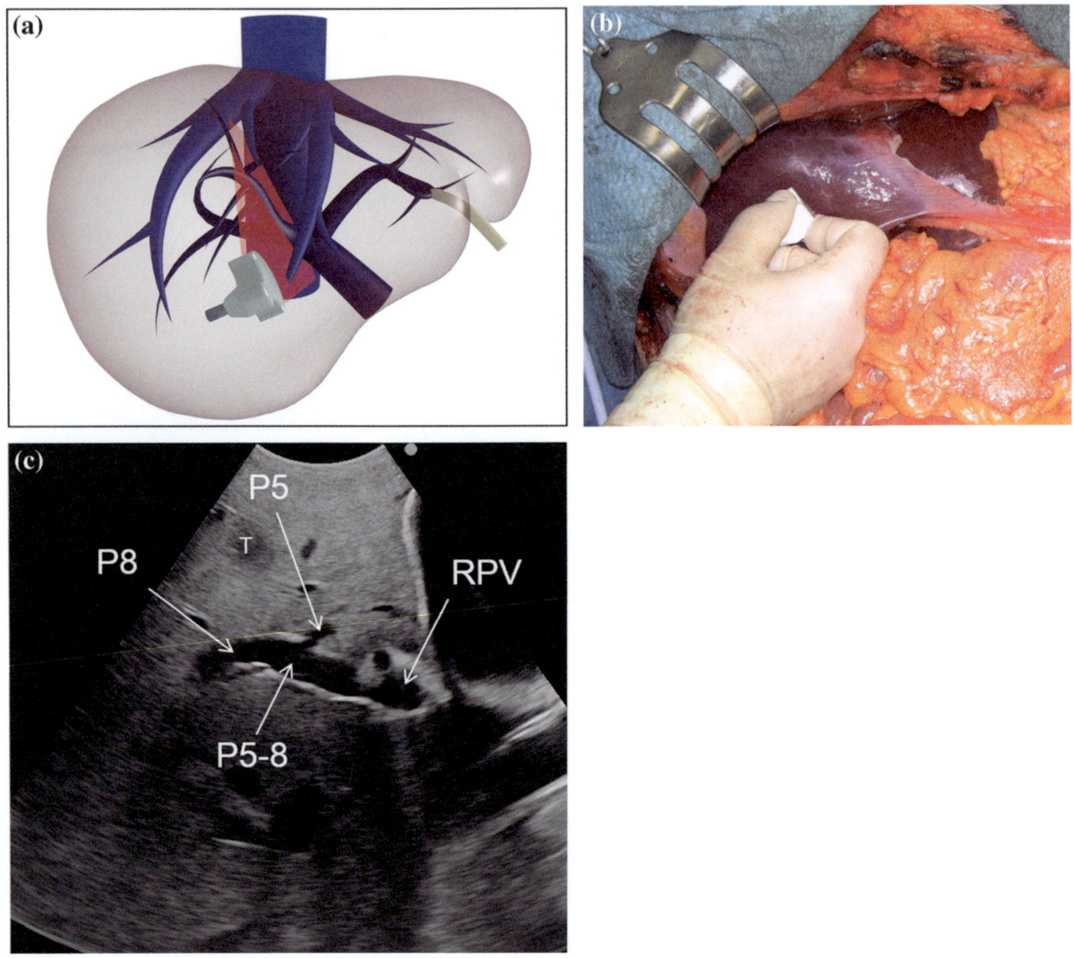

Fig. 3.6 **a** Scan, **b** intraoperative probe position, and **c** IOUS image; right portal vein (*RPV*); portal branch to segments 5 and 8 (right anterior section) (*P5-8*); portal branch to segment 5 (*P5*); portal branch to segment 8 (*P8*); tumor (*T*)

In starting the liver exploration from the hepatic veins, there is the need to tilt upward the probe to meet the plane of the hepatocaval confluence or inversely to position the probe at the hepatocaval confluence. The latter should be done despite the general recommendation not to dissect in the first exploration the falciform ligament to avoid the insertion of air and artifacts at the caval confluence (Fig. 3.28). Furthermore, this complicates exploring the liver with minimal movement of the probe.

Generally, there is no fixed position in exploring the liver, but in certain areas one can find landmarks more frequently and more easily from which to start the exploration. For example, the portal bifurcation can also be well visualized by placing the probe close to the caval confluence with the scanning view almost perpendicular to the liver surface (Fig. 3.29a, b). Encountering glissonean pedicles by IOUS can drive the exploration of the entire organ just by tilting the probe (Fig. 3.3a, b).

Starting form the main portal bifurcation (Fig. 3.2a, b), one can follow with the probe on the right the portal branches of first (Fig. 3.4a, b), second (Fig. 3.5a, b), and third order (Figs. 3.6a–c, 3.7a–c, 3.8a–c, 3.9a–c) and the right hemiliver can be fully explored. Then, moving back to the main

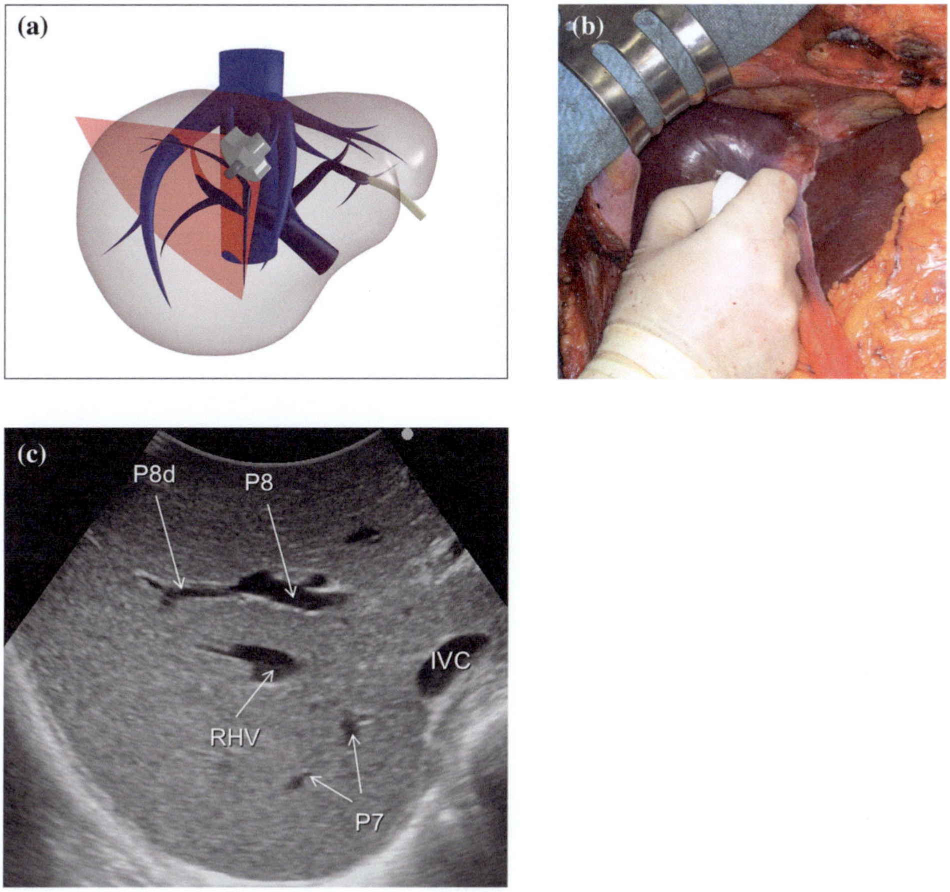

Fig. 3.7 Scan (**a**), intraoperative probe position (**b**), and IOUS image (**c**); inferior vena cava (*IVC*); right hepatic vein (*RHV*); portal branch to segment 8 (*P8*); portal branch to subsegment 8 dorsal (*P8d*); portal branches to segment 7 (*P7*)

bifurcation, the same is done for the left hemiliver (Figs. 3.10a–c, 3.11a, b, 3.12a, b, 3.13a, b, 3.14a, b). Peculiarities can thus be recognized and perfectly depicted, such as the branching pattern of segment 8 with its dorsal and ventral branches, e.g., one of the branches to the dorsal portion of segment 8 appears in IOUS as crossing above the right hepatic vein (*RHV*): this way, following the portal branching pattern, the operator will be able to clarify a common misunderstanding. Accordingly, IOUS is able to properly address to segment 8 that portion of the liver and any lesion in it (Fig. 3.30) located on the right side of the RHV, rather than, as generally and wrongly done, to segment 7.

Advancing to the left side, the umbilical portion and its segmental branches can be followed with IOUS (Figs. 3.10a–c, 3.11a, b, 3.12a, b, 3.13a, b, 3.14a, b). Peculiarities of the branching pattern of segment 4 can now be explored (Figs. 3.11a, b, 3.12a, b). The portal branches to segment 4 are generally divided into two groups: those for the superior and those for the inferior portion and IOUS can precisely estimate their origin and trajectories. Similarly,

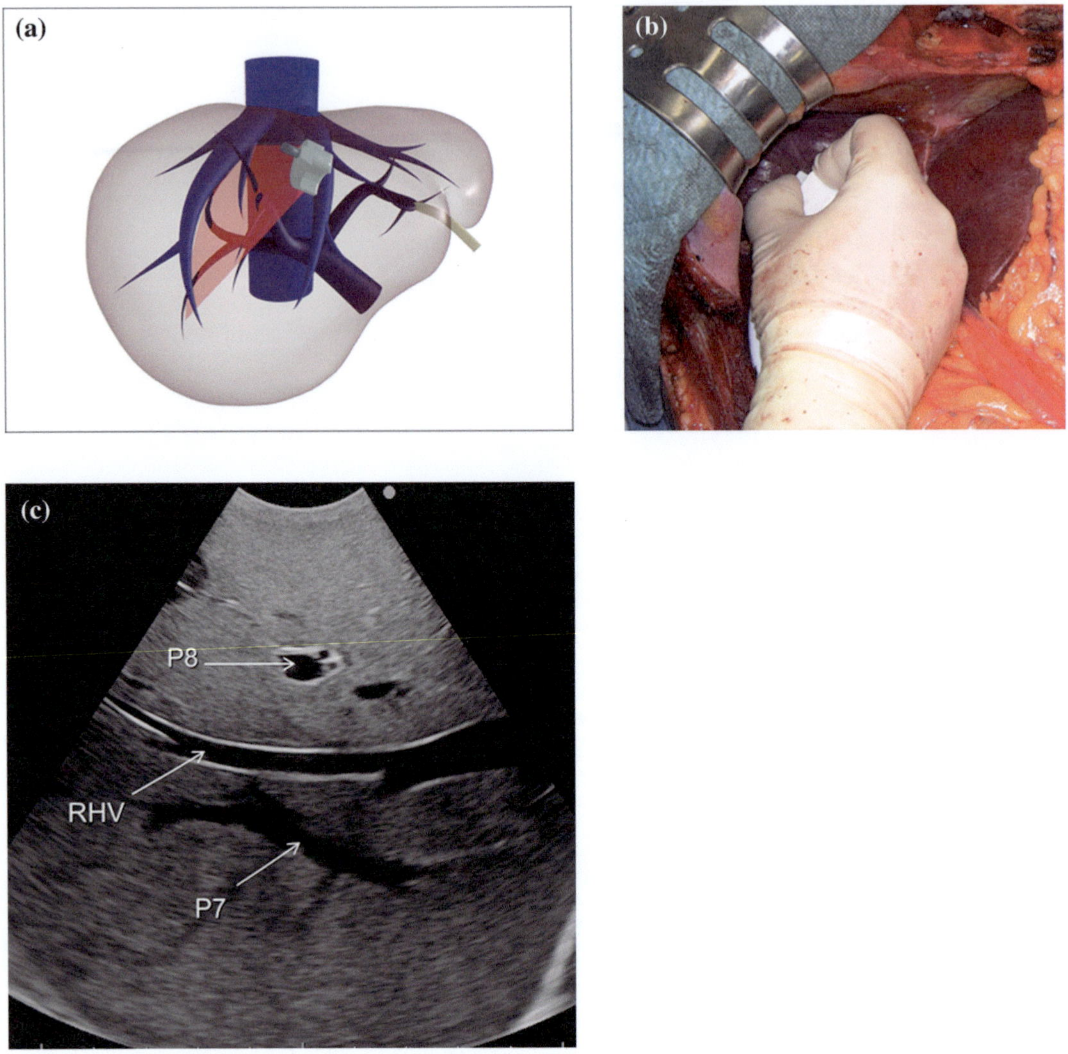

Fig. 3.8 Scan (**a**), intraoperative probe position (**b**), and IOUS image (**c**); right hepatic vein (*RHV*); portal branch to segment 8 (*P8*); portal branch to segment 7 (*P7*)

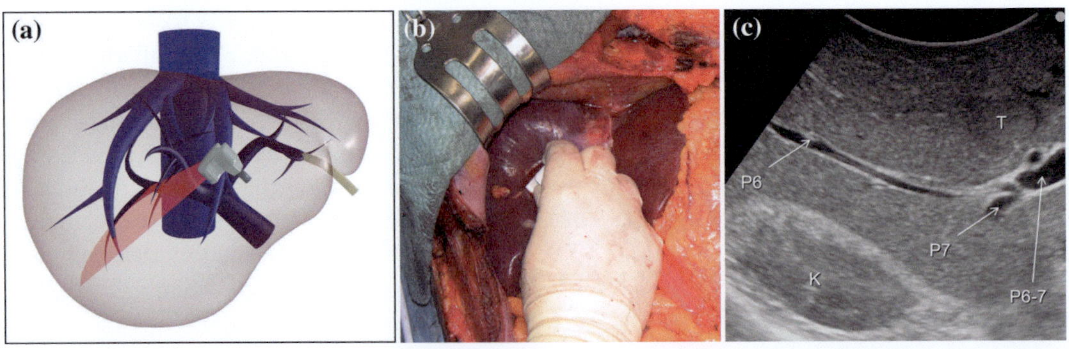

Fig. 3.9 Scan (**a**), intraoperative probe position (**b**), and IOUS image (**c**); kidney (*K*); portal branch to segments 6 and 7 (*P6-7*) (right posterior section); portal branch to segment 6 (*P6*); portal branch to segment 7 (*P7*)

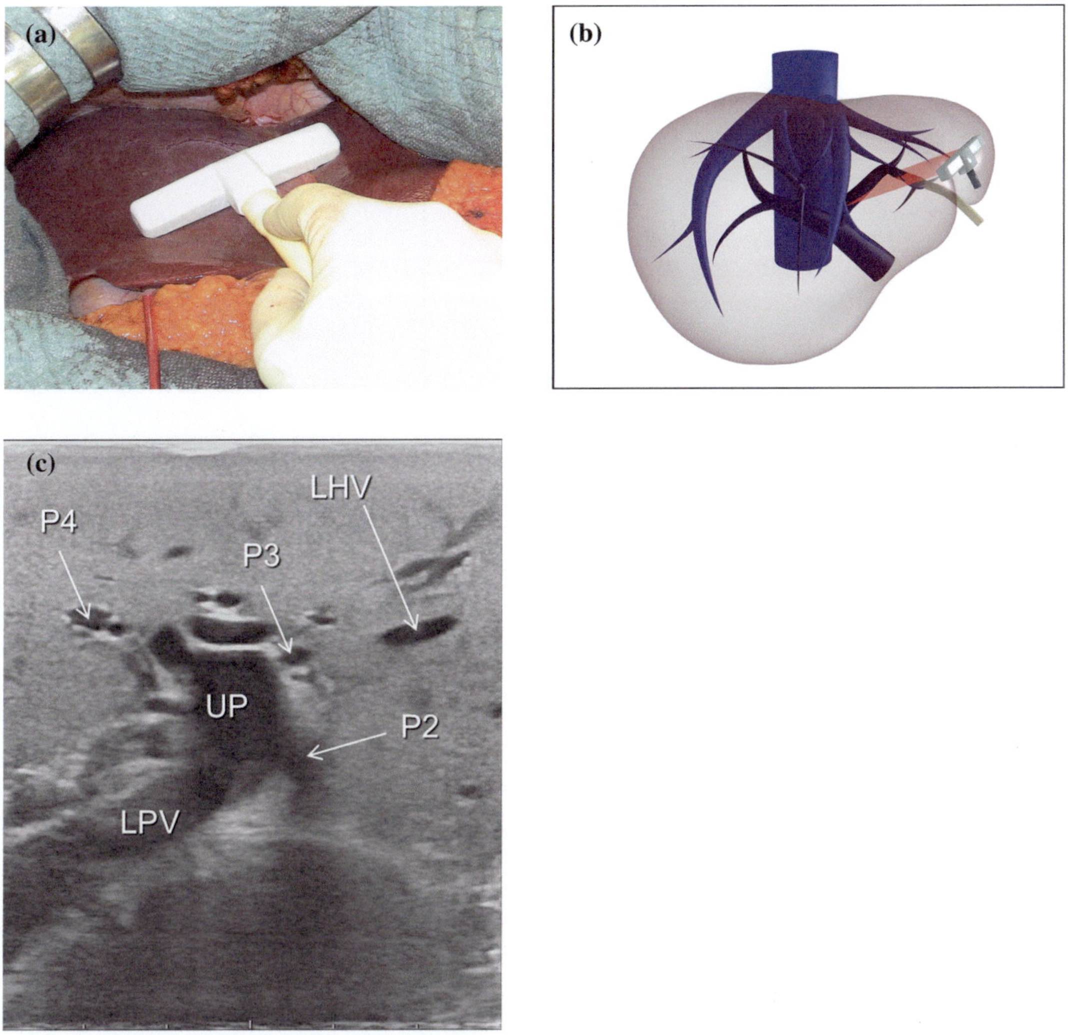

Fig. 3.10 Intraoperative probe position (**a**), scan (**b**), and IOUS image (**c**); left hepatic vein (*LHV*); left portal vein (*LPV*); portal branch to segment 2 (*P2*); portal branch to segment 3 (*P3*); portal branch to segment 4 (*P4*); umbilical portion (*UP*)

those pedicles feeding segments 2 (Fig. 3.14a, b) and 3 (Fig. 3.13a, b) can be disclosed.

Between those feeding segments 2 and 3 the LHV should appear (Figs. 3.14a, b, 3.17). At this point, as mentioned, the exploration of the hepatic veins is initiated moving toward the hepatocaval confluence (Fig. 3.18), and from there disclosing each hepatic vein along their entire length. It is worth to be recalled, that from the hepatocaval confluence, bending the probe downward, the entire segment 1 is explored which is demarcated by the curved plane described by the hepatic veins and posteriorly by the IVC (Fig. 3.25).

Once the main portal bifurcation is scanned, tilting the probe slightly upward allows to disclose the intrahepatic biliary tree within the glissonian pedicle even if not dilated (Fig. 3.31a–d). The particular peculiarity of the biliary tree to be taken into account is their branching pattern: indeed, the confluences of segmental and sectional ducts are closer to the

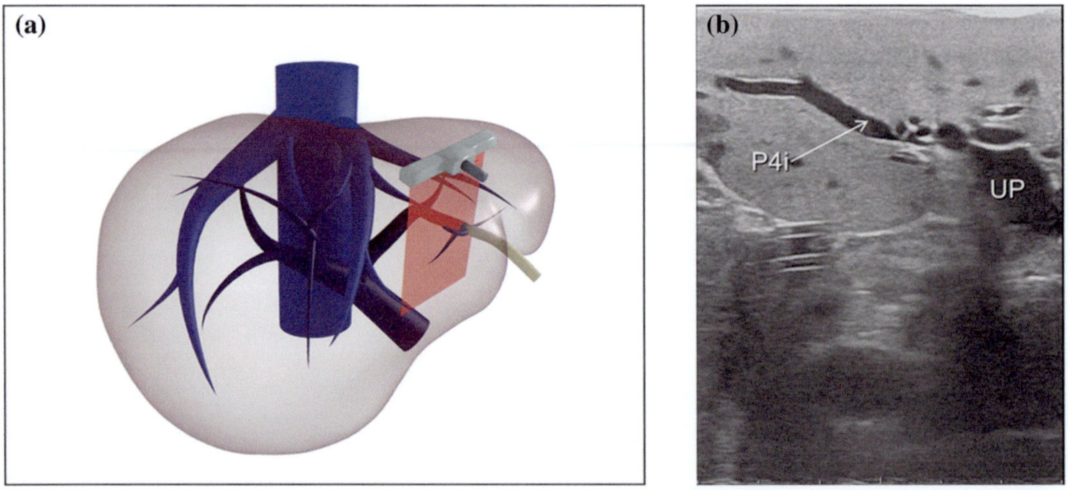

Fig. 3.11 Scan (**a**), and IOUS image (**b**); portal branch to segment 4 inferior (*P4i*); umbilical portion (*UP*)

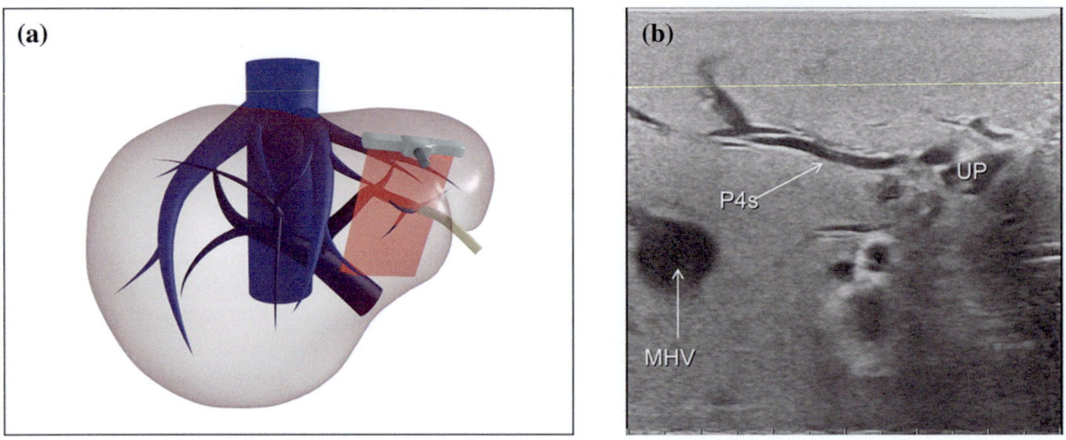

Fig. 3.12 Scan (**a**) and IOUS image (**b**); middle hepatic vein (*MHV*); portal branch to segment 4 superior (*P4s*); umbilical portion (*UP*)

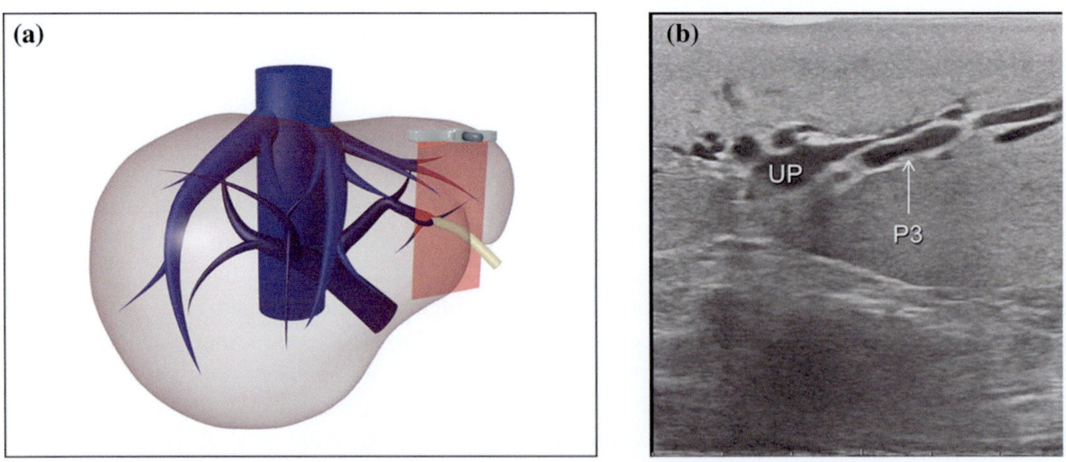

Fig. 3.13 Scan (**a**) and IOUS image (**b**); portal branch to segment 3 (*P3*); umbilical portion (*UP*)

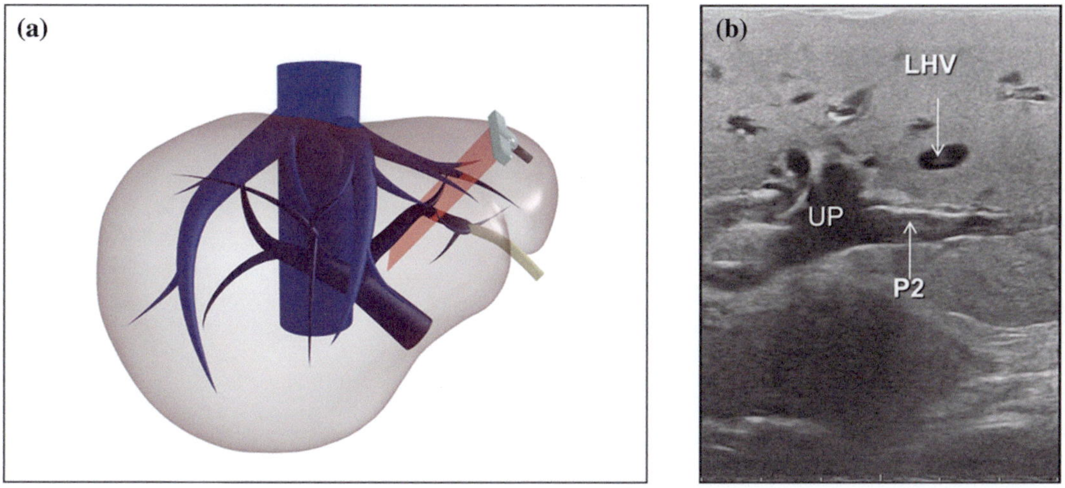

Fig. 3.14 Scan (**a**) and IOUS image (**b**); left hepatic vein (*LHV*); portal branch to segment 2 (*P2*); umbilical portion (*UP*)

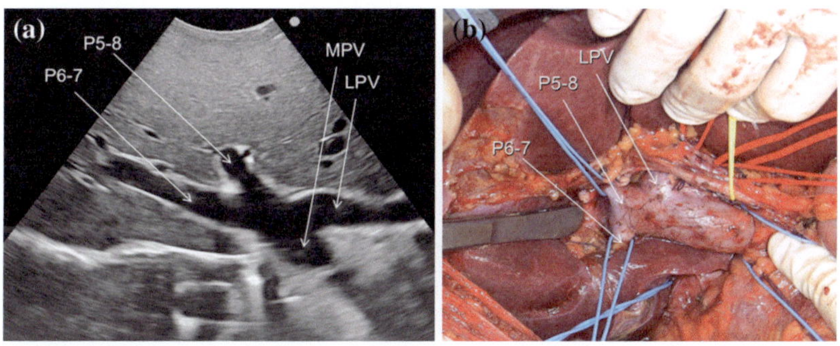

Fig. 3.15 Portal trifurcation by IOUS (**a**), and on the surgical field (**b**); left portal vein (*LPV*); main portal vein (*MPV*); portal branch to segments 5 and 8 (*P5-8*) (right anterior section); portal branch to segments 6 and 7 (*P6-7*) (right posterior section)

hilum as compared to the portal branches, and for that reason it is possible with one single scan to visualize more than a segmental bile duct. This is necessary to recognize aberrant (normally existing but assuming an unusual anatomical feature) and accessory (usually not existing) ducts, which may occur with rates ranging up to one-fifth of the patients: this indicates the crucial relevance of their recognition. For this reason, any hepatectomy should involve a careful IOUS exploration of the biliary tree to allow the surgeon to become aware of variants, which may be relevant for the scheduled procedure or in case of any variation of the strategy bearing the risk of biliary damage. A typical variant occurring in 13–19 % of patients and represented by the confluence of the right posterior sectional bile duct (B6-7)) into the left bile duct (Fig. 3.32a, b) rather than in the right as usually the case [2]. This variant if unrecognized during a left hepatectomy may cause the accidental division of B6-7 leaving the right posterior section of the liver undrained.

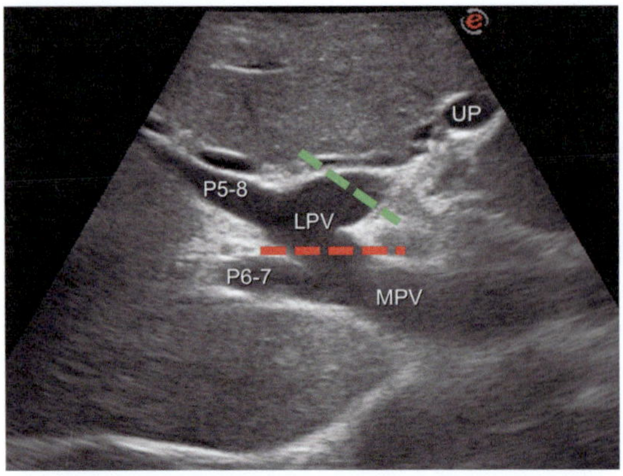

Fig. 3.16 IOUS image of a particular branching pattern in which the right portal vein does not exist and the right anterior portal branch (*P5-8*) originates from the left portal vein (*LPV*) after the origin from the main portal vein (*MPV*) of the right posterior portal branch (*P6-7*). This variant, if not recognized during a left hepatectomy, bears the risk of ligating the left portal vein before the origin of *P5-8* (*red dotted line*) rather than after (*green dotted line*), leading to a left trisectionectomy; this latter, since unexpected, could potentially lead to insufficient remaining liver and consequently hepatic failure; umbilical portion (*UP*)

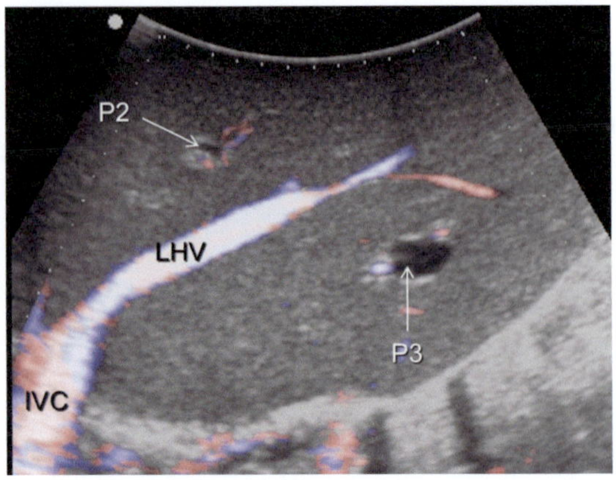

Fig. 3.17 Proceeding with IOUS, having disclosed all segmental portal branches including segments 2 (*P2*) and 3 (*P3*), the left hepatic vein (*LHV*) appears, and moving towards its confluence into the inferior vena cava (*IVC*) the hepatic veins are explored

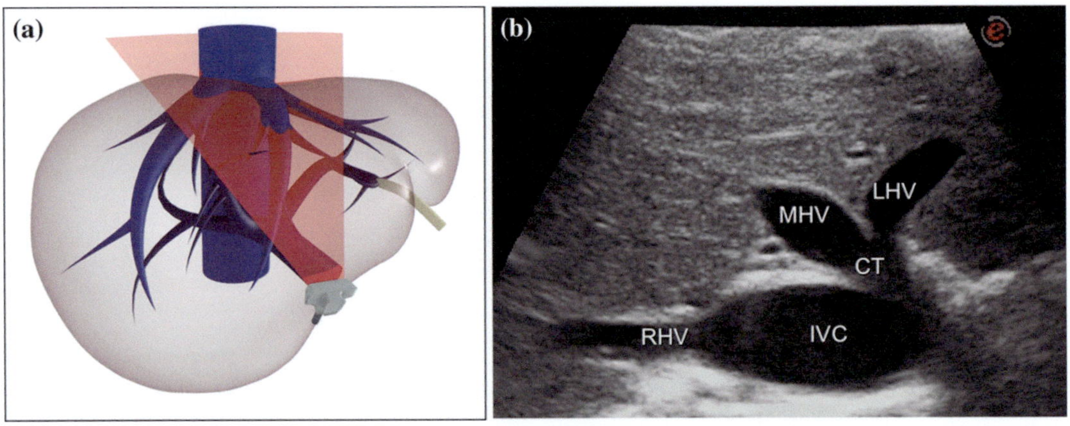

Fig. 3.18 Scan (**a**) and IOUS image obtained with a micro-T-shaped probe (**b**) revealing the caval confluence; common trunk (*CT*); inferior vena cava (*IVC*); left hepatic vein (*LHV*); middle hepatic vein (*MHV*); right hepatic vein (*RHV*)

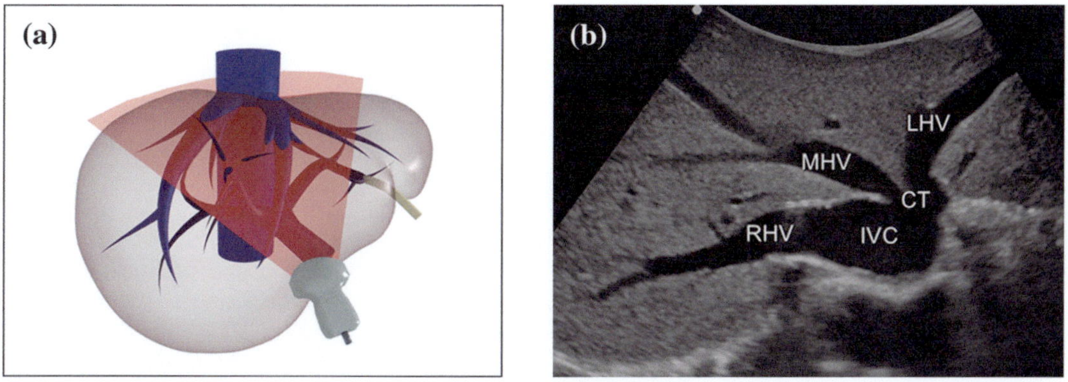

Fig. 3.19 Scan (**a**) and IOUS image obtained with a convex probe (**b**) showing the caval confluence; common trunk (*CT*); inferior vena cava (*IVC*); left hepatic vein (*LHV*); middle hepatic vein (*MHV*); right hepatic vein (*RHV*)

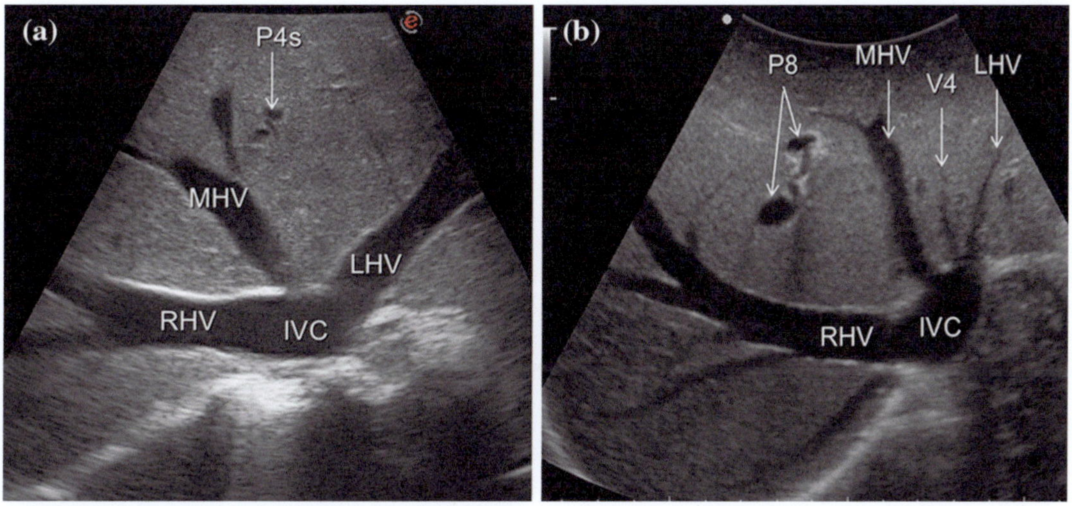

Fig. 3.20 **a** IOUS of a caval confluence in which there is no common trunk between the middle (*MHV*) and the left hepatic vein (*LHV*), and another (**b**) in which other than the absence of a common trunk there is the scissural vein (*V4*) flowing directly into the inferior vena cava (*IVC*); portal branch to segment 4 superior (*P4s*); portal branches to segment 8 (*P8*); right hepatic vein (*RHV*)

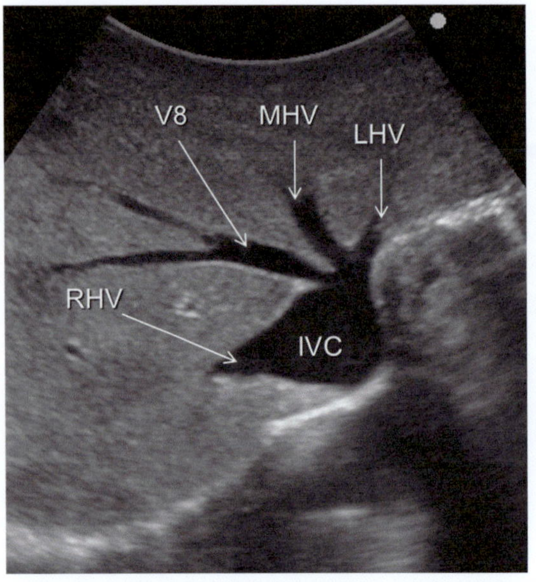

Fig. 3.21 IOUS of a caval confluence in which the branch draining segment 8 (*V8*) flows directly into the inferior vena cava (*IVC*); left hepatic vein (*LHV*); middle hepatic vein (*MHV*); right hepatic vein (*RHV*)

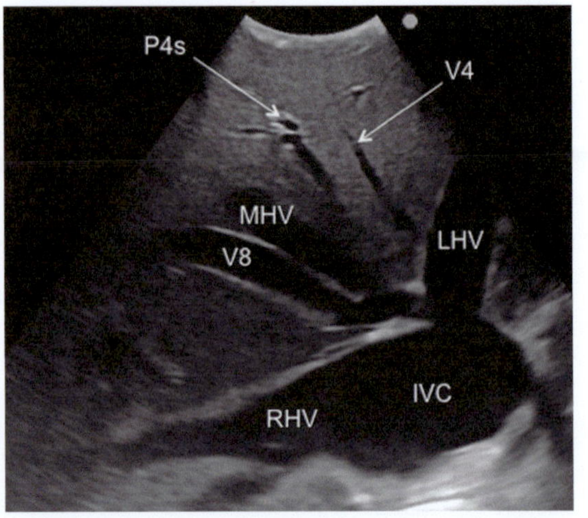

Fig. 3.22 IOUS of a caval confluence in which there is a thick hepatic vein draining segment 8 (*V8*) having the same diameter of the main trunk of the middle hepatic vein (*MHV*); inferior vena cava (*IVC*); left hepatic vein (*LHV*); portal branch to segment 4 superior (*P4s*); right hepatic vein (*RHV*); scissural vein (*V4*)

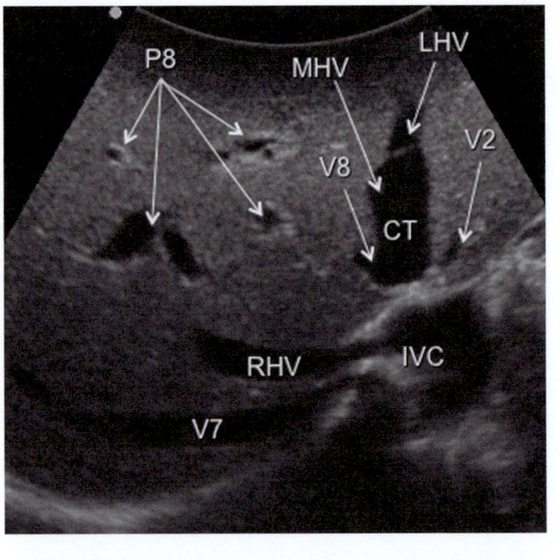

Fig. 3.23 IOUS of a caval confluence in which there is a thick hepatic vein draining segment 7 (*V7*) and flowing directly into the inferior vena cava (*IVC*), and a thick and dominant common trunk (*CT*) between the left (*LHV*) and the middle hepatic vein (*MHV*) into which flows, just in the proximity of its confluence into the *IVC*, the hepatic veins draining segments 8 (*V8*) and 2 (*V2*); portal branches to segment 8 (*P8*); right hepatic vein (*RHV*)

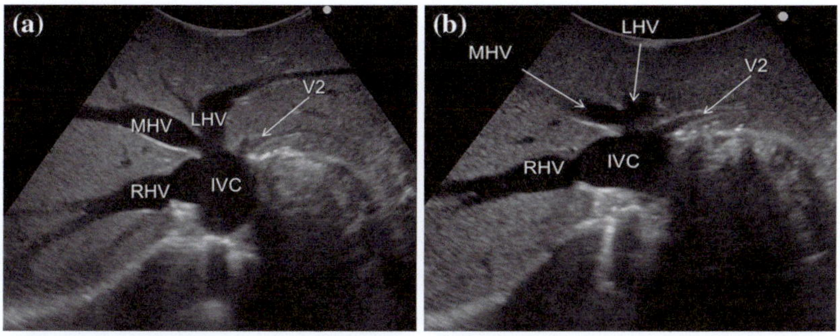

Fig. 3.24 IOUS of two conditions in both cases of which there is a left hepatic vein (*LHV*) and, separately, a hepatic vein draining segment 2 (*V2*) into the inferior vena cava (*IVC*) (**a**, **b**); middle hepatic vein (*MHV*); right hepatic vein (*RHV*)

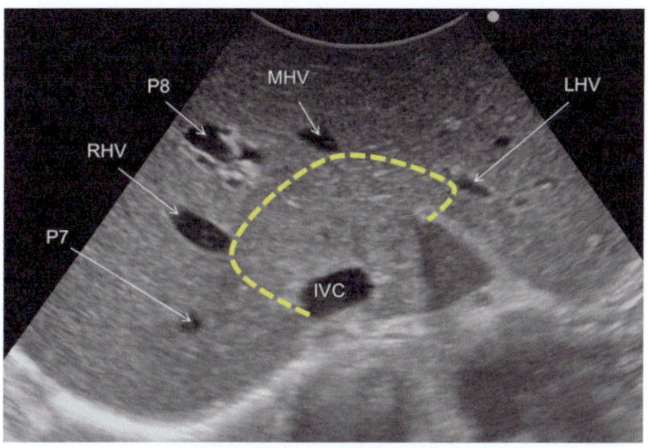

Fig. 3.25 IOUS of the paracaval portion of segment 1 which is that part between the plane connecting the three hepatic veins (*yellow-dotted line*); inferior vena cava (*IVC*); left hepatic vein (*LHV*); middle hepatic vein (*MHV*); portal branch to segment 8 (*P8*); portal branch to segment 7 (*P7*); right hepatic vein (*RHV*)

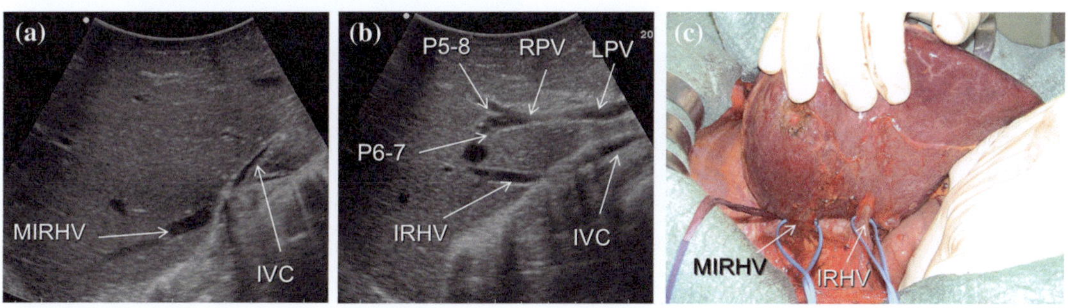

Fig. 3.26 IOUS of the paracaval part. Moving the probe from up- to downward can reveal accessory veins, such as (**a**) the middle inferior right hepatic vein (*MIRHV*) and (**b**) the inferior right hepatic vein (*IRHV*); the latter is recognizable by its typical pattern of flowing into the inferior vena cava (*IVC*) running behind the right portal vein (*RPV*) and the portal branch to the right posterior section (*P6-7*). Once recognized, they can be skeletonized and taped (**c**); left portal vein (*LPV*); portal branch to segments 5 and 8 (*P5-8*) (right anterior section)

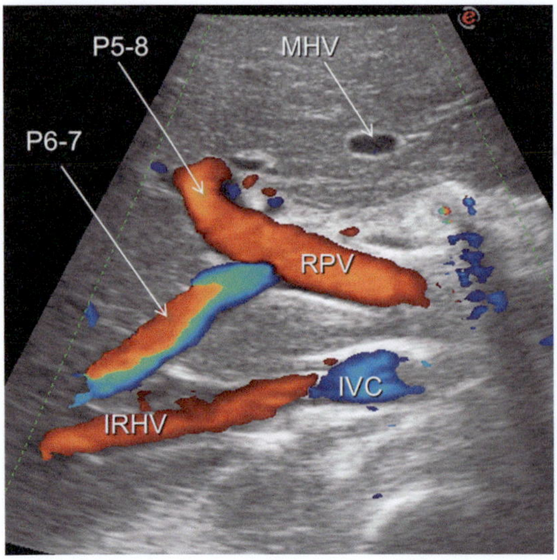

Fig. 3.27 IOUS of the paracaval part in which with the addition of the color-Doppler modality shows a thick inferior right hepatic vein (*IRHV*), which typically runs behind the right portal vein (*RPV*) and the portal branch to the right posterior section (*P6-7*); middle hepatic vein (*MHV*); portal branch to segments 5 and 8 (*P5-8*) (right anterior section)

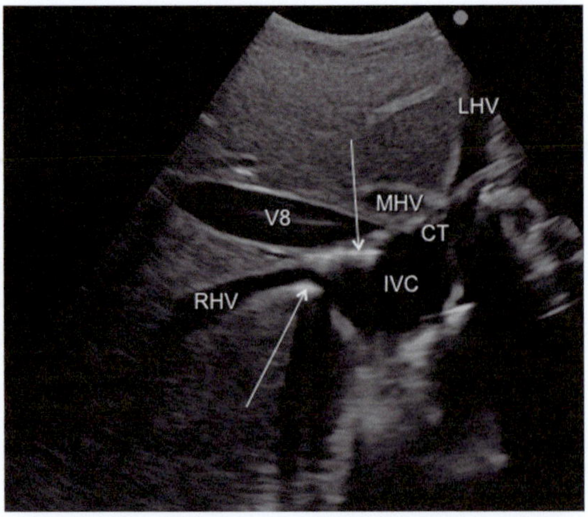

Fig. 3.28 IOUS of the caval confluence after dissecting; artifacts generated by air bubbles (*arrows*) are evident; common trunk (*CT*); inferior vena cava (*IVC*); left hepatic vein (*LHV*); middle hepatic vein (*MHV*); right hepatic vein (*RHV*); thick hepatic vein draining segment 8 (*V8*)

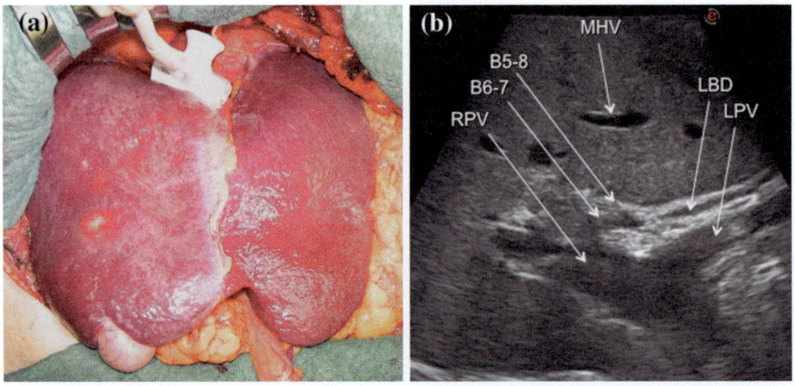

Fig. 3.29 Scanning the liver with the probe positioned cranially (**a**) the portal and biliary bifurcations are visible (**b**); bile duct draining the right posterior section (*B6-7*); bile duct draining the right anterior section (*B5-8*); left bile duct (*LBD*); left portal vein (*LPV*); middle hepatic vein (*MHV*); right portal vein (*RPV*)

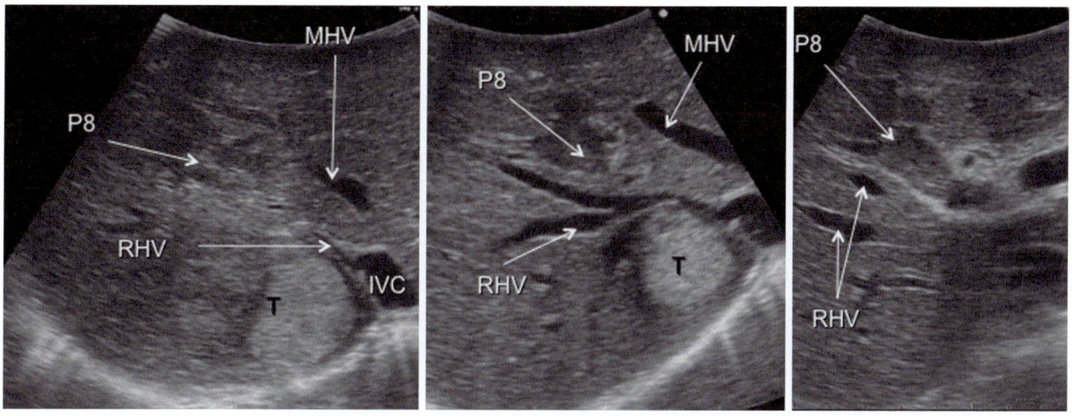

Fig. 3.30 IOUS following the portal branches of the liver. It is possible to properly address any lesion to the correct segment: a lesion (*T*) right-sided to the right hepatic vein (*RHV*) instead of belonging to segment 7, having invaded with a tumor thrombus the portal branch of segment 8 (*P8*) is located in the dorsal portion of segment 8; inferior vena cava (*IVC*); middle hepatic vein (*MHV*); right hepatic vein (*RHV*)

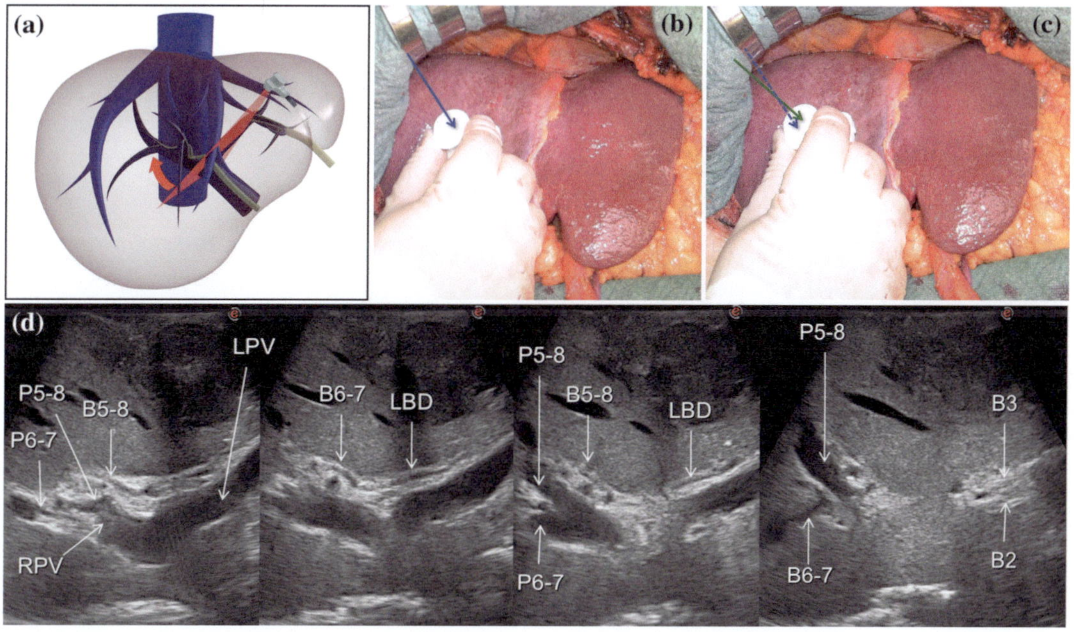

Fig. 3.31 Scan of the liver with the probe visualizing the intrahepatic biliary tree. **a** Once having selected the scan to visualize the main portal bifurcation, it is sufficient to slightly tilt the probe upwards remaining with the scan within the glissonean sheath but just cranially. **b** Movement in the surgical field: the *blue arrow* indicates the scan for the portal branch (*solid and dashed line*), the *green arrow* for the bile duct (note the importance of the movement, not the position of the probe). Moving the probe cranially, i.e., from left to right in (**d**), it is possible to follow the biliary bifurcation from the main to the sectional and even segmental branches taking advantage of anatomical features of the biliary tree with its centripetal branching pattern (close to the main hilar bifurcation) compared to the portal one; bile duct draining the segment 2 (*B2*); bile duct draining the segment 3 (*B3*); bile duct draining the right posterior section (*B6-7*); bile duct draining the right anterior section (*B5-8*); left bile duct (*LBD*); left portal vein (*LPV*); portal branches to the right posterior section (*P6-7*); portal branch to the right anterior section (*P5-8*); right portal vein (*RPV*)

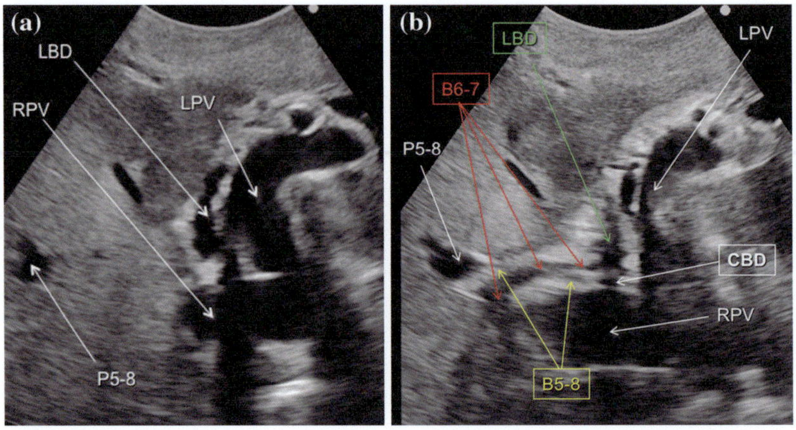

Fig. 3.32 IOUS can clearly disclose not only the normal anatomy of the intrahepatic biliary tree but also important variations, which if unrecognized during hepatic surgery account for potentially life-threatening damage. **a** Left bile duct (*LBD*) visible together with the left (*LPV*) and the right portal vein (*RPV*); **b** tilting upward the probe sheath containing the right posterior bile duct (*B6-7*), and the right anterior bile duct (*B5-8*) appear. However, more importantly the confluence of *B6-7* into the *LBD*, and then the confluence of the latter into the common bile duct (*CBD*) together with B5-8 confirm an important intrahepatic variation of the biliary tree. The inadvertent division of the LBD centrally to the confluence of *B6-7* during a left hepatectomy interrupts the biliary drainage of the right posterior section; right anterior portal branch (*P5-8*)

References

1. Belghiti J, Clavien PA, Gadzijev E et al (2000) The Brisbane 2000 terminology of liver anatomy and resections. HPB (Oxford) 2:333–339
2. Mortelé KJ, Ros PR (2001) Anatomic variants of the biliary tree: MR cholangiographic findings and clinical applications. Am J Roentgenol 177:389–394

Part II
Diagnosis and Staging

Diagnosis and Staging: Intraoperative Ultrasound

4

Guido Torzilli, Matteo Donadon, and Matteo Cimino

Detection and differentiation are the two main targets of IOUS explorations of the liver. IOUS is thus still serves as a reference standard compared to preoperative imaging. However, to make its performance provide the expected results one needs to consider several important aspects which, although basic, if unrecognized could lead to misinterpreting neoplastic or non-neoplastic lesions, normal findings, or artifacts to avoid useless resection and additional risk for the patients.

Proper interpretation of the echogenicity of a lesion is of paramount importance. One rather frequently will encounter simple hepatic cysts which can be recognized quite easily as they appear as anechoic (fully black) (Fig. 4.1a) rather than hypoechoic (Fig. 4.1b), and as having a posterior hyperechoic shadow (Fig. 4.1a) which exists also when they are very small (Fig. 4.2a). Inversely, the latter is absent if the lesion is a solid one as in the case of tiny metastastic fore sites (Fig. 4.2b). However, misinterpretation may result if the IOUS image is not properly adjusted and in particular the gain and the focus are not set in a suitable way. Therefore, the gain of the gray scale should not be too high and, in particular, should be homogeneous and the focus level should not be positioned distant from the level of the target: if not, a cystic lesion can appear as a solid one (echogenic) rather than as liquid (fully anechoic) (Fig. 4.3).

Even the round ligament appearing in a transverse scan as a hyperechoic target lesion may resemble a solid tumor (Fig. 4.4): its origin from the umbilical portion, its linear shape once the scan is sagittal would disclose its real nature. A frequent source of misinterpretation is represented by the so-called skip-areas, which are portions of the liver with different intracellular distribution of lipids resulting in areas with different echogenicity [1]. These areas are typically located around the gallbladder (Fig. 4.5) or around the main portal pedicles (Fig. 4.6): their shape, the fact that vessels are passing through without distortions, and, not last, the mentioned typical locations should ensure their proper interpretation. There is an artifact being a true optical illusion which is called the mirror effect: in cases where a lesion is just anterior to other structures being a barrier for the diffusion of the ultrasonic waves, a reflection of the lesion itself can appear posteriorly, mimicking the reflection of an image in front of a mirror both without (Fig. 4.7a, b) and with contrast enhancement (Fig. 4.8).

IOUS allows the detection of new lesions in around 30 % of cirrhotic patients [2]. However, most of the nodules detected by IOUS in these patients are not really tumors: in this way, IOUS

G. Torzilli (✉) · M. Donadon · M. Cimino
Department of Hepatobiliary Surgery,
Humanitas Research Hospital-IRCCS,
University of Milan-School of Medicine,
Via A. Manzoni 56, 20089 Rozzano, MI, Italy
e-mail: guido.torzilli@humanitas.it;
guido.torzilli@unimi.it

G. Torzilli (ed.), *Ultrasound-Guided Liver Surgery*,
DOI: 10.1007/978-88-470-5510-0_4, © Springer-Verlag Italia 2014

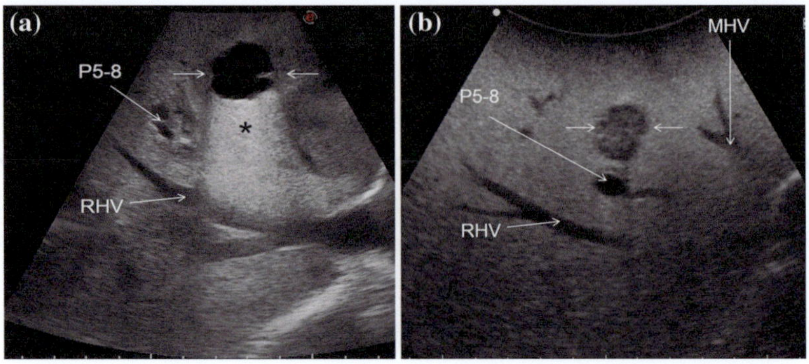

Fig. 4.1 **a** Simple hepatic cyst (*arrows*) with its typical posterior echo (*) and the echofree (*black*) content; **b** clear visibility of hypoechoic metastases (*arrows*) in a so-called ''bright'' (fatty) liver; middle hepatic vein (*MHV*); portal branch to the right anterior section (*P5-8*); right hepatic vein (*RHV*)

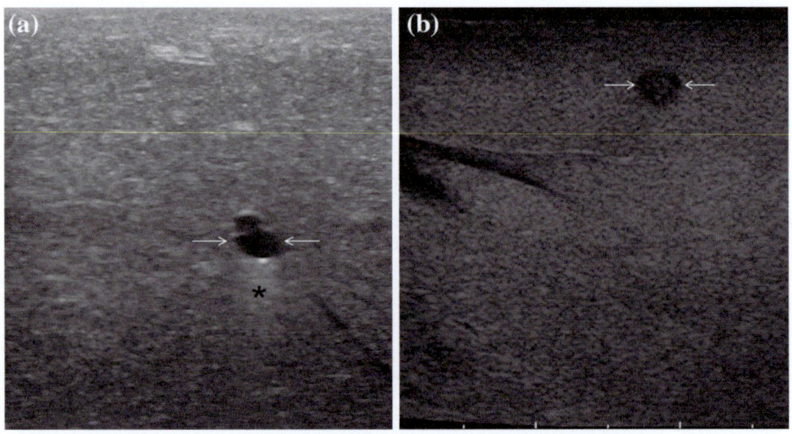

Fig. 4.2 A small, simple hepatic cyst (*arrows*) with its typical posterior echo (*) and the echo-free (*black*) content (**a**), compared to a tiny metastasis (*arrows*) (**b**)

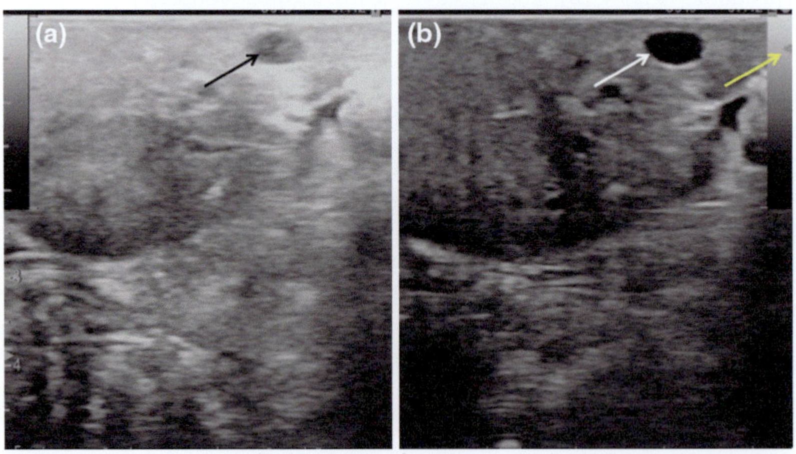

Fig. 4.3 **a** Importance of the regulation of the image setting especially if the focus is not adequately set (too deep for this particular case) and the gain too (too bright) where a cyst (*black arrow*) can mimic a solid lesion, while **b** once the ultrasound system is properly regulated (*yellow arrow* showing the focus level) the same lesions (*white arrow*) shows the typical features of a cysts as previously described

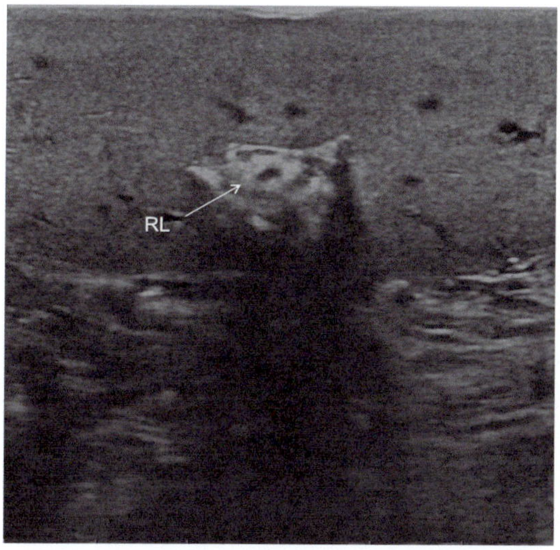

Fig. 4.4 Importance of understanding the anatomical structures and the need during ultrasound exploration of using several axes in investigating a lesion in order to avoid misinterpretation of its nature; otherwise, even the round ligament (*RL*) could mimic a target lesion

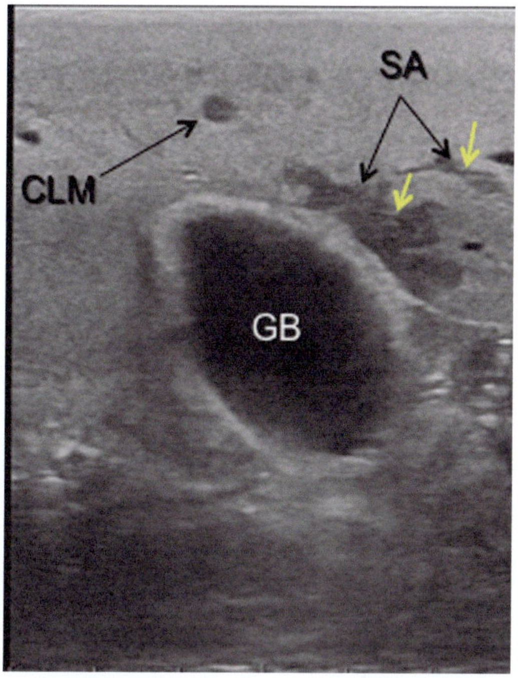

Fig. 4.5 The different appearance of skip-areas (*SA*) also referred to as focal steatosis, and a colorectal liver metastasis (*CLM*): while the SA is located in a typical position—adjacent to the gallbladder (*GB*)—and moreover assumes bizarre shapes with thin vessels (*yellow arrows*) passing through without being interrupted or deviated, the CLM is sharp and rounded

introduces the risk of overestimating the tumor stage (Fig. 4.9). Indeed, except for those nodules with mosaic ultrasonographic patterns (Fig. 4.10a), which are malignant in 84 % of cases, only 24–30 % of hypoechoic nodules (Fig. 4.10b), and 0–18 % of those hyperechoic (Fig. 4.10c) are neoplasm [2, 3]. To overcome this problem even biopsy may not be adequate. The only nodule which can be easily differentiated intraoperatively from an HCC or a liver metastasis is the small hemangioma which is often discovered primarily by IOUS: it has a typical ultrasonographic pattern and moreover when compressed changes its size and appearance (Fig. 4.11a, b). This is based essentially on the different stiffness of the hemangioma compared to other lesions. Stiffness measurements are advantageous in this respect. In fact, intraoperative elastography can afford lesion differentiation based on tissue elasticity expressed on the IOUS screen by differences in colors (Fig. 4.12a, b). Therefore, some authors have introduced a classification for differentiating HCC from metastastic nodules based on their tissue elasticity at intraoperative elastography [4]. In this sense, other authors have proposed the use of elastography to check in real time the completeness of intraoperative tumor ablation [5]. Chapter 5 describes how CEIOUS is starting to play an important role in this respect, and most likely will become more relevant in the near future.

IOUS has long been known to be advantageous for detecting CLM in patients undergoing liver surgery. Detection of additional disease may change the surgical approach to allow complete extirpation of all disease and may contribute to improved outcomes. From 10 to 40 % of patients with colon cancer do not have palpable colorectal liver metastases (CLM) [6, 7]: thus, IOUS exploration of the liver remains crucial. However, the real impact of IOUS varies widely among series, ranging from 2–3 % [8, 9] to 16–20 % [10–12]. This variability probably depends on the ultrasound equipment used, surgeon experience in ultrasonography, and

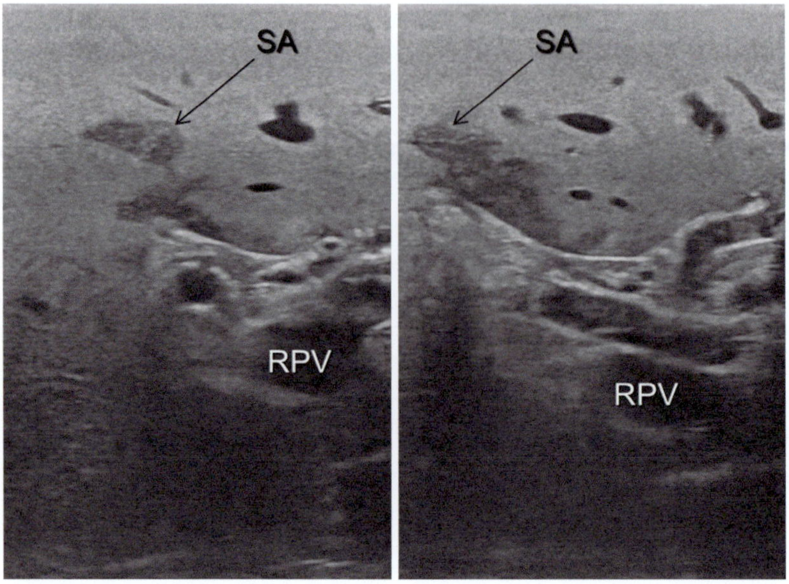

Fig. 4.6 Another typical location of skip-areas (*SA*): also located adjacent to the main glissonian sheaths; right portal vein (*RPV*)

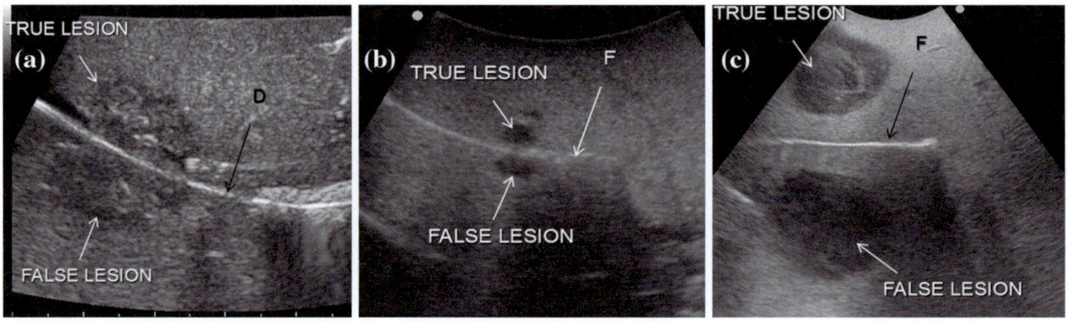

Fig. 4.7 A classic artifact called *mirror effect* consisting of a real image and a virtual one caused by a reflecting interface such as diaphragm-lung (**a**), liver-finger for tiny (**b**) and large lesions (**c**); diaphragm (*D*); finger (*F*)

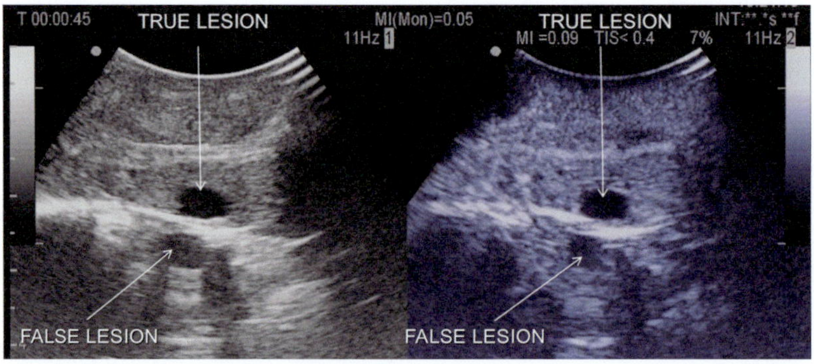

Fig. 4.8 A mirror effect evident also by CEIOUS

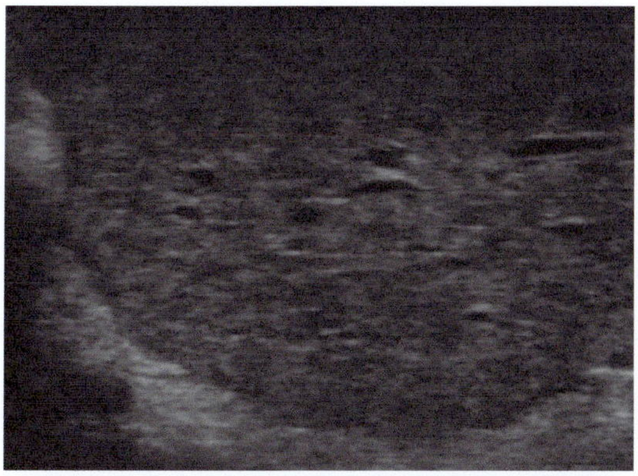

Fig. 4.9 Cirrhotic liver with an inhomogeneous pattern due to the presence of an uncountable number of hypoechoic (*dark*) nodules

rigorousness of both the preoperative cross-sectional imaging and the IOUS protocol. However, an important role is also played by the degree and relevance to which the obtained IOUS information is applied on the surgical strategy (see Chap. 7). Indeed, if a strict parenchyma-sparing approach is favored [13], the attention paid to disclose any eventual new CLM is probably more pronounced than in case of preference of a conventional surgical approach, such as major right or left hepatectomy. In addition to aspects of technology, experience, and surgical approach, another important factor is tumor echogenity: indeed, a hypoechoic CLM (Fig. 4.13a) is better visualized than a

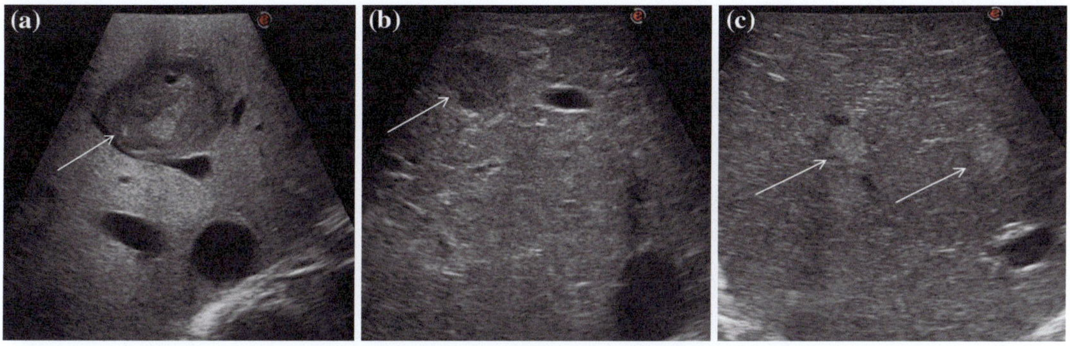

Fig. 4.10 **a** Nodule (*arrow*) with a mosaic pattern in IOUS; **b** nodule (*arrow*) with a hypoechoic pattern in IOUS; **c** two nodules (*arrows*) with a hyperechoic pattern in IOUS

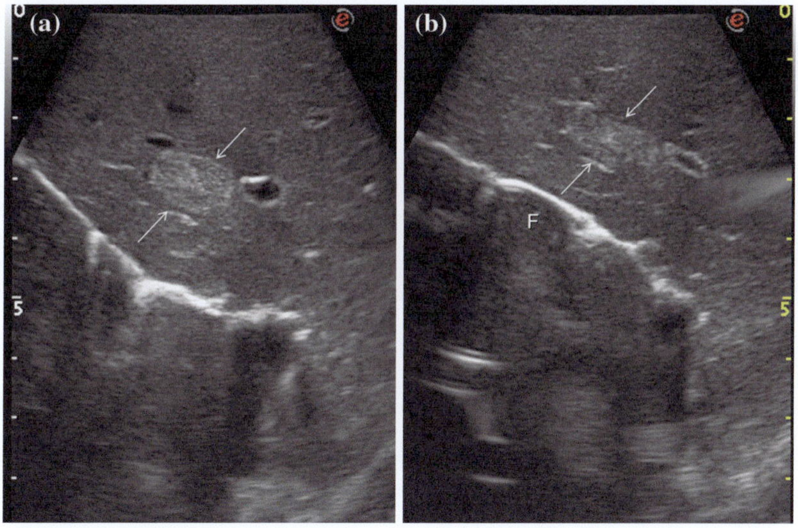

Fig. 4.11 Hemangioma diagnosis: **a** an hemangioma (*arrows*) with hyperechoic (*bright*) pattern, typical for this kind of lesion but not specific enough; **b** the lesion once compressed under IOUS guidance changes its shape and thickness (*arrows*)—this finding together with its echogenicity lead to the diagnosis of hemangioma; surgeon's fingertip (*F*)

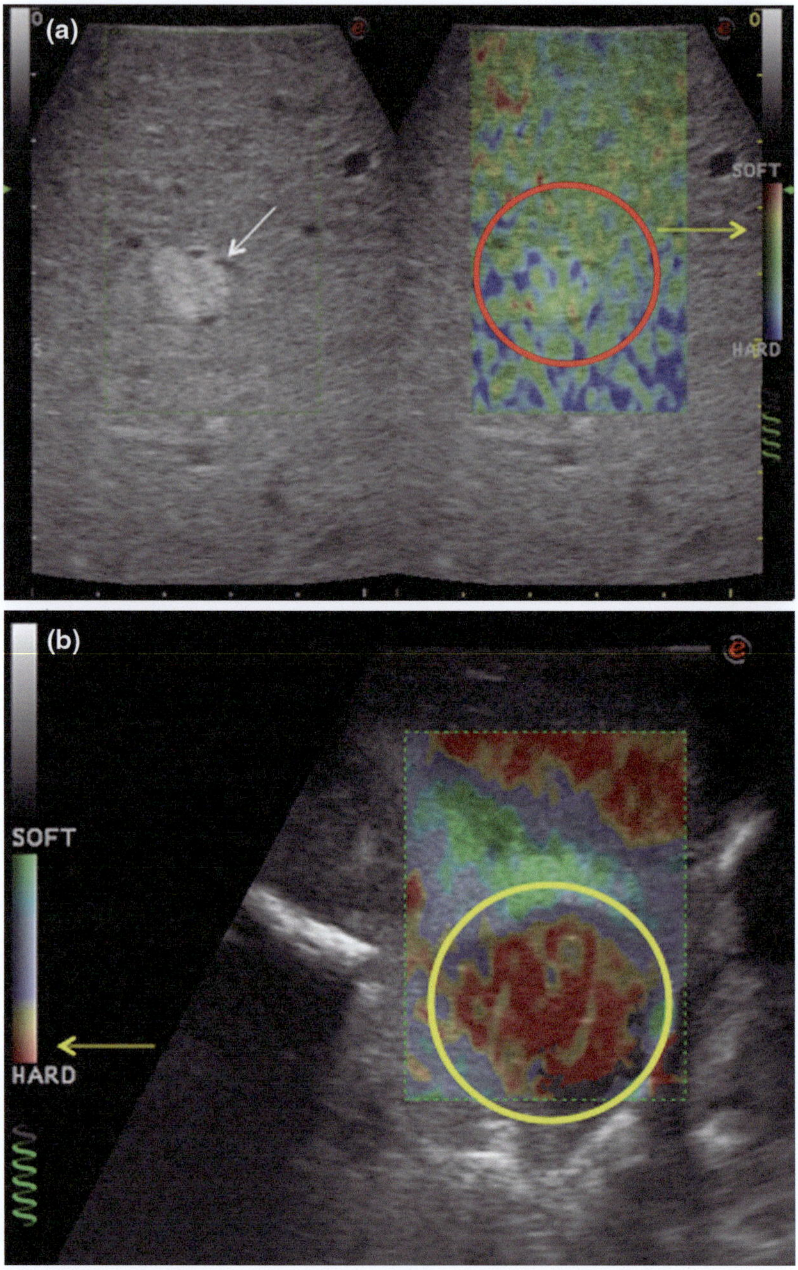

Fig. 4.12 The potential value of elastography in estimating tissue stiffness in reference to a color scale displayed on the side of each image; **a** hemangioma (*arrow*) expected to be soft, compressible as in Fig. 4.11; on the right, its softness is confirmed by elastography (*red circle*) according to the color scale (*yellow arrow*); **b** upon elastography of a metastastic tumor (*yellow circle*); the increased stiffness of the latter is confirmed by elastography, according to the color scale (*yellow arrow*)

hyperechoic (Fig. 4.13b) or isoechoic (Fig. 4.13c) lesion; and though the three patterns occur in approximately 40, 20, and 40 % of patients, respectively, the rate of new lesions have been shown to be 18, 9, and 3 % [10]. This discrepancy may impact both radicality and even long-term outcome, and, other than tumor biology per se, it could be a reason of the still high rate of early recurrence [14]. Thus, there is the potential for improving the detection power of IOUS for CLM particularly for those patients bearing isoechoic lesions, this particularly being the case for CEIOUS (Fig. 4.14a, b).

A further problem in CLM detection is related to the changes in the echogenicity of the lesions induced by chemotherapy. Some lesions

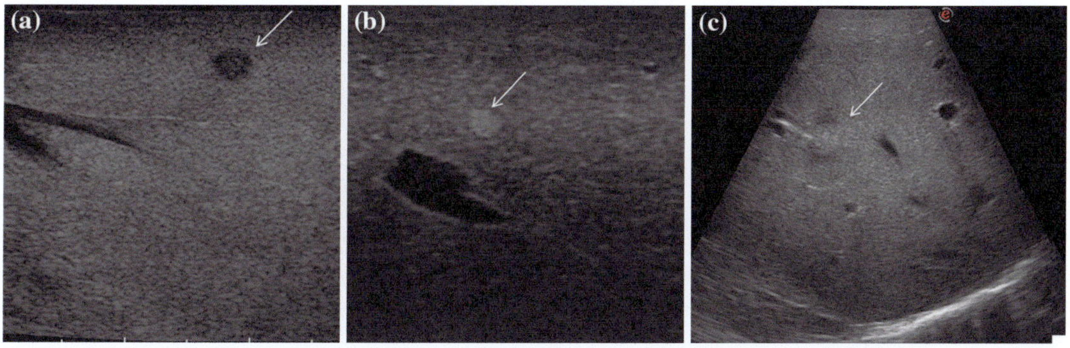

Fig. 4.13 **a** Colorectal liver metastases with a hypoechoic pattern (*arrow*) in IOUS; **b** colorectal liver metastases with a hyperechoic pattern (*arrow*) in IOUS; **c** colorectal liver metastases with an isoechoic pattern (*arrow*) in IOUS

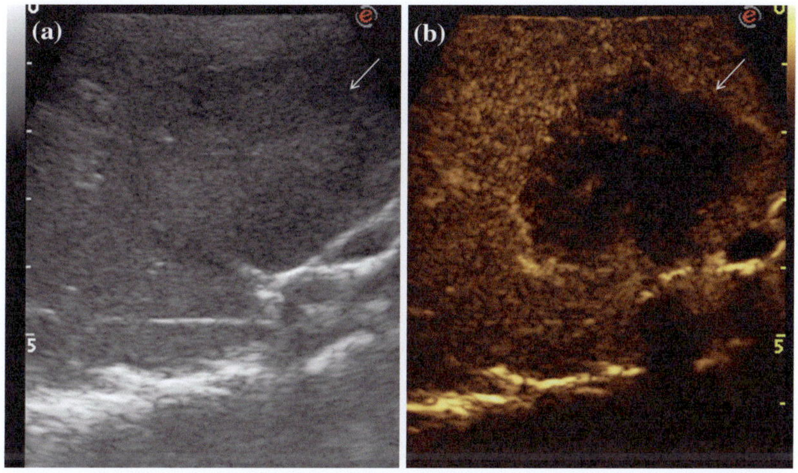

Fig. 4.14 Relatively extensive colorectal liver metastases (*arrows*) with an isoechoic pattern (**a**) in IOUS and (**b**) CEIOUS, with enhanced visibility and more clear edges

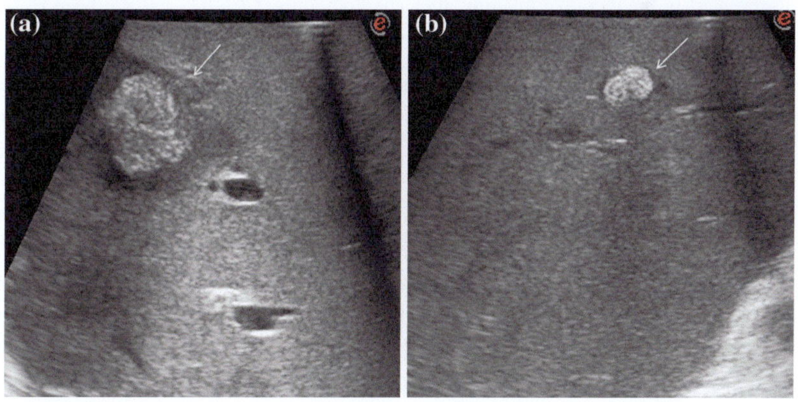

Fig. 4.15 IOUS of (**a**) medium or (**b**) tiny calcified colorectal liver metastases (*arrows*) as appearing after chemotherapy

shift to a calcified pattern: although this change does not mean absence of residual tumors [15], it still helps to localize them intraoperatively. Indeed, calcified lesions appear well visible at IOUS due to the typical hyperechoic pattern (Fig. 4.15a, b). More problematic is the not rare

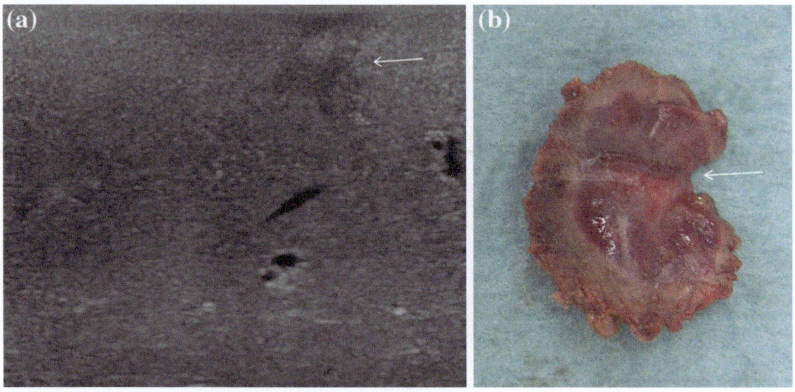

Fig. 4.16 IOUS of colorectal metastases (*arrow*) having disappeared in preoperative imaging after chemotherapy (**a**), and resulting on the specimen as a scar (*arrow*) (**b**)

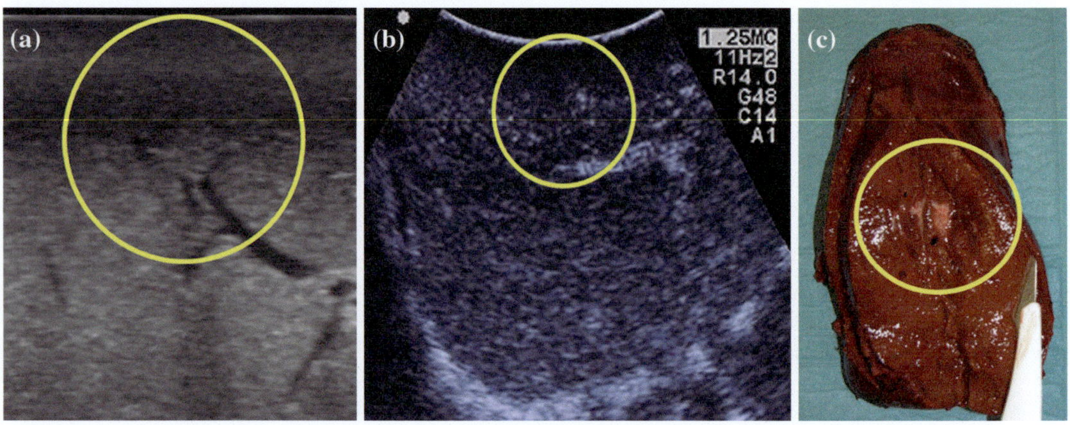

Fig. 4.17 IOUS (**a**), CEIOUS (**b**) and specimen (**c**) of a residual scar of a colorectal metastasis (*yellow circle*) having disappeared in preoperative imaging after chemotherapy. CEIOUS has not been of value here

disappearance of the lesions after chemotherapy [16], which are difficult to locate intraoperatively even by IOUS. Indeed, while up to 80 % of the CLM may have disappeared, it still may contain some viable tumoral tissue which can be the source of postsurgical relapse [17], and IOUS has only been able to disclose this in 60–70 % of cases [18] (Fig. 4.16a, b). Whether CEIOUS may eventually improve the detection rate is not clear, but early attempts in this respect have been disappointing (Fig. 4.17a–c).

Focal lesions which liver surgeons now more frequently need to address are biliary tumors. They may generally be divided into peripheral, intrahepatic, and perihilar cholangiocarcinomas. Their incidence has recently increased, possibly due to certain risk factors [19]. Intrahepatic ones in the mass-forming variant can be assimilated both by IOUS (Fig. 4.18a–c) and CEIOUS (Fig. 4.19) as a CLM. The perihilar variant, called Klatskin tumor [20], is mostly isoechoic upon IOUS being presenting by the concentrically distributed dilated bile ducts (Fig. 4.20a, b). This latter feature together with the intramural and perineural growth pattern of this tumor, as later described in Chap. 9, limits the utility of IOUS for resection guidance.

As mentioned in Chap.3, another limitation to IOUS exploration which definitely needs to be taken into account is that hard and irregular

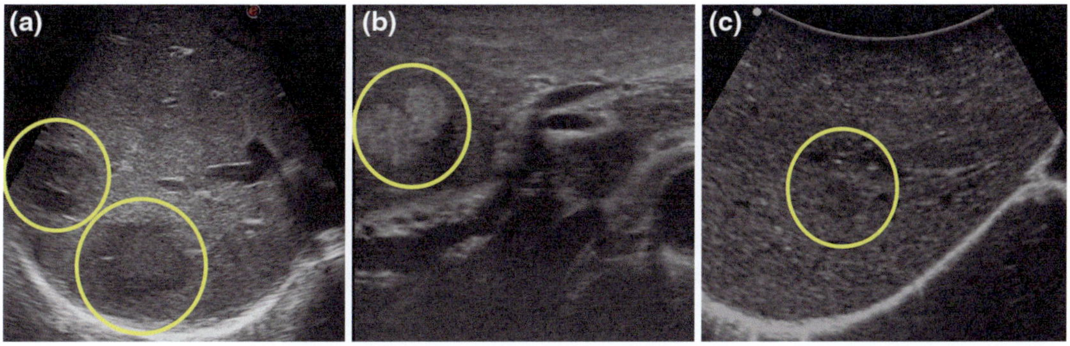

Fig. 4.18 IOUS of mass-forming cholangiocarcinoma (*yellow circles*) which can assume hypoechoic (**a**), hyperechoic (**b**) and almost isoechoic (**c**) patterns

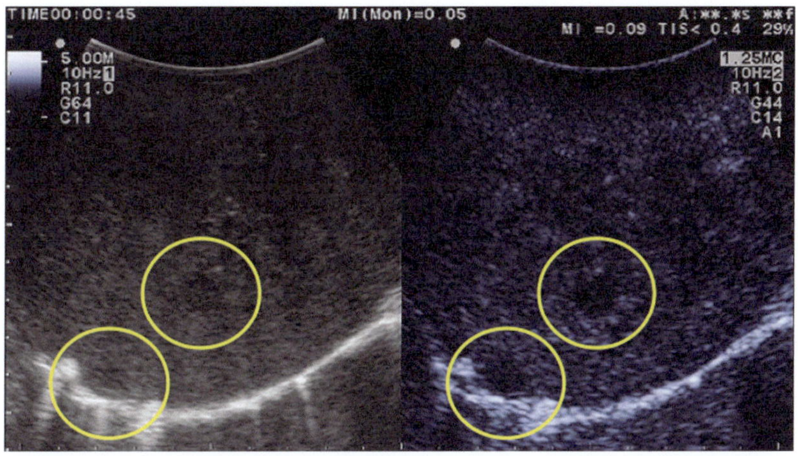

Fig. 4.19 CEIOUS (*right*) of two tiny mass-forming cholangiocarcinomas (*yellow circles*), which recall the pattern of colorectal liver metastases (see Chaps. 5 and 6)

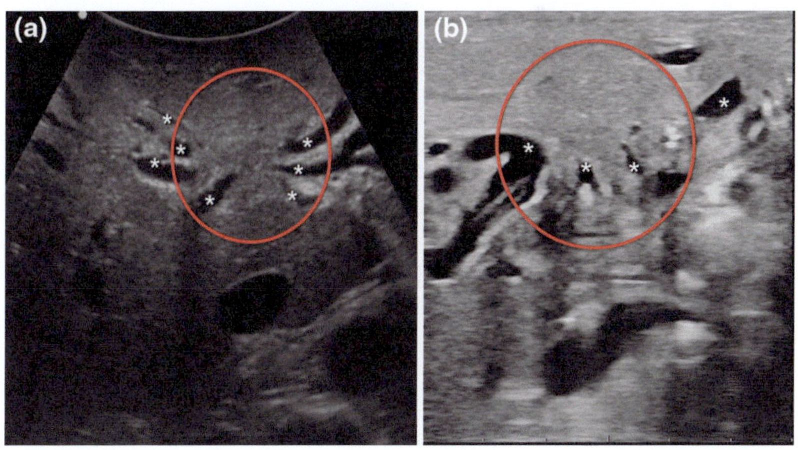

Fig. 4.20 IOUS of perihilar cholangiocarcinoma (*red circles*), which is generally isoechoic (**a**, **b**), and detectable for the dilated bile ducts (*) rather than for its edges

surfaces of a cirrhotic liver (Fig. 4.21a), scars of previous operations (Fig. 4.21b), ablations, or other tight postsurgical adhesions may impair the chance to feel tiny superficial lesions by palpation or to visualize them by IOUS as they may locally prevent the adherence of the probe

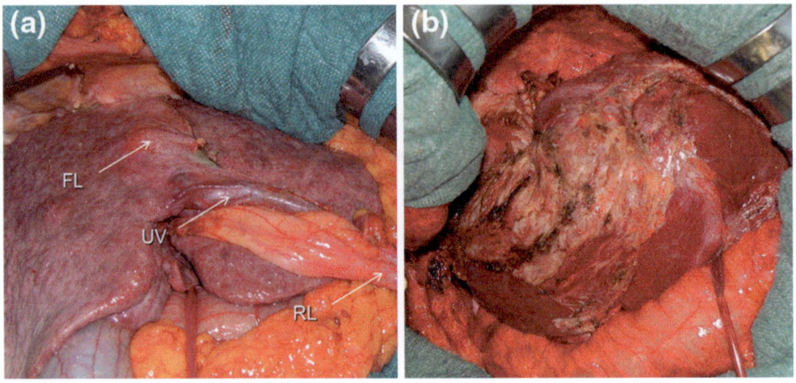

Fig. 4.21 Cirrhosis (**a**) and scars (**b**) leading to an irregular liver surface being a potential source of artifacts in IOUS; falciform ligament (*FL*); round ligament (*RL*); umbilical vein (*UV*)

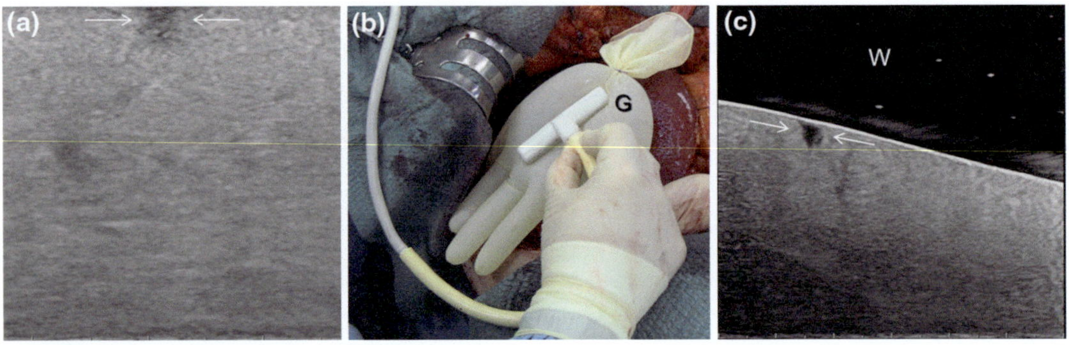

Fig. 4.22 A tiny lesion (*arrows*) appearing upon direct-contact IOUS (**a**) and how, once a glove filled with deaerated sterile water is interposed between the probe and the liver surface (**b**), the lesion itself becomes clearer (*arrows*) in IOUS; glove (*G*); water (*W*)

to the liver surface. As already mentioned in Chap. 1, condoms or gloves filled with deaerated water may aid in detecting these lesions by IOUS (Fig. 4.22a–c). The real novelty here is the recent introduction in the surgical practice of fluorescent imaging with indocyanine green (ICG) as fluorescent source [21, 22]. The near-infrared light penetrates the human tissue by about 5–10 mm, and the ICG (used in several centers as routine liver function test) is injected intravenously approx. 3 days before surgery. During laparotomy the liver is explored for detecting any sign of fluorescence on its surface by means of a fluorescent imaging system consisting of a control unit and a camera unit. The specimen itself, once removed, is also explored for undisclosed fluorescent areas. Ishizawa et al. [21] thus detected 13 out of 91 lesions by ICG-fluorescent imaging, with a sensitivity of 100 % for HCC and 93 % for CLM. Similarly, in a smaller series and referred just to carriers of HCC, Gotoh et al. [22] revealed all new lesions by ICG-fluorescent imaging. These promising results warrant further experience. The staining pattern differs from histology and tumor differentiation: CLM and poorly differentiated HCC retain ICG at the periphery, while well-differentiated HCC is fully stained. Certainly, the main limitation of this technique is that it can only be applied for lesions located on the liver surface and on cut surfaces once the specimen has been removed.

References

1. Caturelli E, Costarelli L, Giordano M et al (1991) Hypoechoic lesions in fatty liver. Quantitative study by histomorphometry. Gastroenterology 100:1678–1682
2. Kokudo N, Bandai Y, Imanishi H et al (1996) Management of new hepatic nodules detected by intraoperative ultrasonography during hepatic resection for hepatocellular carcinoma. Surgery 119:634–640
3. Takigawa Y, Sugawara Y, Yamamoto J et al (2001) New lesions detected by intraoperative ultrasound during liver resection for hepatocellular carcinoma. Ultrasound Med Biol 27:151–156
4. Kato K, Sugimoto H, Kanazumi N et al (2008) Intraoperative application of real-time tissue elastography for the diagnosis of liver tumours. Liver Int 28:1264–1271
5. Van Vledder MG, Boctor EM, Assumpcao LR et al (2010) Intra-operative ultrasound elasticity imaging for monitoring of hepatic tumour thermal ablation. HPB (Oxford) 12:717–723
6. Machi J, Isomoto H, Kurohiji T et al (1991) Accuracy of intraoperative ultrasonography in diagnosing liver metastasis from colorectal cancer: evaluation with postoperative follow-up results. World J Surg 15:551–556
7. Agrawal N, Fowler AL, Thomas MG (2006) The routine use of intraoperative ultrasound in patients with colorectal cancer improves the detection of hepatic metastases. Colorectal Dis 8:192–194
8. Rydzewski B, Dehdashti F, Gordon BA et al (2002) Usefulness of intraoperative sonography for revealing hepatic metastases from colorectal cancer in patients selected for surgery after undergoing FDG PET. Am J Roentgenol 178:353–358
9. Tamandl D, Herberger B, Gruenberger B et al (2008) Adequate preoperative staging rarely leads to a change of intraoperative strategy in patients undergoing surgery for colorectal cancer liver metastases. Surgery 143:648–657
10. Van Vledder MG, Pawlik TM, Munireddy S et al (2010) Factors determining the sensitivity of intraoperative ultrasonography in detecting colorectal liver metastases in the modern era. Ann Surg Oncol 17:2756–2763
11. Conlon R, Jacobs M, Dasgupta D et al (2003) The value of intraoperative ultrasound during hepatic resection compared with improved preoperative magnetic resonance imaging. Eur J Ultrasound 16:211–216
12. Sietses C, Meijerink MR, Meijer S et al (2010) The impact of intraoperative ultrasonography on the surgical treatment of patients with colorectal liver metastases. Surg Endosc 24:1917–1922
13. Torzilli G, Procopio F, Botea F et al (2009) One-stage ultrasonographically guided hepatectomy for multiple bilobar colorectal metastases: a feasible and effective alternative to the 2-stage approach. Surgery 146:60–71
14. Yoshidome H, Kimura F, Shimizu H et al (2008) Interval period tumor progression: does delayed hepatectomy detect occult metastases in synchronous colorectal liver metastases? J Gastrointest Surg 12:1391–1398
15. Goyer P, Benoist S, Juliè C et al (2012) Complete calcification of colorectal liver metastases on imaging after chemotherapy does not indicate sterilization of diseases. J Visc Surg 149:e271–e274
16. Auer RC, White RR, Kemeny NE et al (2010) Predictors of a true complete response among disappearing liver metastases from colorectal cancer after chemotherapy. Cancer 116:1502–1509
17. Benoist S, Brouquet A, Penna C et al (2006) Complete response of colorectal liver metastases after chemotherapy: does it mean cure? J Clin Oncol 24:3939–3945
18. Ferrero A, Langella S, Russolillo N et al (2012) Intraoperative detection of disappearing colorectal liver metastases as a predictor of residual disease. J Gastrointest Surg 16:806–814
19. Palmer WC, Patel T (2012) Are common factors involved in the pathogenesis of primary liver cancers? A meta-analysis of risk factors for intrahepatic cholangiogarcinoma. J Hepatol 57(1):69–76
20. Klatskin G (1965) Adenocarcinoma of the hepatic duct at its bifurcation within the porta hepatis. An unusual tumor with distinctive clinical and pathological features. Am J Med 38(2):241–256
21. Ishizawa T, Fukushima N, Shibahara J et al (2009) Real-time identification of liver cancers by using indocyanine green fluorescent imaging. Cancer 115:2491–2504
22. Gotoh N, Yamada T, Ishikawa O et al (2009) A novel image-guided surgery of hepatocellular carcinoma by indocyanine green fluorescence imaging navigation. J Surg Oncol 100:75–79

5 Diagnosis and Staging: Contrast-Enhanced Intraoperative Ultrasound (CEIOUS) Using Intravascular Contrast Agents

Guido Torzilli, Matteo Donadon, and Guido Costa

Tumor echogenicity and background liver appearance in IOUS (i.e., cirrhotic, steatotic) can affect our ability to recognize tiny lesions. It has been shown that small metastases can be better recognized if they are hypoechoic rather than isoechoic [1]. Another drawback of IOUS is its limitations in differentiating new lesions according to their echogencity. Based on these two well-known limitations, some authors have tried to find a solution by introducing additional analytical features, as, e.g., the modifications that can be induced on the ultrasound image by injecting a contrast agent.

In the early 1990s, attempts were made using carbon dioxide as a contrast agent for IOUS. However, the need for arterial catheterization made this technique too invasive [2]. The introduction of contrast agents injected intravenously generated new interest in this technique. The first generation consisted of gas-filled microbubbles with a galactose shell, which was both intravascular and somehow hepatospecific accumulating in Kupffer cells. For the ultrasonic visualization of this agent, insonation at a high acoustic pressure was applied intermittently to allow both a vascular and a hepato-specific phase. However, this resulted in collapse of the microbubbles and generated scattered ultrasound waves visualized on the US system in the vascular phase as flashes, not allowing a continuous ultrasound observation. Furthermore, in the postvascular phase, scanning of the liver was limited to one swing of the ultrasonic probe because all the microbubbles that accumulated in the hepatic parenchyma had collapsed by this time. The introduction of a second generation of pure intravascular contrast agents , providing real-time continuous monitoring of the contrast enhancement, has led to widespread use of this modality in ultrasound examination [3, 4].

The gas-filled microbubbles of these agents tolerate low acoustic pressures, enabling continuous observation during the arterial phase and repeated scanning during the late phase. We first introduced this new approach in an intraoperative pilot study on 20 patients [5], establishing their use by CEIOUS in surgery for both HCC and CLM. Recently, the introduction of contrast agents combining the intravascular features of second-generation contrast agents with the hepato-specific features of first-generation contrast agents taken up by Kupffer cells has shown further improvements in this technique, as discussed further in Chap. 6.

G. Torzilli (✉) · M. Donadon · G. Costa
Department of Hepatobiliary Surgery,
Humanitas Research Hospital-IRCCS,
University of Milan-School of Medicine,
Via A. Manzoni 56, 20089 Rozzano, MI, Italy
e-mail: guido.torzilli@humanitas.it;
guido.torzilli@unimi.it

G. Torzilli (ed.), *Ultrasound-Guided Liver Surgery*,
DOI: 10.1007/978-88-470-5510-0_5, © Springer-Verlag Italia 2014

5.1 Technique

Still, second-generation intravascular contrast agents are only available in the European countries. As described in Chap. 1, the major contrast agent available in Europe is composed of sulfur hexafluoride microbubbles stabilized by a phospholipid shell (SonoVue, Bracco Imaging, Milan, Italy). The machine is set to contrast mode (Fig. 5.1); preferably arranged side-by-side in order to simultaneously show the fundamental IOUS and CEIOUS so as not to loose any eventual targets found by IOUS (Fig. 5.2). The contrast is prepared as a solution by adding the powder and shaking gently to be injected intravenously by the anesthesiologist: 2.4–4.8 ml of SonoVue is rapidly infused per exploration through a peripheral vein advising the surgeons once the injection is started to let them initiate the timer of the ultrasound system and starting the registration of the enhancement process. The amount of contrast agent is established according to the preference of the operator; usually, half sample (2.4 ml), if properly prepared, is sufficient.

5.2 Indications

5.2.1 Hepatocellular Carcinoma

As mentioned for HCC, CEIOUS is now used for characterizing new lesions initially detected by IOUS [6]: the rationale is to check the vascular pattern during contrast enhancement of each new lesion. Since, in the case of HCC, it is very important to identify the arterial vascularization, which lasts from 20 to 30 s, each nodule has to be carefully evaluated, and that demands multiple injections in the presence of multiple nodules.

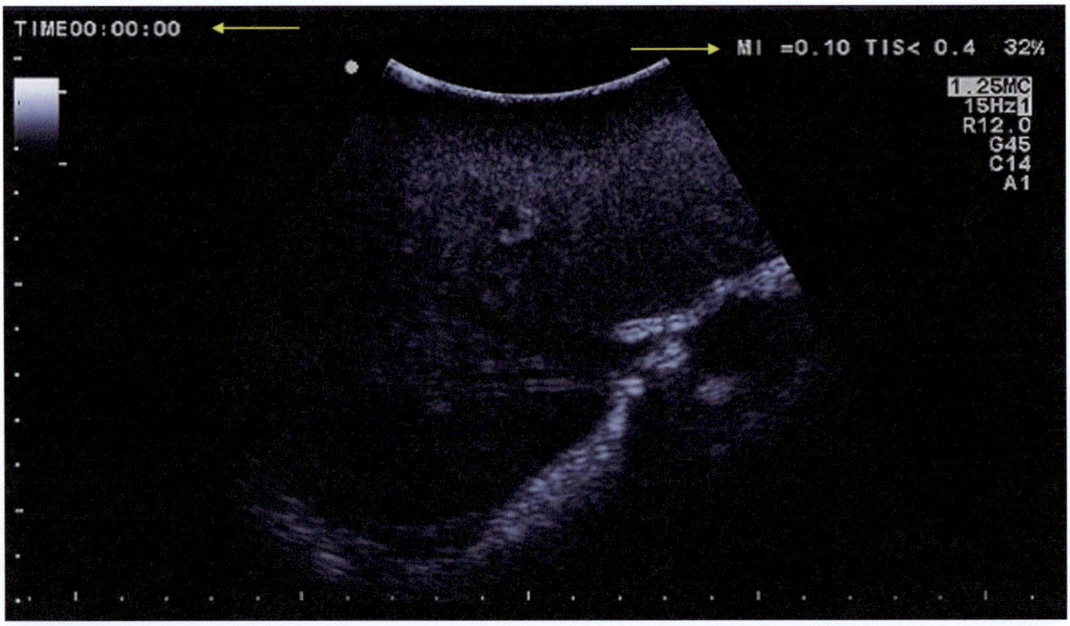

Fig. 5.1 Screen of the ultrasound system regulated by contrast preset. In the *upper right corner*, MI (*yellow arrow*) means mechanical index, which corresponds with the power at which the ultrasound waves intercept the microbubbles composing the contrast agent, which should be below 1, in order not to break the microbubbles and providing the contrast effect of real-time enhancement in ultrasound. In the *upper left corner*, the time (*yellow arrow*) elapsing from injection of the contrast agent by the anesthesiologist into a peripheral vein

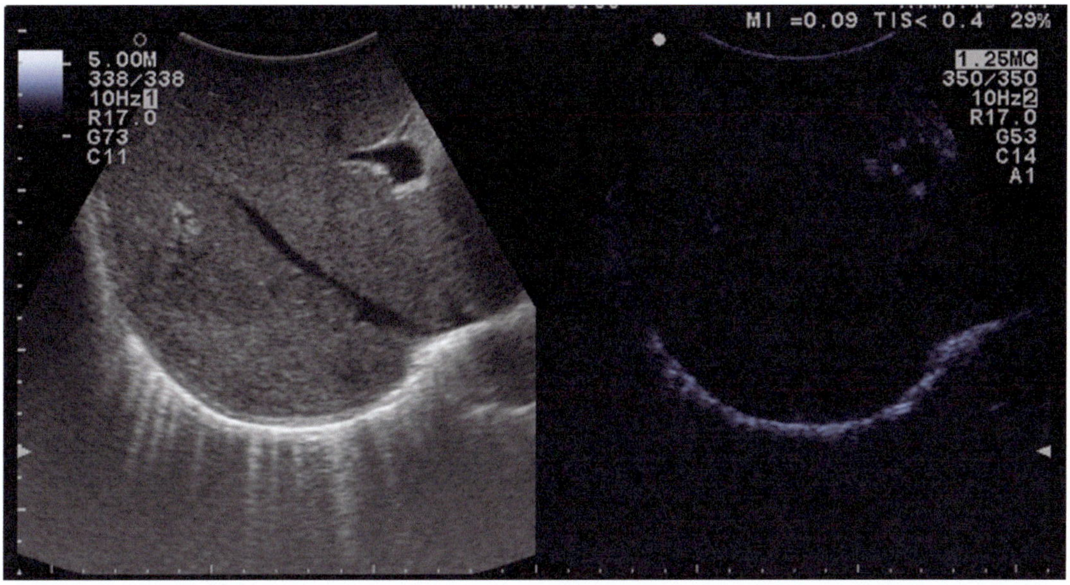

Fig. 5.2 The screen of the ultrasound system can be set to combine on the same image the preset for B-mode (*left*) and contrast (*right*)

This may no longer be necessary with the use of hepato-specific contrast agents (see Chap. 6).

Tumor vascularity is a criterion for differentiating regenerative or dysplastic nodules from the HCC well correlated with the histological evidence of a progressive increase in unpaired arteries from dysplastic to neoplastic nodules in a cirrhotic liver [7]. However, the pattern of vascular enhancement is not sufficient for clearly differentiating malignant from nonmalignant nodules in a cirrhotic liver. Percutaneous contrast-enhanced ultrasound (CE-US) provides a 95 % specific differential diagnosis of focal liver lesions [4]; this rate is, however, referred to another type of lesion if compared to the target of CEIOUS. Intraoperative exploration profits from the higher resolution of US done in direct contact with the liver. Therefore, nodules detected by IOUS are usually smaller than 1 cm: here, vascularity as a criterion for differential diagnosis is less specific. However, some improvements compared with conventional IOUS can be expected. Our preliminary experience showed that CEIOUS can provide remarkable findings, either by the additional information on nodular vascularity in patients with HCC, or by detecting nodules that were not visible in IOUS in patients with CLM [5]. For patients with HCC, we introduced a classification of the pattern of enhancement by CEIOUS of the lesions detected in IOUS from which surgical decision-making can be established (Fig. 5.3) [6]. Briefly, any lesion with a pathologic behavior should appear as hypoechoic in the late phase and with an arterial phase in which it is fully enhanced prior to the remnant liver parenchyma (Fig. 5.4a), or with just inner vessels visualized in it (Fig. 5.4b): this kind of lesions are removed. Those lesions which disappear once the contrast enhances the liver are not considered neoplastic, and those are not removed (Fig. 5.5). With these criteria

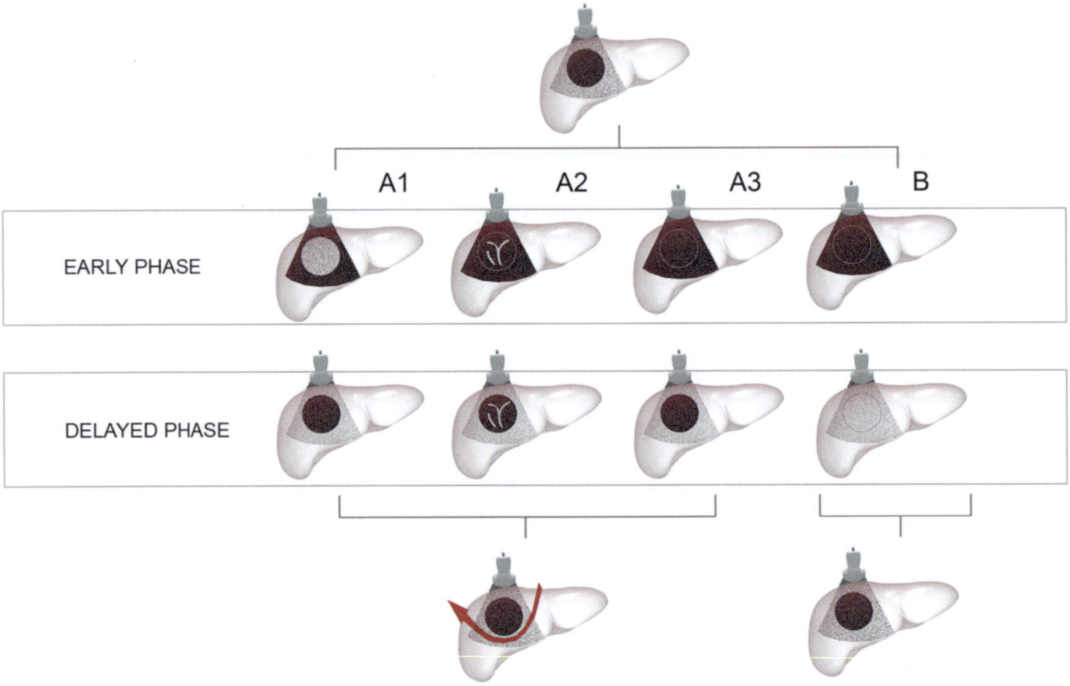

Fig. 5.3 Classification of patterns of enhancement in CEIOUS of those lesions detected in IOUS during surgery for HCC. Lesions having a class A pattern, featured by a hypervascular enhancement in early phase (*A1-2*), or any hypoechoic pattern in the delayed phases (*A1-3*), has to be resected; while lesions showing a class B pattern of enhancement are not removed

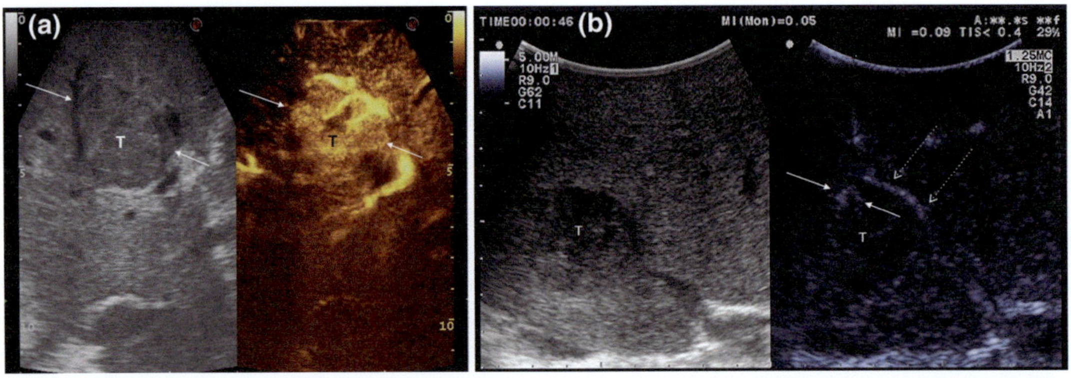

Fig. 5.4 **a** At an early stage, the lesion (*T*) on the right assumes contrast prior to the surrounding tissue showing a nodular arterial enhancement (A1 pattern); **b** while this lesion is not fully enhanced in the arterial phase but just shows inner vessels (*arrows*) originating from a perinodular basket of arteries (*dashed arrows*), and flowing into the nodule itself (A2 pattern)

we obtained a specificity of 69 % by CEIOUS [6]. This value is not very high especially when compared with that reported for CE-US [4]. However, as mentioned above, the small size of the lesions targeted by CEIOUS could explain this discrepancy: for these tiny nodules, there

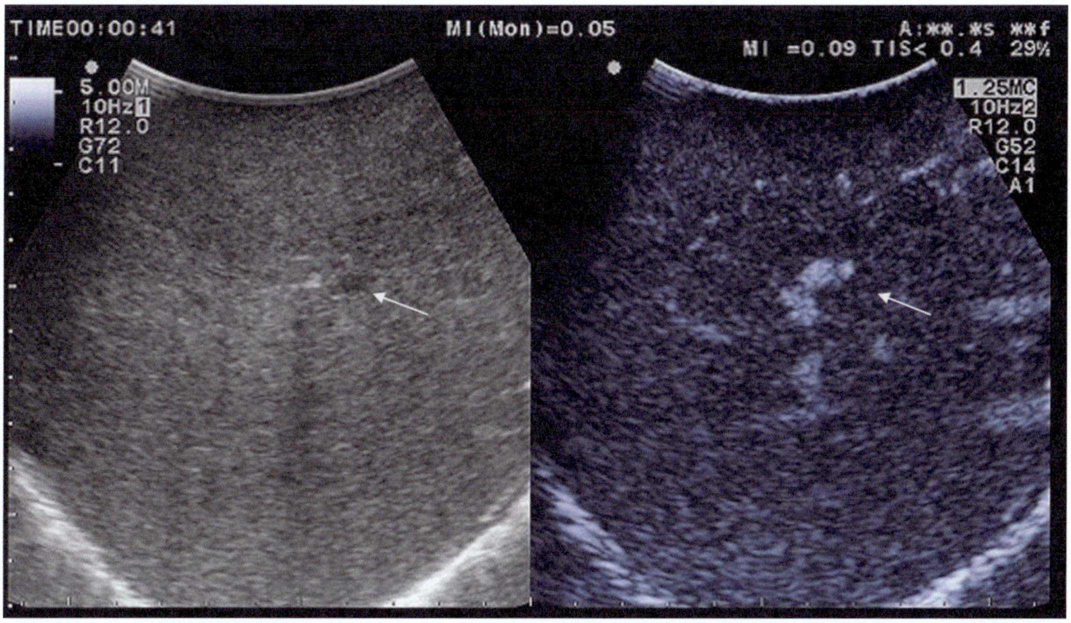

Fig. 5.5 In the delayed phase, the lesion visible on the left in B-mode exploration (*arrow*) is no longer detectable on the right by CEIOUS (*arrow*) (B pattern)

are limits to the use of neo-vascularity as a criterion for differentiating between malignant and benign lesions, which are independent from the method we use. Therefore, CEIOUS can be helpful in a certain percentage of nodules but not in all: in this respect the rate of 69 % of specificity is encouraging as it means that we can provide proper information with this new technique in seven out of ten lesions we detect at the time of laparotomy. For the remaining three, even histology may be lacking. Indeed, we are aware that there is no common agreement between pathologists in East and West on the definition of early HCC and dysplastic lesions [8]. The possible new perspective provided by the new contrast agent, is, as mentioned, still the object of extensive analyses (see Chap. 6).

5.2.2 Colorectal Liver Metastases

Echogenicity impacts detection of CLM [1], as previously mentioned. Therefore, a modality that would improve lesion visibility, and enhancing detection, was needed: CEIOUS addresses this main goal in the case of CLM. In the 1990s, in half of the patients undergoing surgery for CLM the surgical strategy was modified by IOUS findings [9]. However, more recently, progress in preoperative imaging has reduced this rate: in fact, some authors have recently reported that merely 4 % of operative decision-making has been modified by IOUS [10]. By adding CEIOUS to IOUS exploration, operation decision-making has been affected in 38 % of patients with CLM [11]: if this discrepancy in the rates of modified surgical

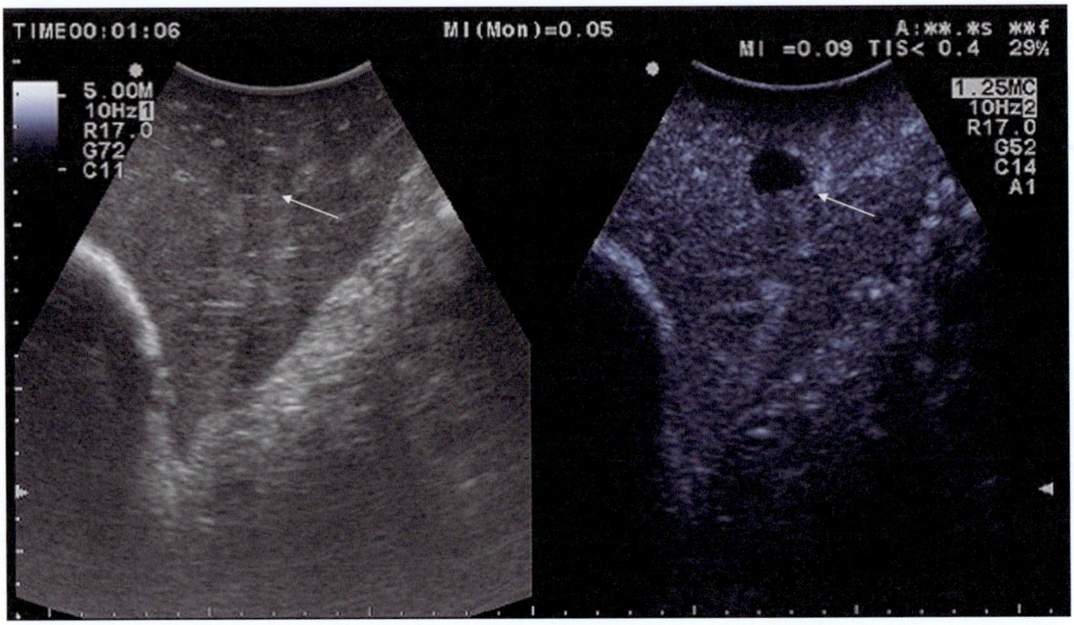

Fig. 5.6 In the delayed phase, the CLM visible as hypoechoic in B-mode exploration on the left (*arrow*) may lead to the assumption of a so-called ''black-hole'' pattern in CEIOUS (*arrow*)

strategy among series is partially motivated by the different surgical approach, which by latest experience is featured by more parenchymal sparing procedures (see Chap. 7), probably CE-IOUS is playing a role too. By using CE-US, CLM has shown a so-called ''black-hole'' effect (Fig. 5.6): the metastastic nodule in the late phase (2–5 min after injection) remains unenhanced and then becomes black in comparison with the surrounding enhanced liver parenchyma. Therefore, CEIOUS allows better nodule visibility. However, with growing experience, we paradoxically witnessed a decrease in the rate of detectable new lesions from 44–77 % in the first two reports [12, 13] to 17–19 % in the most recent reports [11, 14]. The clinical impact of CEIOUS thus seems to progressively decrease with the improvement of preoperative imaging. However, looking at the number of new lesions detected by IOUS, the latter explanation may not be convincing. Indeed, the 16 % of new lesions detected by IOUS in the first report [12] has been substantially confirmed by more recent experience [11, 14]. Technologically, the improvements in IOUS can explain the still high rate of new lesions detected intraoperatively. However, technological improvements in CE-IOUS have been observed in the last years, too, with the introduction of new contrast agents (see Chap. 6). However, initial data do not substantially differ from those mentioned above. Therefore, the decrease observed in the impact of CEIOUS in clinical practice probably means that a steady state has been reached for this method in the case of CLM: therefore, the definition of useful criteria for selective use of CEIOUS seems justified.

In our experience, multinodularity (Fig. 5.7) and isoechogenicity (Fig. 5.8) seem to affect the detection power of IOUS for CLM, and, the latter, as mentioned in Chap. 4, may even impact patient prognosis after surgery [1]. In this

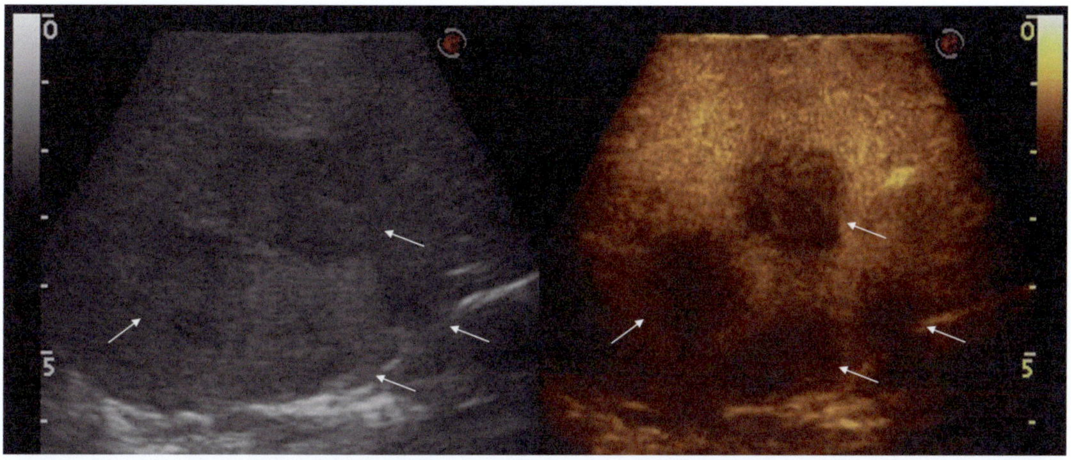

Fig. 5.7 In the delayed phase, the ''black-hole'' effect significantly increases the visibility of CLM (*arrows*) by CEIOUS (*right*) compared to the B-mode (*left*) even in the case of large nodules (*arrows*): this is very useful in case of multiple nodules, particularly when isoechoic, as shown here

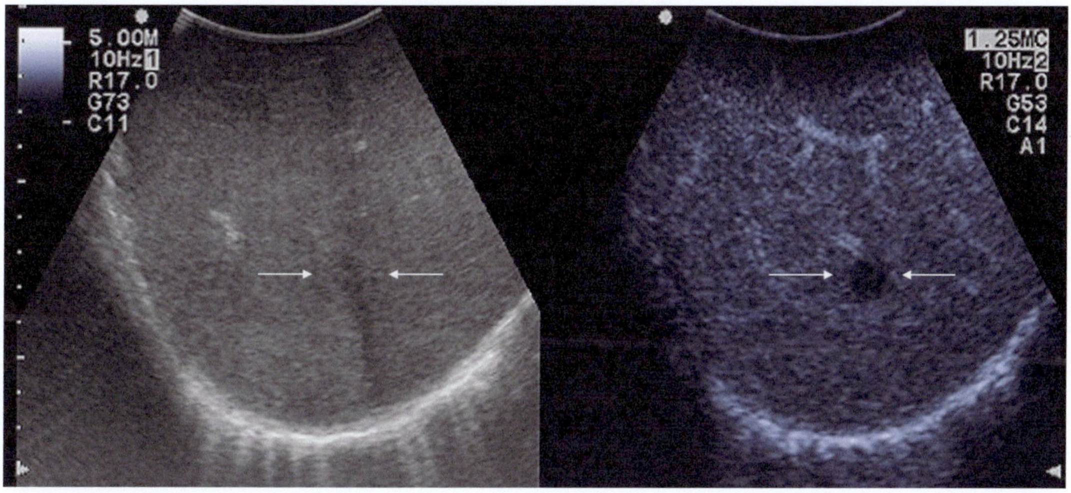

Fig. 5.8 In the case of a tiny isoechoic lesion in B-mode (*arrows on the left*), CEIOUS enhances significantly its detectability (*arrows on the right*)

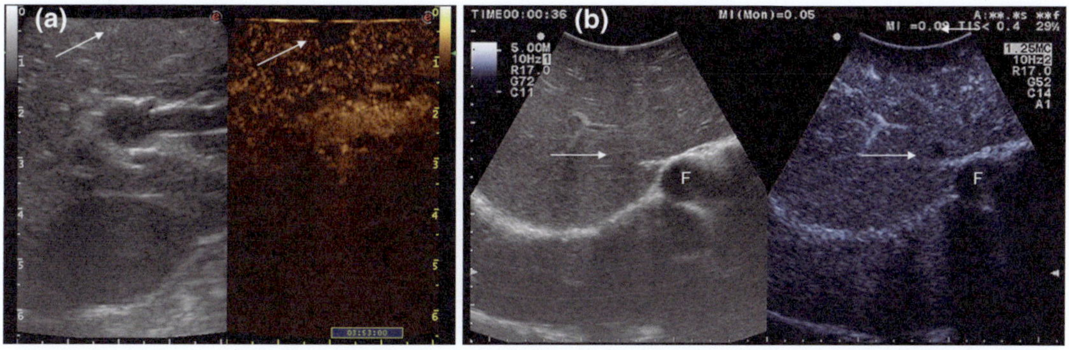

Fig. 5.9 **a** CEIOUS makes lesions visible (*arrow on the right*) that otherwise are not visible in B-mode (*arrow on the left*); **b** combination of finger palpation (*F*) and CEIOUS further facilitates the detection of small lesions (*arrow on the right*) otherwise invisible by IOUS (*arrow on the left*)

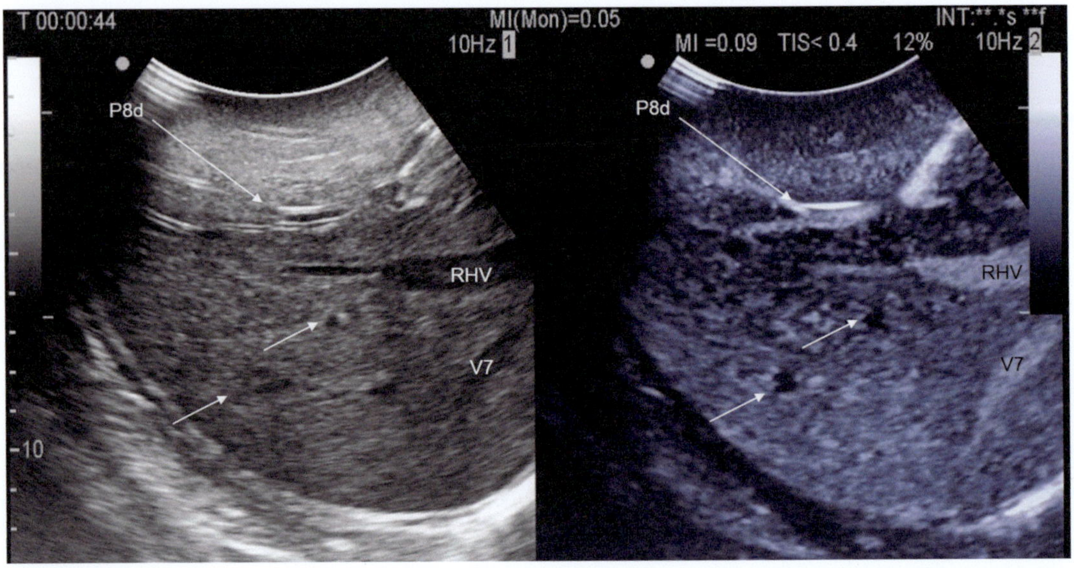

Fig. 5.10 In the case of multiple tiny isoechoic lesions in B-mode (*arrows on the left*), CEIOUS allows their detection (*arrows on the right*); portal branch feeding subsegment 8 dorsal (*P8d*); right hepatic vein (*RHV*); hepatic vein draining segment 7 (*V7*)

respect, CEIOUS seems to be able to play a role in limiting their significance in terms of risk of missed lesions aiding in the detection of otherwise undetectable small CLM (Fig. 5.9a, b). This is particularly the case for patients with multiple lesions (Fig. 5.10). However, a condition where the application of CEIOUS is useless is evidence of bright liver in IOUS, which correlates with the effects of intracellular fat amount and distribution [15], and accounts for 10 % of our patients [11]. In these cases, the visibility of CLM, which is generally hypoechoic, is enhanced by the brightness of the surrounding liver parenchyma mimicking the effect of contrast enhancement (Fig. 5.11). As a confirmation, we never detected new CLM by CEIOUS in those patients with bright liver in IOUS.

CEIOUS may also be employed to aid in detecting CLM positively treated after chemotherapy, although, in this sense results are still inconclusive [16, 17]. Actually, tiny shrunk CLM, sometimes appearing as linear defects, may not be visible by CEIOUS, while being evident upon careful IOUS with high-frequency probes (Fig. 5.12).

Scars may not become evident at palpation of tiny CLM and may generate artifacts which mask them in IOUS, while being detectable in CEIOUS (Fig. 5.13).

Care should be taken in the case of patients with CLM in a liver bearing cystic lesions. In fact, these latter appear similar to CLM during the delayed phases of contrast enhancement: however, the cysts should have been already mapped into the liver upon basic exploration (see Chap. 4), and the CLMs known prior to surgery should have been already differentiated from the cysts themselves. Therefore, any new "black hole" detected in the liver in different locations from those where cysts were eventually detected should be considered as suspicious for malignancy. This example further stresses the usefulness of keeping a side-by-side modality of exploration having the possibility of

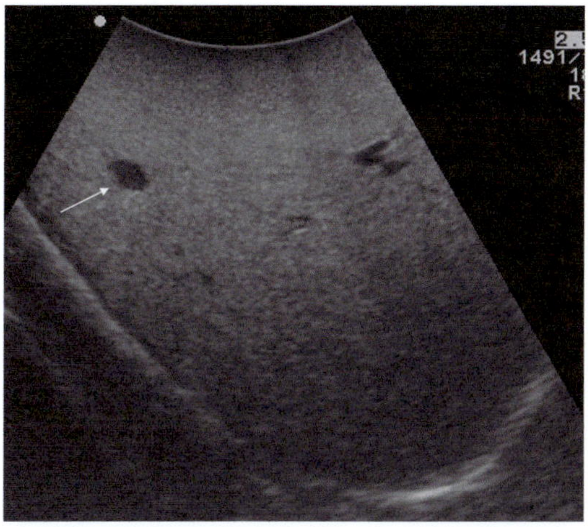

Fig. 5.11 Identifying a lesion, even if small (*arrow*), is satisfactory per se if the lesion is hypoechoic and the liver appears as a "bright liver"

simultaneously visualizing both the IOUS and CEIOUS images, allowing to recognize both CLM and cysts.

5.3 Resection Guidance

The echogenicity may affect detection power [1]. This reduces the operator's ability to depict the tumor burden and can make it more difficult to judge the relationship between a tumor and an adjacent vessel. As also further elaborated in Chaps. 7 and 8, this impacts both surgical strategy and resection guidance. Thus, CEIOUS, which allows improved visualization of tumor margins even of main lesions, supports a

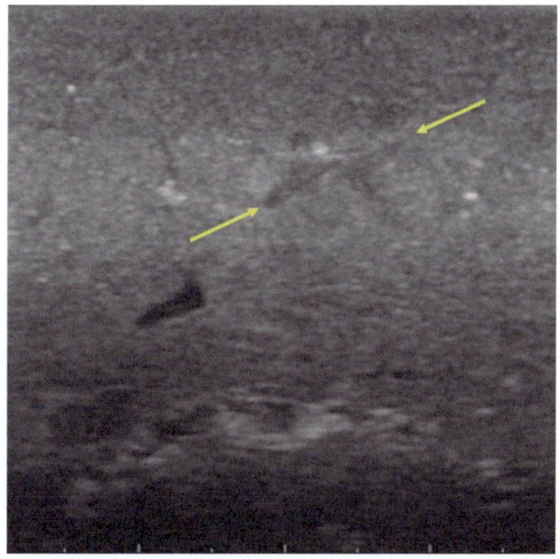

Fig. 5.13 Lesions almost disappeared after chemotherapy and are only bearly visible in IOUS (*arrows*): the detection of these lesions is facilitated by having available in the operating room the images obtained prior to chemotherapy, which would show the baseline of the disease presentation

superior definition of tumor-vessel relationships. CEIOUS facilitates outlining the resection area and determining the dissection plane, resulting in easier resection guidance (Fig. 5.14a–d). Our experience has shown this to be the case in 1/5 of patients with CLM [11].

The precise correlation between palpatory and IOUS findings can be checked by exploring the liver in positioning the probe on the opposite side of the lesion while the latter is palpated with the left hand (see Chap. 2): this maneuver can be repeated during contrast enhancement (Fig. 5.15).

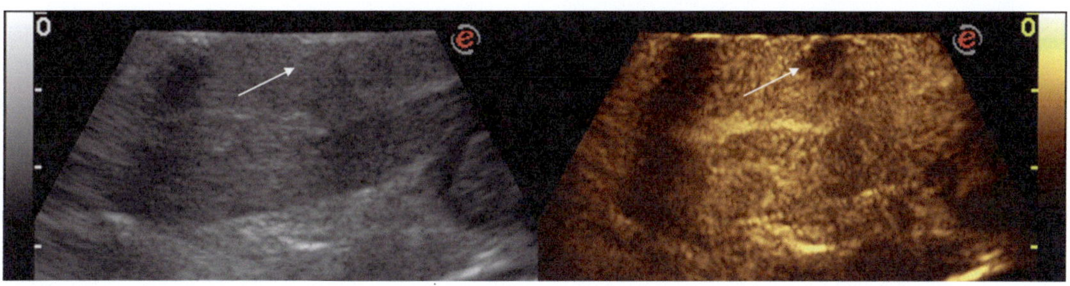

Fig. 5.12 Sometimes in a liver with an irregular surface, as, e.g., due to scars resulting from previous operations, shadowing echoes on the screen (*arrow on the left*) may mask lesions which do become evident in CEIOUS, however (*arrow on the right*)

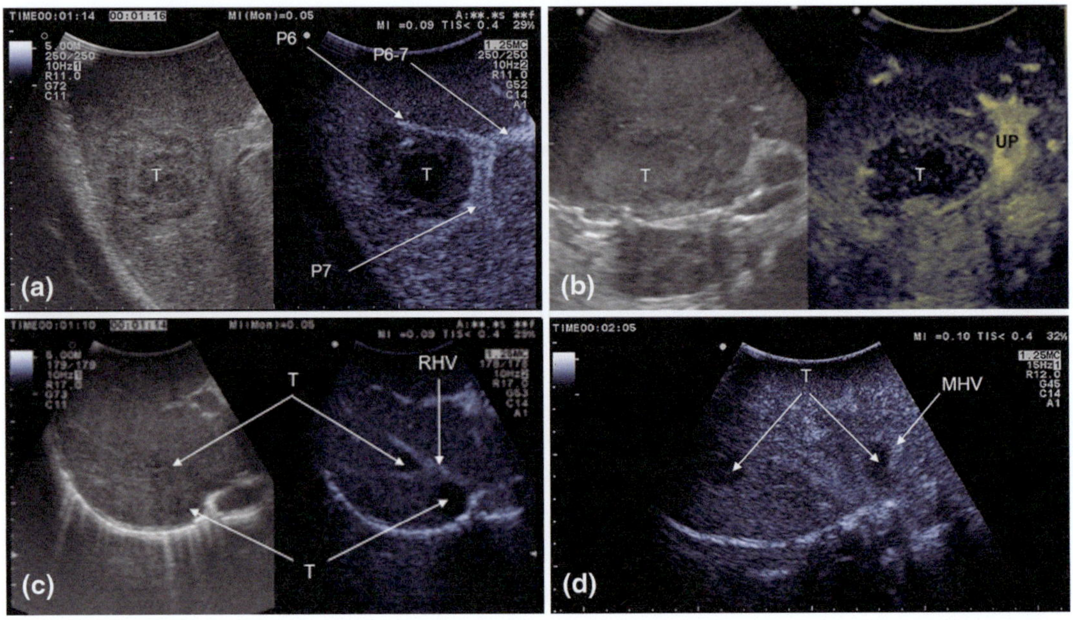

Fig. 5.14 **a** CEIOUS enhances lesion visibility may better defining the tumor–vessel relationship as for this CLM located between the portal branch to segment 6 (*P6*) and that of segment 7 (*P7*); **b** similarly, in this case, the relation of the lesion (*T*) with the umbilical portion is well disclosed by CEIOUS (*right*), compared to the B-mode image (*left*); **c** in this case the two lesions (*T*) are not well visible by IOUS, and consequently also their tumor–vessel relationship remains undisclosed (*left*), although they are evident in CEIOUS (*right*); **d** in this CEIOUS image of two lesions (*T*), one remains in contact with the middle hepatic vein (*MHV*); right hepatic vein (*RHV*)

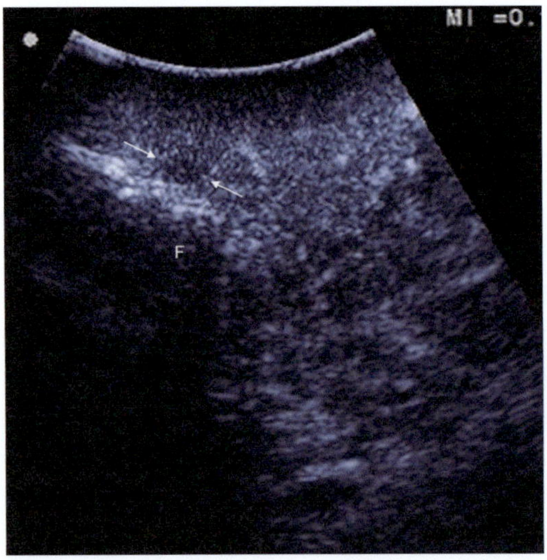

Fig. 5.15 Palpation (*F*) and CEIOUS may help in precisely locating tiny lesions (*arrows*)

References

1. Van Vledder MG, Pawlik TM, Munireddy S et al (2010) Factors determining the sensitivity of intraoperative ultrasonography in detecting colorectal liver metastases in the modern era. Ann Surg Oncol 17(10):2756–2763
2. Takada T, Yasuda H, Uchiyama K et al (1990) Contrast-enhanced intraoperative ultrasonography of small hepatocellular carcinomas. Surgery 107:528–532
3. Blomley MJ, Albrecht T, Cosgrove DO et al (1999) Improved imaging of liver metastases with stimulated acoustic emission in the late phase of enhancement with the US contrast agent SH U 508A: early experience. Radiology 210(2):409–416
4. Quaia E, Calliada F, Bertolotto M et al (2004) Characterization of focal liver lesions with contrast-specific US modes and a sulfur hexafluoride-filled microbubble contrast agent: diagnostic performance and confidence. Radiology 232(2):420–430

5. Torzilli G, Del Fabbro D, Olivari N et al (2004) Contrast-enhanced ultrasonography during liver surgery. Br J Surg 91:1165–1167
6. Torzilli G, Palmisano A, Del Fabbro D et al (2007) Contrast-enhanced intraoperative ultrasonography during surgery for hepatocellular carcinoma in liver cirrhosis: is it useful or useless? A prospective cohort study of our experience. Ann Surg Oncol 14:1347–1355
7. Roncalli M, Roz E, Coggi G et al (1999) The vascular profile of regenerative and dysplastic nodules of the cirrhotic liver: implications for diagnosis and classification. Hepatology 30:1174–1178
8. Kojiro M (2010) Pathological diagnosis at early stage: reaching international consensus. Oncology 78(Suppl 1):31–35
9. Kane RA, Hughes LA, Cua EJ et al (1994) The impact of intraoperative ultrasonography on surgery for liver neoplasms. J Ultrasound Med 13:1–6
10. Sahani DV, Kalva SP, Tanabe KK et al (2004) Intraoperative US in patients undergoing surgery for liver neoplasms: comparison with MR imaging. Radiology 232:810–814
11. Torzilli G, Botea F, Procopio F et al (2008) Does contrast-enhanced intraoperative ultrasonography impact radicality of hepatectomies for colorectal cancer liver metastases inspite of modern preoperative imaging? Analysis on a prospective cohort. Eur J Cancer 6:16–23
12. Torzilli G, Del Fabbro D, Palmisano A et al (2005) Contrast-enhanced intraoperative ultrasonography during hepatectomies for colorectal cancer liver metastases. J Gastrointest Surg 9:1148–1153
13. Leen E, Ceccotti P, Moug SJ et al (2006) Potential value of contrast-enhanced intraoperative ultrasonography during partial hepatectomy for metastases: an essential investigation before resection? Ann Surg 243:236–240
14. Schulz A, Dormagen JB, Drolsum A et al (2012) Impact of contrast-enhanced intraoperative ultrasound on operation strategy in case of colorectal liver metastasis. Acta Radiol 53(10):1081–1087
15. Caturelli E, Costarelli L, Giordano M et al (1991) Hypoechoic lesions in fatty liver. Quantitative study by histomorphometry. Gastroenterology 100:1678–1682
16. Ferrero A, Langella S, Russolillo N et al (2012) Intraoperative detection of disappearing colorectal liver metastases as a predictor of residual disease. J Gastrointest Surg 16:806–814
17. Ruzzenente A, Conci S, Iacono C et al (2013) Usefulness of contrast-enhanced intraoperative ultrasonography (CE-IOUS) in patients with colorectal liver metastases after preoperative chemotherapy. J Gastrointest Surg 17(2):281–287

6 Contrast-Enhanced Intraoperative Ultrasound Using Liver-Specific Contrast Agents

Junichi Arita, and Norihiro Kokudo

6.1 Introduction

As already described in the former chapters, the technique of liver surgery has substantially improved over the past few decades, partially because of the invention of IOUS [1].

Recently, second-generation contrast agents for ultrasound have been developed and are now widely used worldwide. The use of this kind of contrast agent in CEIOUS reportedly enhances utility, compared with conventional IOUS. Pure intravascular contrast agents, such as the SonoVue (Bracco Imaging, Milan, Italy) have already been discussed in Chap. 5.

Another second-generation contrast agent for ultrasound, Sonazoid (gaseous perflubutane; GE Healthcare, Norway), first became commercially available in Japan in 2007. This agent has the peculiarity of providing Kupffer imaging, in addition to vascular information regarding the liver and hepatic nodules, and is therefore expected to increase the role of CEIOUS in liver surgery.

In this chapter, the clinical technique of CEIOUS using Sonazoid will be described and the results of this technique in patients with hepatocellular carcinoma (HCC) and patients with liver metastasis from colorectal cancer, which are the two major liver malignancies amenable to hepatic resection, will be presented.

6.2 CEIOUS Procedure

Sonazoid is not only an intravascular contrast agent but additionally has the peculiar characteristic of accumulating in Kupffer cells in the liver [2, 3], thereby enabling Kupffer imaging in addition to demonstrating tumor vascularity [4]. In the Kupffer phase, microbubbles accumulate in Kupffer cells; this causes the liver parenchyma to turn homogenously hyperechoic and clearly delineates any malignant tumor because of the absence of Kupffer cells. This effect lasts up to 2 h [5], enabling repeated screening of the malignant tumors for a long time period prior to hepatic resection. The frame rate is 10–20 Hz. The mechanical index is set at 0.15–0.25 for all CEIOUS procedures. A real-time fundamental B-mode image is displayed simultaneously with a harmonic mode image side-by-side for reference (Fig. 6.1). This technique prevents target lesions from being missed because the harmonic mode image is usually dark before the venous injection

J. Arita (✉)
Department of Digestive Surgery, Cancer Institute Hospital of Japanese Foundation for Cancer Research, 3-8-31, Ariake, Koto-ku, Tokyo 135-8550, Japan
e-mail: jarita-tky@umin.ac.jp

N. Kokudo
Hepato-Biliary-Pancreatic Surgery Division, Department of Surgery, Graduate School of Medicine, University of Tokyo, 7-3-1, Hongo, Bunkyo-ku, Tokyo 113-8655, Japan
e-mail: KOKUDO-2SU@h.u-tokyo.ac.jp

G. Torzilli (ed.), *Ultrasound-Guided Liver Surgery*,
DOI: 10.1007/978-88-470-5510-0_6, © Springer-Verlag Italia 2014

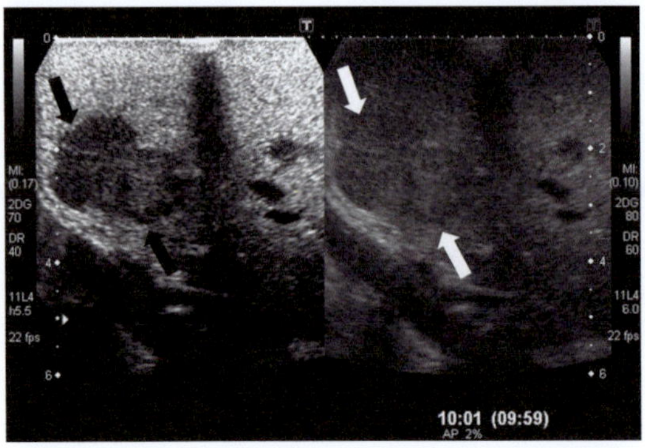

Fig. 6.1 An image obtained during CEIOUS in a patient with colorectal liver metastasis. A harmonic mode image is shown in the *left* side and a fundamental B-mode image is shown in the *right* side simultaneously. A metastatic tumor in the liver is delineated more clearly in the harmonic mode image (*arrows*)

of the contrast agent. Sonazoid is injected through a peripheral vein, and one focal liver lesion is continuously observed in the harmonic mode (vascular phase). The focus point is set at a level just below the approximate bottom of the target focal liver lesion during this phase. Following a pause of approximately 15 min after the vascular phase, ultrasonic observation is re-started to scan the entire liver; this period is defined as the "Kupffer phase". The focus point is set at the approximate bottom of the liver. Malignant tumors appear as hypoechoic areas surrounded by hyperechoic background liver (Fig. 6.1). Repeat scans can be performed during this phase, and unlike CEIOUS using SonoVue, the contrast effect lasts for up to 2 h.

The vascularity of only one focal liver lesion can be examined following an injection of contrast agent. The vascularity of additional focal liver lesion can be examined as follows if this lesion appears hypoechoic during the Kupffer phase. Subsequent to the Kupffer phase scanning, Sonazoid is injected once again while the new target lesion is visualized in the ultrasound image (Fig. 6.2). This procedure enables early enhancement, if present, to be confirmed within the clearly demonstrated hypoechoic lesion. The vascularity of multiple lesions can be examined in this manner; this procedure is known as "defect reperfusion" [6]. The advantage of this technique is that the target lesion is rarely missed because it is clearly delineated as hypoechoic until the injected microbubbles reach the liver parenchyma.

6.3 Hepatocellular Carcinoma

CEIOUS provides surgeons with additional information regarding new lesions found during IOUS. As described in Chap. 5, Torzilli et al. reported the usefulness of CEIOUS using SonoVue as an alternative means of differentiating HCC from benign lesions among such newly identified lesions [7]. Sonazoid, which became commercially available later than SonoVue, is also expected to be useful in a similar manner, especially with its advantage of enabling Kupffer imaging. Kupffer imaging in CEIOUS using Sonazoid is further expected to contribute to searches for new HCC tumors that were missed by IOUS and preoperative imaging studies.

At the University of Tokyo Hospital, we conducted a prospective clinical study assessing the usefulness of CEIOUS in HCC patients [8]. A total of 192 consecutive patients were enrolled. The vascularity of one representative lesion, preferentially a new lesion found during IOUS, was examined after the intravenous injection of Sonazoid (vascular phase). Approximately 15 min after the vascular phase, total liver scanning in the harmonic mode was commenced (Kupffer phase). One additional injection of Sonazoid was allowed to examine the vascularity of another lesion, if necessary. A tentative diagnosis of HCC was made when a lesion was either hypervascular during the vascular phase or hypoechoic during the Kupffer phase (Fig. 6.3). Any lesion that was newly detected during the Kupffer phase of CEIOUS was tentatively diagnosed as HCC. A final diagnosis of HCC was made based on the results of a histological examination or dynamic computed tomography findings obtained during the 12-month postoperative period. During the study period, 79 new lesions were identified during IOUS in 50 patients (26 % of all patients), 17 of

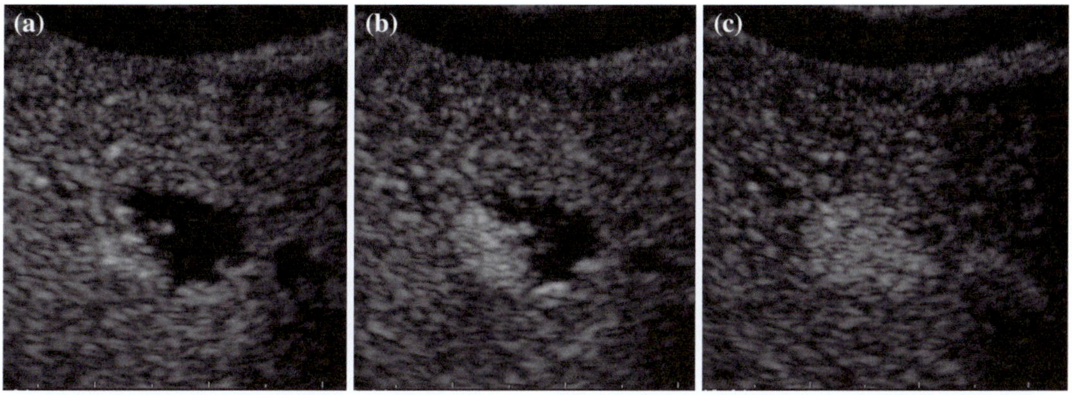

Fig. 6.2 A new hypoechoic lesion was found in segment 4 during the Kupffer phase of CEIOUS in a patient with a classical HCC tumor. It was examined during the vascular phase following a repeat injection of Sonazoid. **a–c** Contrast enhancement appeared in the peripheral part of the lesion and gradually extended toward the center of the lesion. The lesion was occupied with contrast enhancement about 1 min after contrast injection

which (22 %) were finally diagnosed as HCC. The sensitivity, specificity, and accuracy of CEIOUS for differentiating HCC among the 79 IOUS-new lesions were 65, 94, and 87 %, respectively. These figures were considered satisfactory because the median diameter of the 79 lesions was 0.7 cm and all the lesions were considered so obscure that all preoperative imaging studies had missed them. Furthermore, 21 additional new hypoechoic lesions were found in 16 patients, of which 14 lesions (67 %) in 11 patients were finally diagnosed as HCC. Another advantage of the Kupffer phase of CEIOUS is that it sometimes clearly visualizes those HCC tumors which are diagnosed in preoperative images but not seen during conventional IOUS (Fig. 6.4). Surgeons cannot resect such tumors unless they can be seen in CEIOUS. Thus, CEIOUS using Sonazoid appears to enable a more accurate intraoperative staging of patients with HCC.

6.4 Liver Metastasis

After undergoing hepatic resection for CLM, 40 % of all patients experience intrahepatic recurrence [9]. These intrahepatic recurrences theoretically have been present as small or microscopic lesions at the time of the initial hepatectomy. B-mode IOUS is reportedly the most sensitive imaging modality capable of identifying such tiny metastases that have been missed by preoperative imaging studies. Recently, CEIOUS has been reported to be capable of identifying CLM in addition to those identified by IOUS and preoperative imaging studies. Another benefit of CEIOUS is that it delineates CLM with a clearer border, helping surgeons to see the relation between the tumor and neighboring vasculature and to decide on a resectional strategy with greater confidence. Results of CEIOUS using SonoVue for CLM have already been discussed. As discussed, CEIOUS using Sonazoid, providing Kupffer imaging, enables a longer period for screening for hepatic malignant tumors. This advantage may be more enhanced in patients with CLM than in patients with HCC because an examination of vascularity is usually unnecessary for the diagnosis of liver metastasis. A preliminary clinical study has been reported by Nakano et al. [10], in which CEIOUS was performed in 8 patients and one new liver metastasis was identified during the Kupffer phase of CEIOUS in 2 patients.

At the University of Tokyo Hospital, a prospective clinical study was performed to assess the additional value of CEIOUS using Sonazoid

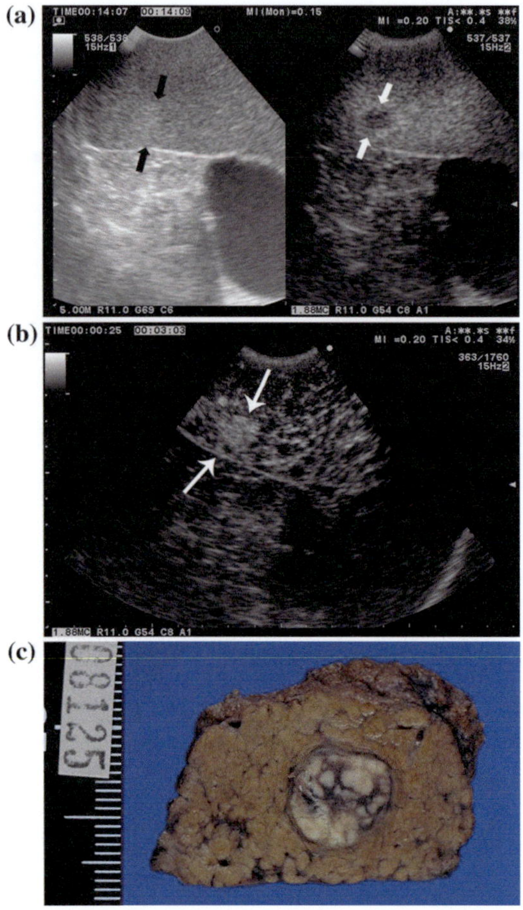

Fig. 6.3 A new focal liver lesion was found during conventional IOUS in segment 6 of the liver and was subsequently examined by CEIOUS. **a** In the left sided fundamental B-mode image, a hyperechoic lesion (*black arrows*) was found in conventional IOUS. In the right sided harmonic mode image obtained about 14 min after Sonazoid injection, the lesion was hypoechoic (*white arrows*), which indicated it was HCC. **b** The vascular phase with the typical arterial wash-in. **c** This lesion was resected and diagnosed as moderately differentiated HCC after pathological examination

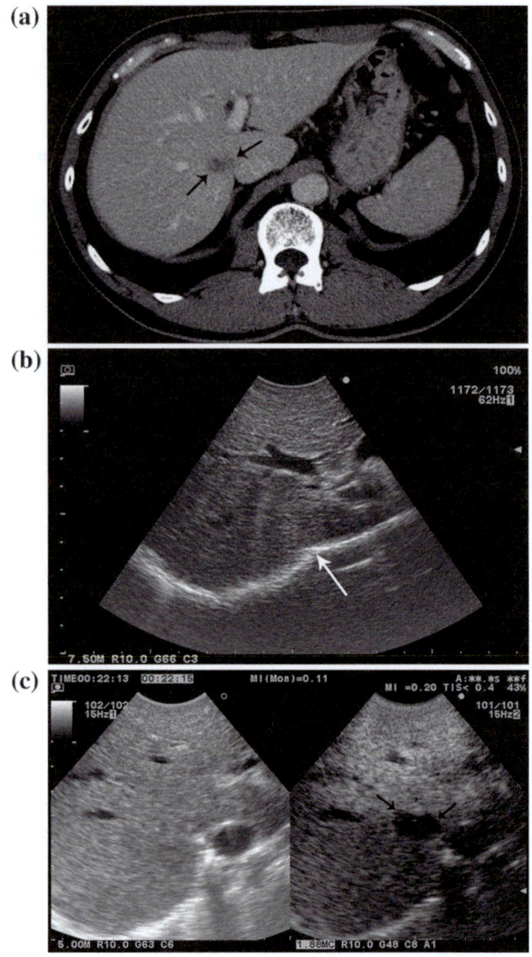

Fig. 6.4 A patient with HCC underwent hepatic resection. **a** A classical HCC tumor in segment 1 was diagnosed by dynamic CT scan (*arrows*). **b** The tumor was hard to see during conventional IOUS. **c** The tumor was clearly visualized by CEIOUS during the Kupffer phase (*arrows*)

in comparison to conventional IOUS in consecutive 102 patients undergoing resections for colorectal liver metastases [11]. Preoperative contrast-enhanced CT or MRI was performed in all patients. A total of 315 liver metastases were identified on preoperative imaging and conventional intraoperative examination including IOUS identified 350 metastases. During the Kupffer phase of CEIOUS, 370 metastases were identified. The 370 tumors included the 23 tumors which were found exclusively by CEIOUS (Fig. 6.5). The sensitivity, specificity, and accuracy of CEIOUS were 97.1, 59.1, and 93.2 %, respectively. The surgical plans were altered more often in patients who received preoperative chemotherapy than in patients who did not (22 % vs. 10 %, $p = 0.071$). Comparing the results of our study with those of others using SonoVue, appears to be satisfactory.

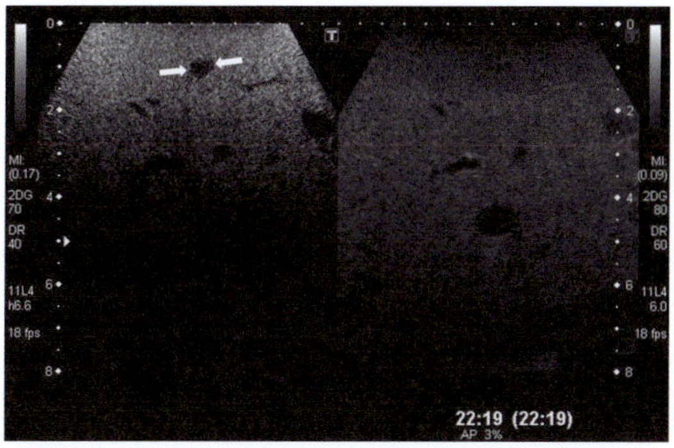

Fig. 6.5 A tiny new liver metastasis was found (*arrows*) in segment 8 during the Kupffer phase of CEIOUS in a patient with 5 colorectal liver metastases in other sites

6.5 Conclusions

Prospective clinical trials have shown that CE-IOUS using the liver-specific contrast agent Sonazoid is of value in patients with HCC and those with colorectal liver metastases, although it is difficult to show the difference in utility compared with use of purely intravascular contrast agents.

References

1. Makuuchi M, Hasegawa H, Yamazaki S, Takayasu K, Moriyama N (1987) The use of operative ultrasound as an aid to liver resection in patients with hepatocellular carcinoma. World J Surg 11(5):615–621
2. Yanagisawa K, Moriyasu F, Miyahara T, Yuki M, Iijima H (2007) Phagocytosis of ultrasound contrast agent microbubbles by Kupffer cells. Ultrasound Med Biol 33(2):318–325
3. Kindberg GM, Tolleshaug H, Roos N, Skotland T (2003) Hepatic clearance of Sonazoid perfluorobutane microbubbles by Kupffer cells does not reduce the ability of liver to phagocytose or degrade albumin microspheres. Cell Tissue Res 312(1):49–54
4. Hatanaka K, Kudo M, Minami Y et al (2008) Differential diagnosis of hepatic tumors: value of contrast-enhanced harmonic sonography using the newly developed contrast agent. Sonazoid Intervirol 51(Suppl 1):61–69
5. Watanabe R, Matsumura M, Chen CJ, Kaneda Y, Ishihara M, Fujimaki M (2003) Gray-scale liver enhancement with Sonazoid (NC100100), a novel ultrasound contrast agent; detection of hepatic tumors in a rabbit model. Biol Pharm Bull 26(9):1272–1277
6. Kudo M (2008) Hepatocellular carcinoma 2009 and beyond: from the surveillance to molecular targeted therapy. Oncology 75(Suppl 1):1–12
7. Torzilli G, Palmisano A, Del Fabbro D et al (2007) Contrast-enhanced intraoperative ultrasonography during surgery for hepatocellular carcinoma in liver cirrhosis: is it useful or useless? A prospective cohort study of our experience. Ann Surg Oncol 14(4):1347–1355
8. Arita J, Takahashi M, Hata S et al (2011) Usefulness of contrast-enhanced intraoperative ultrasound using sonazoid in patients with hepatocellular carcinoma. Ann Surg 254(6):992–999
9. Simmonds PC, Primrose JN, Colquitt JL, Garden OJ, Poston GJ, Rees M (2006) Surgical resection of hepatic metastases from colorectal cancer: a systematic review of published studies. Br J Cancer 94(7):982–999
10. Nakano H, Ishida Y, Hatakeyama T et al (2008) Contrast-enhanced intraoperative ultrasonography equipped with late Kupffer-phase image obtained by sonazoid in patients with colorectal liver metastases. World J Gastroenterol 14(20):3207–3211
11. Takahashi M, Hasegawa K, Arita J et al (2012) Contrast-enhanced intraoperative ultrasonography using perfluorobutane microbubbles for the enumeration of colorectal liver metastases. Br J Surg 99(9):1271–1277

Part III
Hepatobiliary Surgery

7 Planning of the Surgical Strategy

Guido Torzilli, Fabio Procopio, and Guido Costa

IOUS exploration of the liver can have a great impact on surgical strategy. However, more recently the impact of IOUS on operative decision making, when compared with those of preoperative imaging techniques, is reported to be just around 4–7 % [1, 2]. The problem of the impact of IOUS on operative decision making depends on two main factors: the surgical policy of each specific team, and the type of tumor. The relatively low rates reported [1, 2] are also partially motivated by surgical policy: since a considerable number of patients undergo major hepatectomies, new nodules detected by IOUS in the same hemiliver would not have modified the surgical strategy (Fig. 7.1a). Recently, it has been shown how major hepatectomies are carried out in a minority of patients even in extremely complex presentations [3] just because of the extensive use of IOUS guidance for achieving parenchymal sparing resections: in this respect, detection of new nodules warrant a change of the surgical strategy (Fig. 7.1b).

IOUS allows an accurate three-dimensional reconstruction of the relationship between the tumor, the portal branches, and hepatic veins: this is a prerequisite for defining a surgical strategy based on a new principle. The insights gained from IOUS, rather than allowing a safer removal of large amounts of liver parenchyma as conventionally recommended [4, 5], can be thought as aiming at maximizing the conservation of the liver vascular skeleton, while still involving oncological radicality. This approach per se implies leaving enough liver with proper inflow and outflow. For these targets, exposure carried out for staging the disease intraoperatively is often not sufficient. Planning a surgical strategy, one needs to assemble all available inspective, tactile, and ultrasound information and the liver exposure and mobilization need to be accordingly carried out. To better determine the tumor-vessel relationship in a three-dimensional setting, the position of the surgeon's left hand as well as the tumor should be depicted in the IOUS images (Fig. 7.2a, b) similarly as it will be described for resection guidance: the palpation feedback and IOUS image need to be assembled in the surgeon's mind for determining the best approach for tumor removal. Also, knowledge of the liver inflow and outflow by IOUS is crucial for determining the feasibility of new surgical procedures that are otherwise unfeasible: for this purpose an adequate surgical field, with proper liver mobilization, can allow maneuvers of vessel compression or taping indispensable—all information needed to decide whether or not a certain approach is feasible. A first prerequisite is an adequate liver exposure and mobilization, as further detailed in Chap. 8 focusing on resection guidance.

G. Torzilli (✉) · F. Procopio · G. Costa
Department of Hepatobiliary Surgery,
University of Milan-School of Medicine,
Humanitas Research Hospital-IRCCS,
Via A. Manzoni 56, 20089 Rozzano, MI, Italy
e-mail: guido.torzilli@humanitas.it;
guido.torzilli@unimi.it

G. Torzilli (ed.), *Ultrasound-Guided Liver Surgery*,
DOI: 10.1007/978-88-470-5510-0_7, © Springer-Verlag Italia 2014

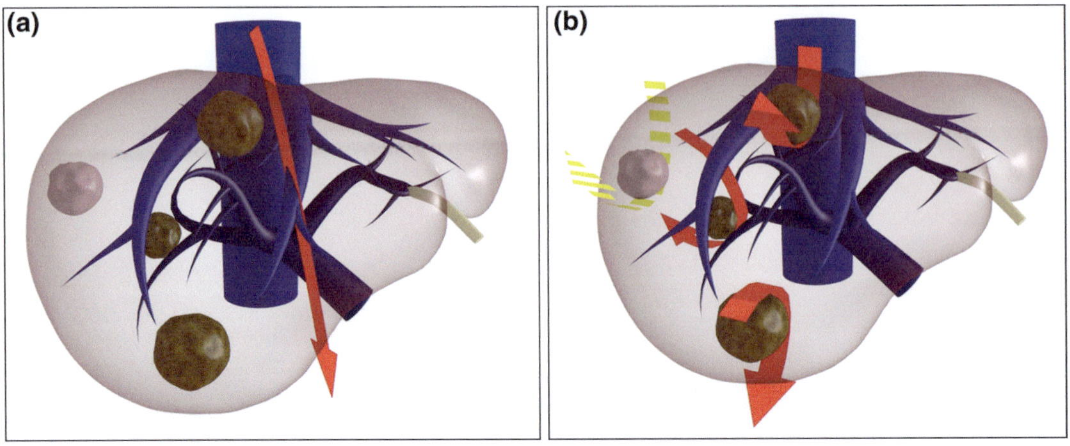

Fig. 7.1 **a** An eventual new lesion (transparent) would not modify the surgical strategy if the chosen operation is a right hepatectomy (*red line* representing the dissection plane); **b** an eventual new lesion (transparent) would modify the surgical strategy if the chosen operation is multiple resection (*red line* representing the dissection planes and the *dashed yellow* the additional one)

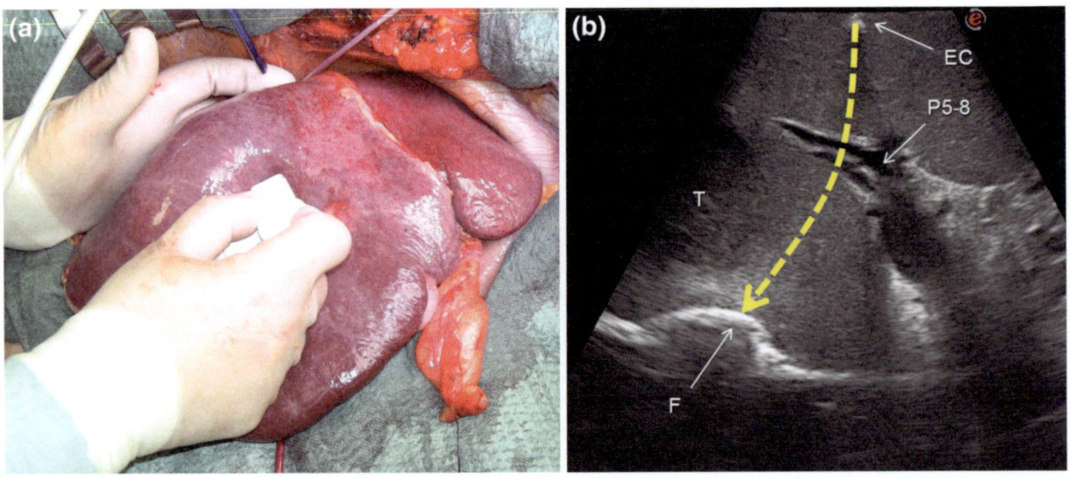

Fig. 7.2 **a** The surgeon's fingertip and the probe act simultaneously to draw the ideal dissection plane to be followed; **b** the corresponding IOUS image in which the *yellow dashed line* indicates the ideal plane connecting the fingertip (*F*) and the shadow generated by the electrocautery (*EC*) interposed between the liver surface and the probe; portal branch to the right anterior section (*P5-8*); tumor (*T*)

7.1 Tumor–Vessel Relationship

Depending on the tumor–vessels relationship, specific and original operations can be performed [6–8]. IOUS easily allows the surgeon to recognize if an HCC is separated by some normal parenchyma from the vessel, or if it is in contact with the vessel without invading its wall, or conversely, whether the HCC has invaded the vessel wall, whether it determines the proximal bile duct dilation, or is associated with a tumor thrombus [9]. Also, determination of the relationship between a CLM and intrahepatic vascular structure is precisely definable by IOUS: in this respect, if the vessel wall is found to be intact, also the circumferential extent of the contact is relevant for deciding on a resection sparing the vessel in contact with the CLM [3]. Based on these features, the decision whether the vessel should be resected or not is taken and a precise surgical strategy can be defined.

7.1.1 Tumor in Contact with a Glissonian Pedicle

The glissonian pedicle in contact with a capsulated HCC is spared in case of integrity of the vessel wall in IOUS without any sign of bile duct dilation (Fig. 7.3a–d) [9]. Similarly, the pedicle can be spared when it is in contact with a CLM once IOUS has confirmed the integrity of the vessel wall and bile duct dilation is ruled out, and the extent of contact is up to two-third of the pedicle circumference (Fig. 7.4a–d) [3]. In case of bile duct dilation (Fig. 7.5a, b), invasion of the vessel wall (Fig. 7.6a, c), and, for CLM, contact wider than two-thirds of pedicle circumference (Fig. 7.6b, c), the glissonian triad has to be divided. Of course, the pedicle has to be also sacrificed in case of a tumor thrombus in the

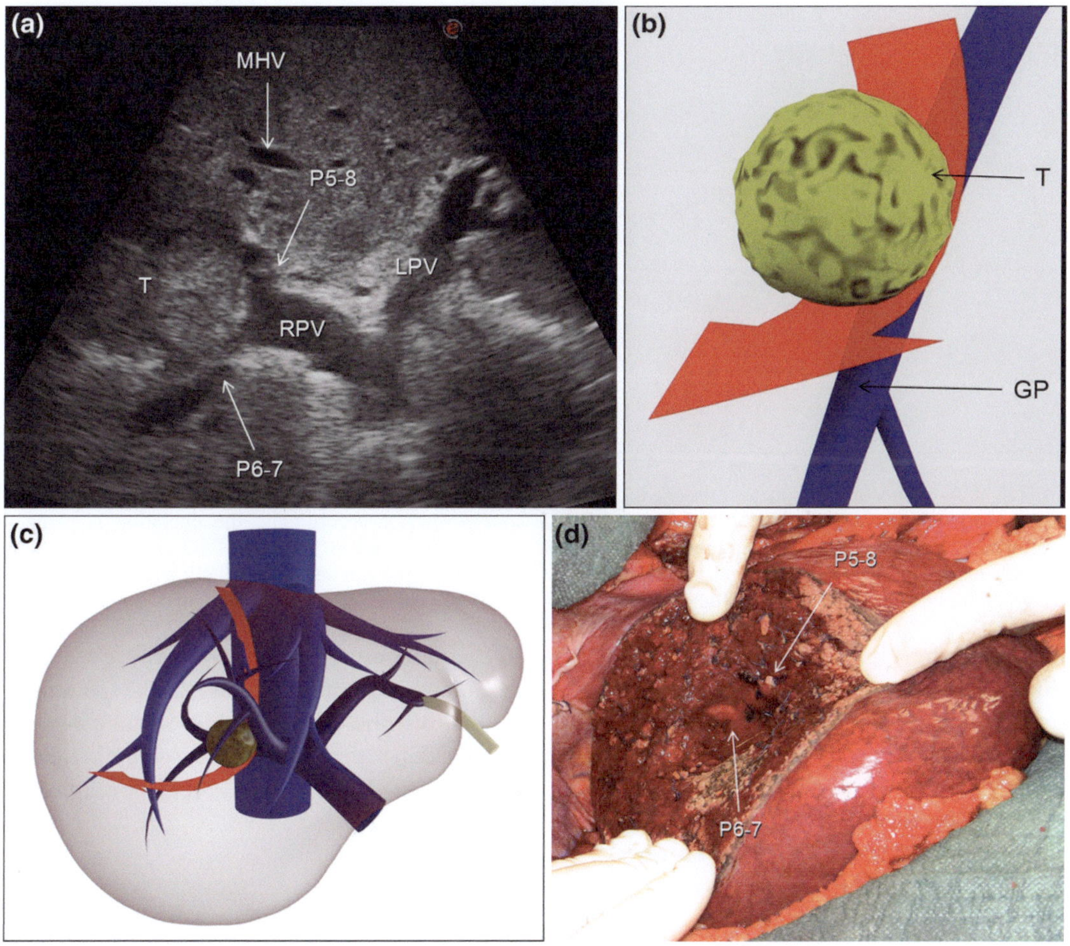

Fig. 7.3 **a** An HCC (*T*) located at the bifurcation between the portal branch to the right anterior section (*P5-8*) and that to the right posterior (*P6-7*); **b** schematically this lesion could be classified as shown and as consequence a detachment of T from the glissonian pedicle (*GP*) would be feasible, and the drawn dissection line (*red arrow*) is planned; **c** accordingly, the operation is planned; **d** finally, the roots of P5-8 and P6-7 are exposed on the cut surface; left portal vein (*LPV*); middle hepatic vein (*MHV*); right portal vein (*RPV*)

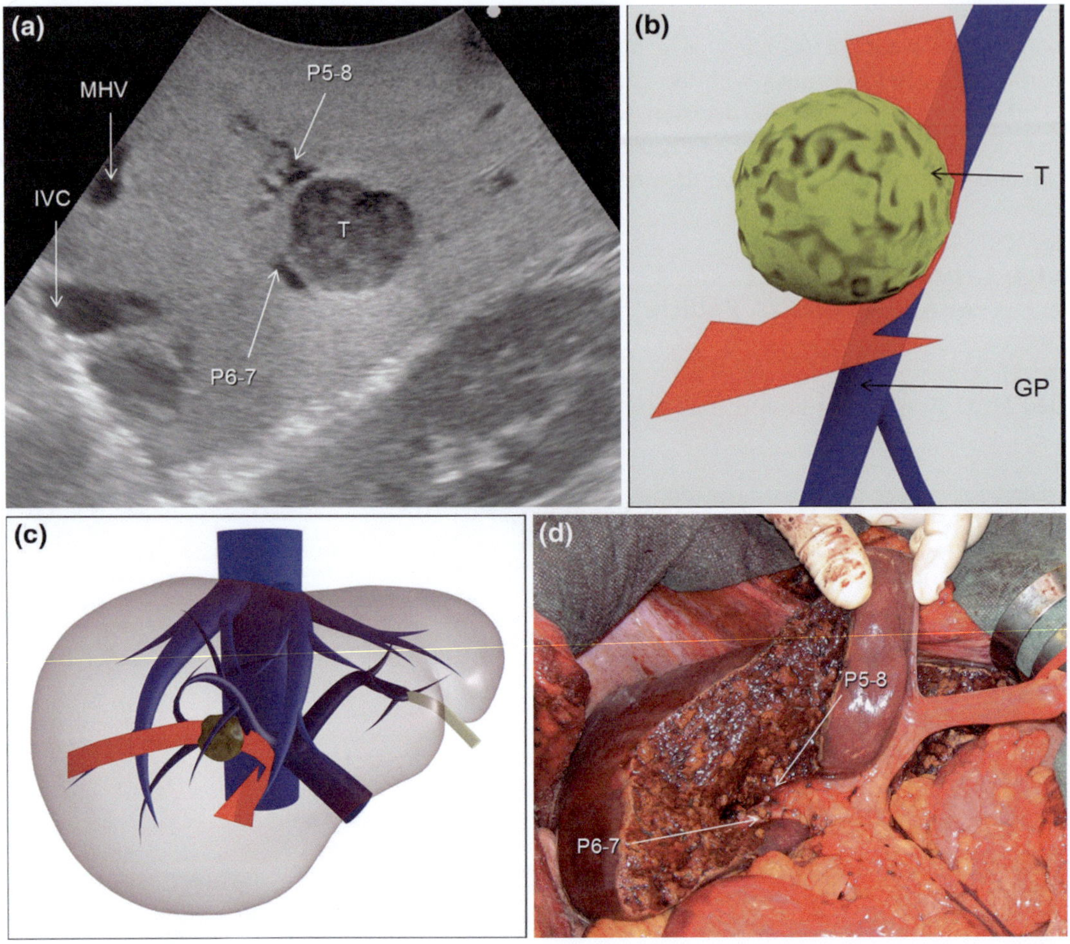

Fig. 7.4 **a** A colorectal liver metastasis (*T*) located at the bifurcation between the portal branch to the right anterior section (*P5-8*) and that to the right posterior (*P6-7*); **b** schematically this lesion can be classified as shown and accordingly a detachment of T from the glissonian pedicle (*GP*) is feasible; the dissection line is planned (*red arrow*); **c** accordingly, the operation is planned; **d** finally, the roots of P5-8 and P6-7 are exposed on the cut surface: inferior vena cava (*IVC*); middle hepatic vein (*MHV*)

portal branch (Fig. 7.7a, b), in the bile duct (Fig. 7.8a, b), or in both (Fig. 7.9). In these cases, extension of the hepatectomy is always considered.

7.1.1.1 Conservative Resection of Centrally Located Tumors

The principal output of this approach is to make feasible small-size resections even in the presence of a tumor in contact with first- or second-order portal branches, which can be represented schematically by a new resection planning as shown in Fig. 7.10. That becomes feasible by performing more complex dissection under strict IOUS guidance (Fig. 7.11a–e), and even standardizing procedures based on the pattern of lesion distribution and IOUS tumor–vessel relationships: this is the case for the so-called *lower inferior hepatectomy* (Fig. 7.12a–p) and *liver tunnel* (Fig. 7.13a–f).

7.1.2 Tumor in Contact with an Hepatic Vein

The hepatic vein is usually spared when in contact with an encapsulated HCC having the integrity of the vessel wall in IOUS (Fig. 7.14a–c). Initially

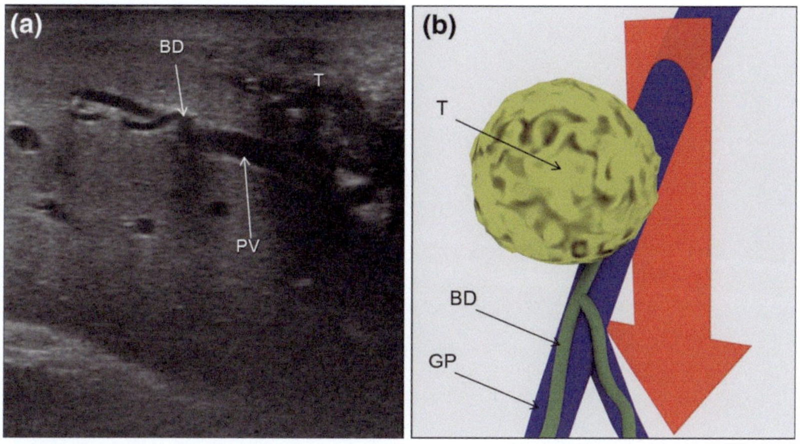

Fig. 7.5 **a** This picture shows a colorectal liver metastases (*T*) in contact with a glissonian pedicle (*GP*) and determining bile duct dilation (*BD*); **b** schematically this lesion can be classified as shown; accordingly, a detachment of T from GP is not feasible; the dissection line (*red arrow*) is planned; portal vein (*PV*)

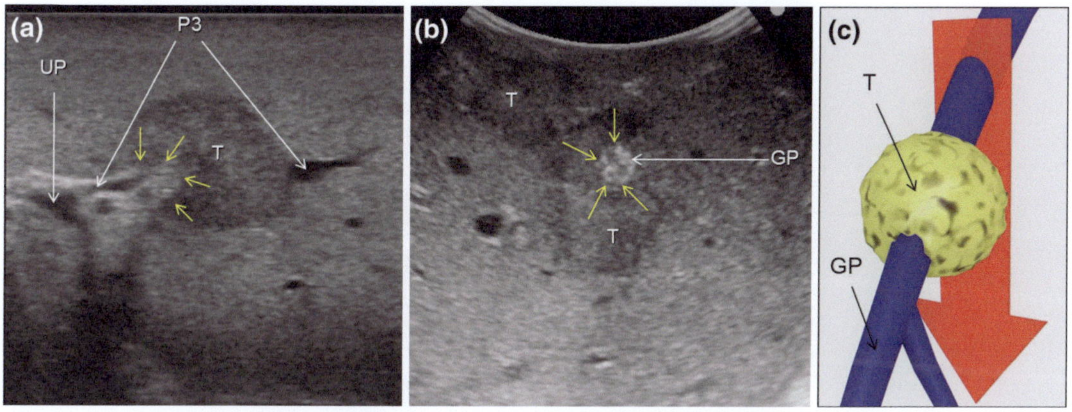

Fig. 7.6 **a** A colorectal liver metastasis (*T*) invading (*yellow arrows*) the glissonian pedicle of segment 3 (*P3*); **b** a colorectal liver metastasis (*T*) in extensive contact (*yellow arrows*) with a glissonian pedicle (*GP*); **c** schematically these lesions can be classified as shown and, accordingly, a detachment of T from the GP is not feasible; the dissection line (*red arrow*) is planned; umbilical portion (*UP*)

for the CLM, its contact was considered an indication for hepatic vein resection. Nowadays, the vein is spared when it is in contact with a CLM, but the integrity of the vessel wall is confirmed at IOUS, and the contact extension is less than two-thirds of the vein's circumference (Fig. 7.15a, b): this allows sparing procedures, which lead to otherwise unfeasible operations (Fig. 7.16a–h). When the nondetachable contact extension achieves almost 2/3, there are no communicating veins (CV), but sparing is recommended due to the association of other simultaneous resections, if part of the vessel wall is still free of tumor, patching is carried out and color-flow IOUS (CFIOUS) is used to check the patency of the vein (Fig. 7.17a–c). In presence of tumor thrombus (Fig. 7.18a–c), invasion of the vessel wall (Fig. 7.19a), and, for CLM, contact wider than two-thirds of the vein's circumference (Fig. 7.19b), the hepatic vein has to be divided (Fig. 7.19c). In these cases, extension of the hepatectomy is not compulsorily considered even if the hepatic vein is invaded at its caval confluence (last 4 cm). An extension of the resection to the entire liver parenchyma theoretically drained by the hepatic vein to be resected, is considered

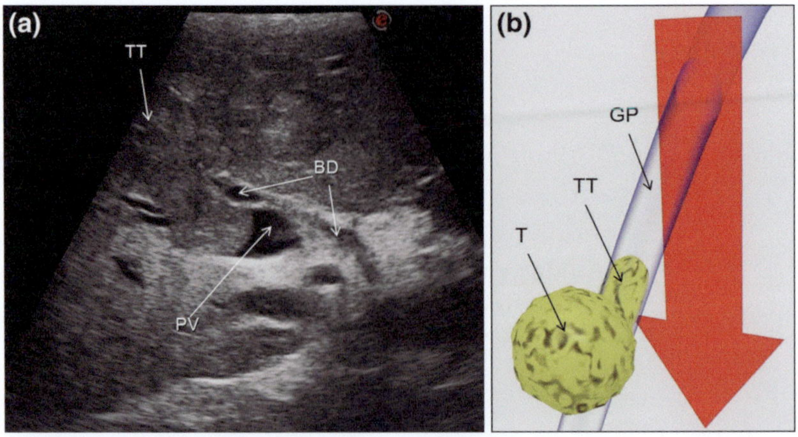

Fig. 7.7 **a** An HCC (*T*) invading the portal vein (*PV*) with a tumor thrombus (*TT*); **b** schematically this lesion can be classified as shown and, accordingly, a detachment of T from the glissonian pedicle (*GP*) is not feasible; the dissection line (*red arrow*) is planned; bile duct (*BD*)

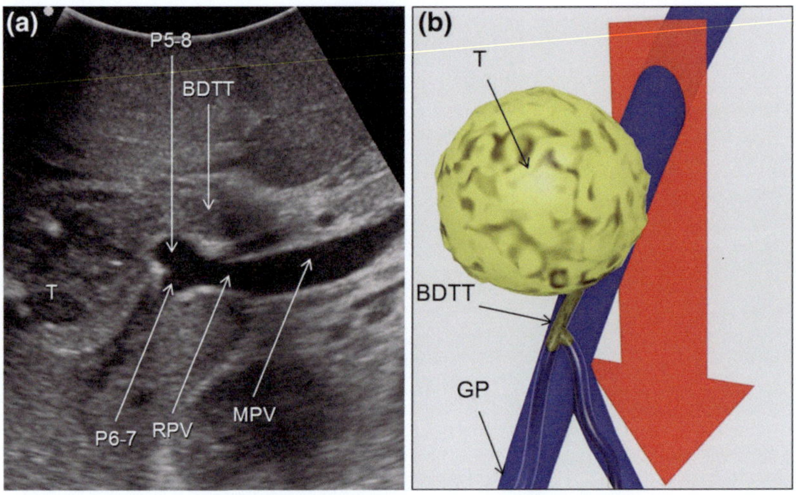

Fig. 7.8 **a** An HCC (*T*) invading the bile duct with a tumor thrombus (*BDTT*); **b** schematically this lesion can be classified as shown and, accordingly, a detachment of T from the glissonian pedicle (*GP*) is not feasible; the dissection line (*red arrow*) is planned; main portal vein (*MPV*); portal branch to the right anterior section (*P5-8*); portal branch to the right posterior section (*P6-7*); right portal vein (*RPV*)

only if one of the following ultrasonographic signs is missing:

- Presence of accessory hepatic veins in IOUS as an inferior right hepatic vein (IRHV) concomittantly with an invasion of the right hepatic vein (RHV) at the caval confluence (Fig. 7.20a–d);
- CFIOUS showing hepatopetal (Fig. 7.21) rather than hepatofugal blood flow (Figs. 7.22 and 7.23) in the feeding portal branch once the hepatic vein to be resected is clamped [10] by means of encirclement or more simply by vein compression at its extrahepatic route using the fingertip (see also Chap. 8) [11];
- Communicating veins (CV) connecting adjacent hepatic veins (Fig. 7.24). CVs are rarely visible without CFIOUS (Fig. 7.25), but more frequently by means of flow analyses, which is becoming progressively more sensitive, both trying to disclose their presence just exploring the liver or by clamping or finger compressing the hepatic vein at the caval confluence.

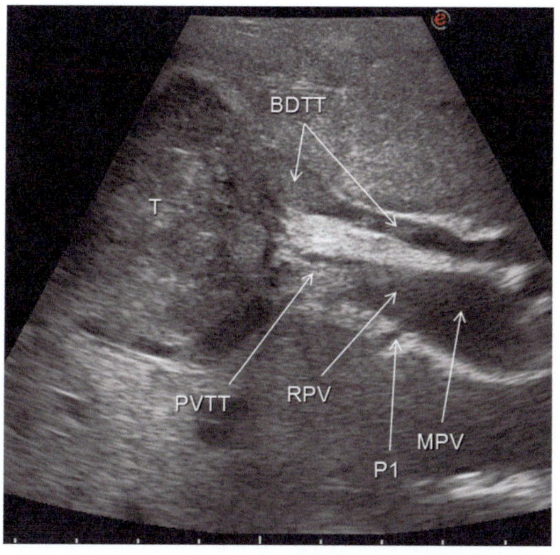

Fig. 7.9 An HCC (*T*) invading the bile duct (*BDTT*) and also the portal vein (*PVTT*) with a tumor thrombus: main portal vein (*MPV*); portal branch to segment 1 (*P1*); right portal vein (*RPV*)

Initially, CVs were considered a relatively infrequent event, based on studies performed in patients undergoing living-donor liver transplantation (LDLT) which intraoperatively occurred in 1/5–1/3 of donors [12]; a recent study has shown that 80 % of patients with CLM at the hepatocaval confluence have CVs detectable by IOUS [13]. This finding justifies new parenchyma-sparing procedures even in resecting the hepatic vein (Fig. 7.26a–d).

Adopting these criteria, we have been able to minimize the rate of major hepatectomy and to devise new procedures as described in the following.

7.1.2.1 Systematic Extended Right Posterior Sectionectomy

Systematic extended right posterior sectionectomy (SERPS) is a surgical technique allowing the systematic sparing of parts of the right

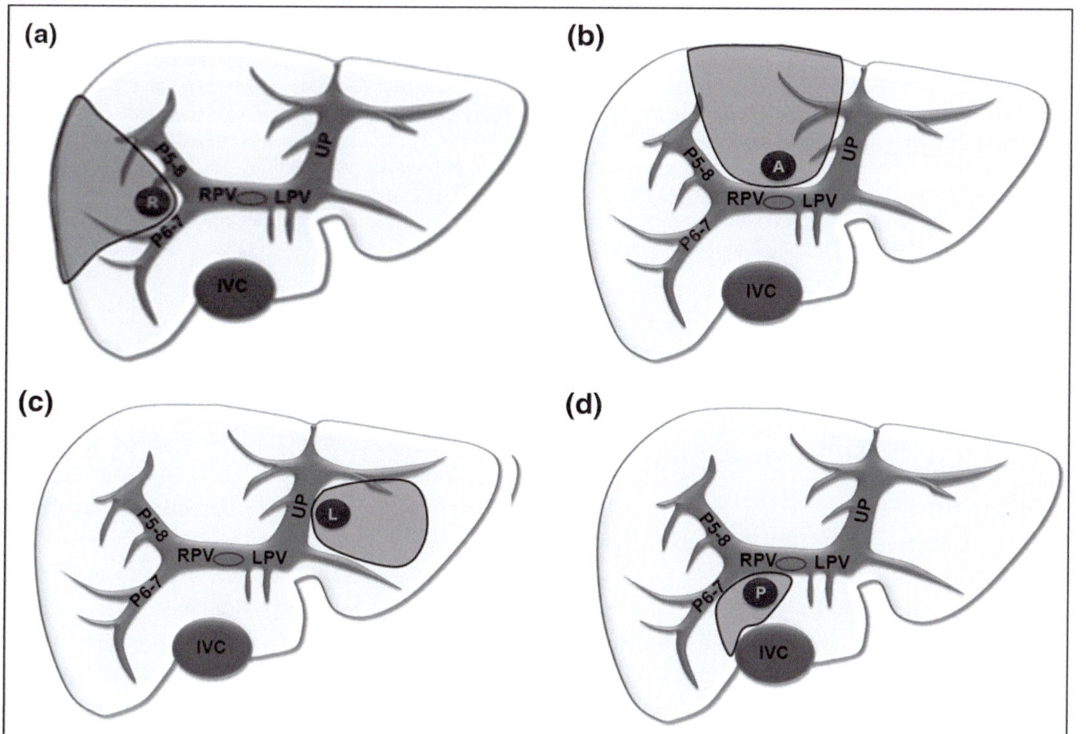

Fig. 7.10 Resection areas (*gray*) adopted for lesions centrally located due to contact with the first- or second-order glissonian pedicles in (**a**) on the right (*R*), in (**b**) anteriorly (*A*), in (**c**) on the left (*L*), and in (**d**) posteriorly (*P*); inferior vena cava (*IVC*); left portal vein (*LPV*); portal branch to the right anterior section (*P5-8*); portal branch to the right posterior section (*P6-7*); right portal vein (*RPV*); umbilical portion (*UP*)

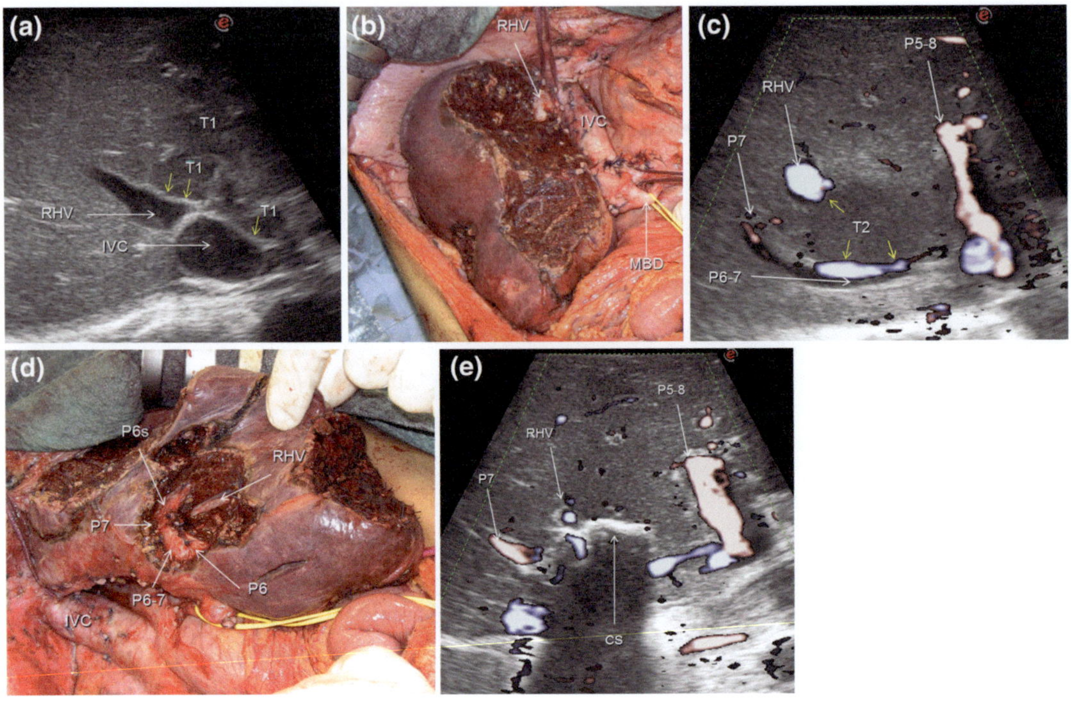

Fig. 7.11 **a** IOUS image of a huge confluent colorectal liver metastasis (*T1*) occupying entirely the left liver, segment 1, and part of the right anterior section, being in contact (*yellow arrows*) with the right hepatic vein (*RHV*) at its confluence into the inferior vena cava (*IVC*); **b** the cut surface after left hepatectomy extended to segment 1 and the right anterior section; **c** IOUS precisely discloses the presence of a lesion (*T2*) in contact (*yellow arrows*) with the RHV, and the portal branch to the right posterior section (*P6-7*) to which in part is lying posteriorly; **d** finally, the cut surface is showing the RHV, and branches to segment 6 (*P6*), 6 superior (*P6s*), and 7 (*P7*); **e** by IOUS, examining from the opposite side of the cut surface (*CS*), it is possible to verify the emptiness of the space previously occupied by the lesion and simultaneously the patency of the detached vessels; portal branch to the right anterior section (*P5-8*)

anterior liver section in the presence of tumors (example of a qualifying presentation shown in Fig. 7.27a–c) and as further elaborated in the following paragraph [6].

Eligibility Criteria

Patients suitable for SERPS have tumors presenting:

(a) invasion of the RHV close to the hepatocaval confluence (within 4 cm), with other lesions involving segment 6 and eventually segment 7 (Fig. 7.28a–g).
(b) invasion of the RHV close to the hepatocaval confluence (within 4 cm), without other lesions involving segment 6, but without IRHV, and with hepatofugal portal blood flow at CFIOUS in the portal branch to segment 6 (P6) when RHV is clamped (Fig. 7.29a–i): if an IRHV is present or, if not, anyway, the flow direction in P6 remains hepatopetal, because of CV or a middle hepatic vein (MHV) draining segment 6 (Fig. 7.30a, b), resection of segments 7 and 8 together with RHV is carried out [14] rather than SERPS. Therefore, SERPS is applied in this presentation just as alternative to segment 7 and segment 8 resection in those patients who would not present sufficient outflow for segments 5 and 6 once RHV is divided.
(c) contact with the right anterior glissonean sheat, and a relation with the right posterior having at least one of the following features: contact with dilation of bile duct draining the

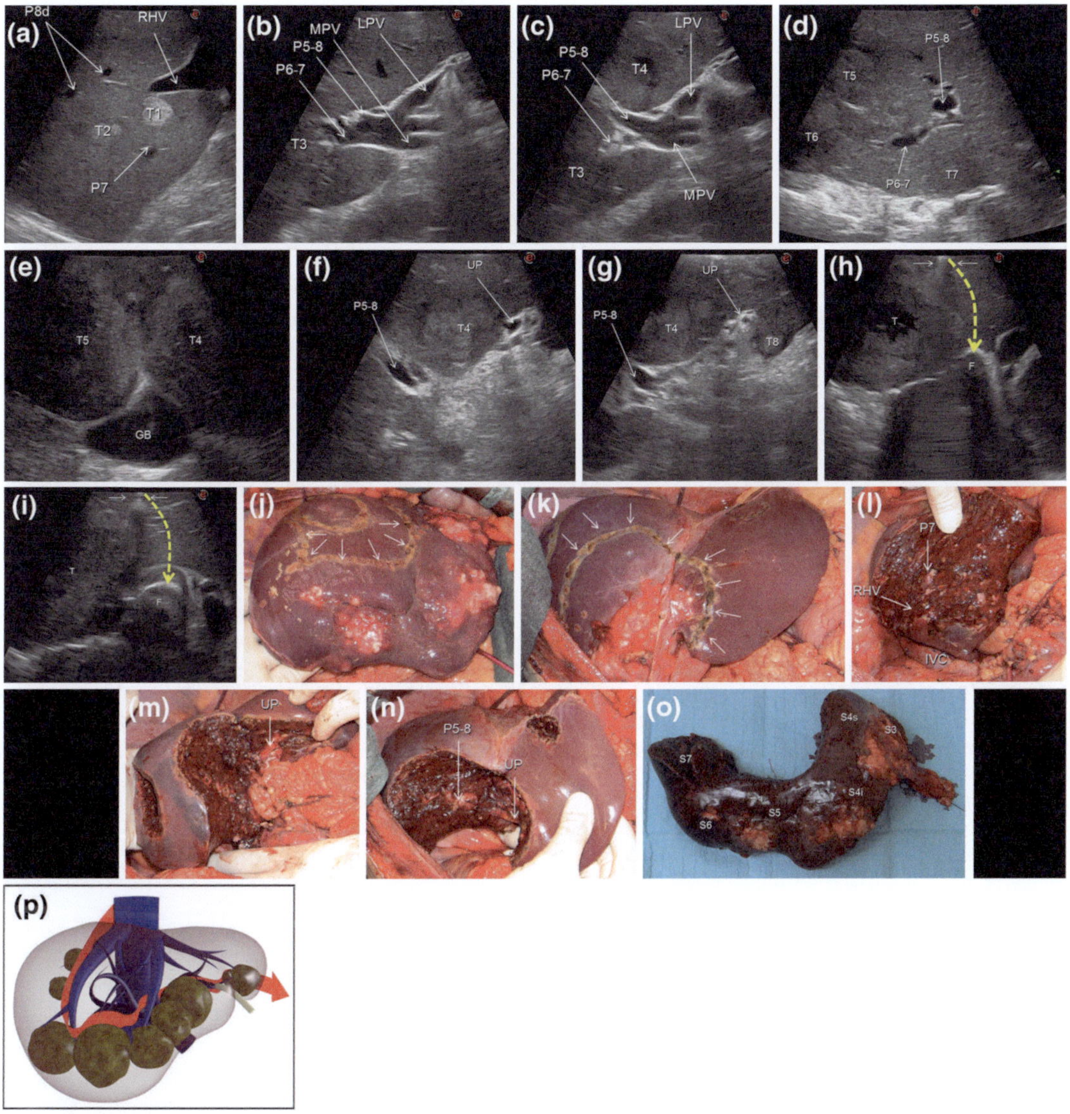

Fig. 7.12 **a** IOUS image of two colorectal liver metastases (*T1*, *T2*) in segment 7; **b** IOUS image of a colorectal liver metastasis (*T3*) below the root of the branch for the right posterior section (*P6-7*); **c** IOUS image of a colorectal liver metastasis (*T3*) below the root of P6-7 and another (*T4*) just in front of the left portal vein (*LPV*) and the branch for the right anterior section (*P5-8*); **d** IOUS image of two colorectal liver metastases (*T5*, *T6*) adjacent to P6-7 and P5-8, and another (*T7*) in the caudate process of segment 1; **e** IOUS image of two colorectal liver metastases (*T4*, *T5*) above the gallbladder (*GB*); **f** IOUS image of a colorectal liver metastasis (*T4*) between P5-8 and the umbilical portion (*UP*); **g** IOUS image of the colorectal liver metastasis described in (**f**) (*T4*), and of another located in segment 3 (*T8*); **h**, **i** two phases of the procedure performed for disclosing by IOUS the margins of the wide resection area by using the probe, the electrocautery (*white arrows*), and the finger (*F*) for planning the dissection plane (*yellow dashed arrows*); **j**, **k** the margins (*arrows*) once drawn on the liver surface; **l**, **m**, **n** the cut surface at the end of the resection; **o** specimen removed; **p** the schema of the procedure carried out and denominated lower inferior hepatectomy with the dissection plane detailed in *red*; inferior vena cava (*IVC*); main portal vein (*MPV*); right hepatic vein (*RHV*); portal branch to segment 7 (*P7*); portal branches to segment 8 dorsal (*P8*); segment 3 (*S3*); segment 4 inferior (*S4i*); segment 4 superior (*S4s*); segment 5 (*S5*); segment 6 (*S6*); segment 7 (*S7*)

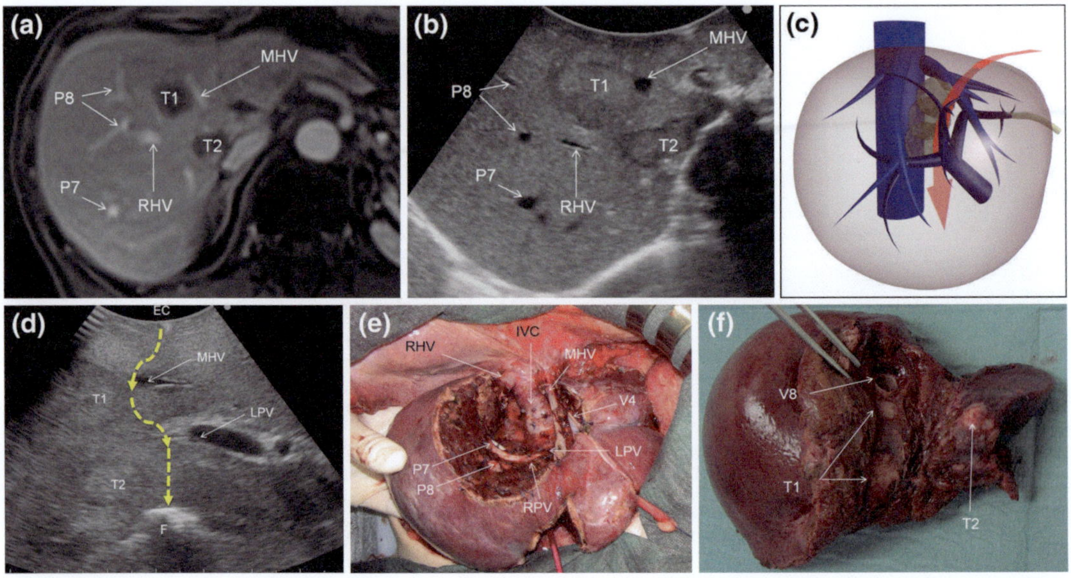

Fig. 7.13 **a** MRI image of two colorectal liver metastases in segment 8 (*T1*) and 1 (*T2*); **b** IOUS image of *T1* and *T2*, which compose a sort of cascade of lesions from segment 8 to 1; **c** main dissection plane (*red arrow*) followed for removing the two lesions: indeed T1 and T2 occupy an area disclosed in the schema by the transparent lesions, where any large and/or multiple lesions in our opinion justify a so-called ''liver tunnel'' parenchyma-sparing procedure; **d** IOUS image of the dissection (*dashed yellow arrows*) followed for removing these two lesions; **e** the cut surface resulting at the end of the resection: so-called ''liver tunnel''; **f** specimen with tumor exposure of the metastases (*T1*, *T2*), which correspond to the portions of the lesions in contact with the middle hepatic vein (*MHV*) (*T1*), and the posterior wall of the portal bifurcation (*T2*); electrocautery (*EC*); finger (*F*); inferior vena cava (*IVC*); left portal vein (*LPV*); right hepatic vein (*RHV*); right portal vein (*RPV*); portal branch to segment 7 (*P7*); portal branch to segment 8 (*P8*); hepatic vein draining segment 4 (*V4*); hepatic vein draining segment 8 (*V8*)

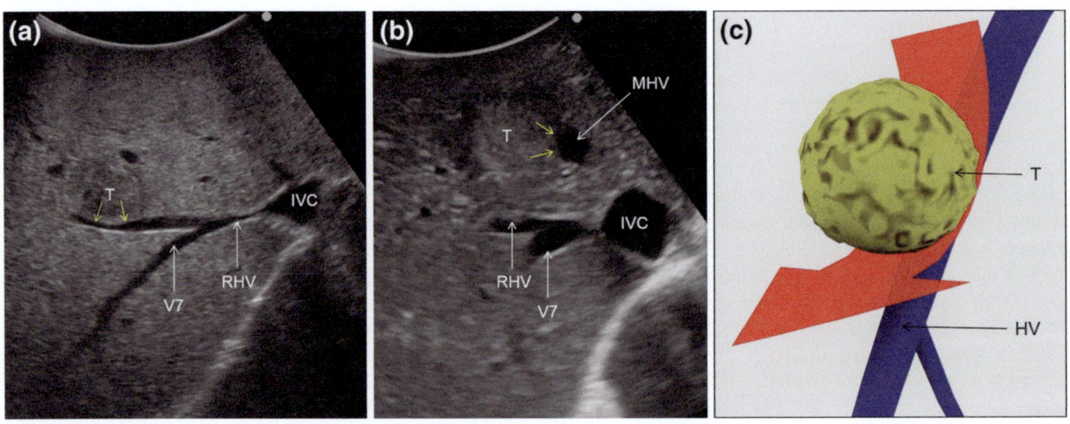

Fig. 7.14 **a** An HCC (*T*) in contact (*yellow arrows*) with the right hepatic vein (*RHV*); **b** an HCC (*T*) in contact (*yellow arrows*) with the middle hepatic vein (*MHV*); **c** schematically these lesions can be classified as shown and in consequence a detachment of the tumor from the hepatic veins (*HV*) may be feasible, and the drawn dissection line (*red arrow*) is planned; inferior vena cava (*IVC*); hepatic vein draining segment 7 (*V7*)

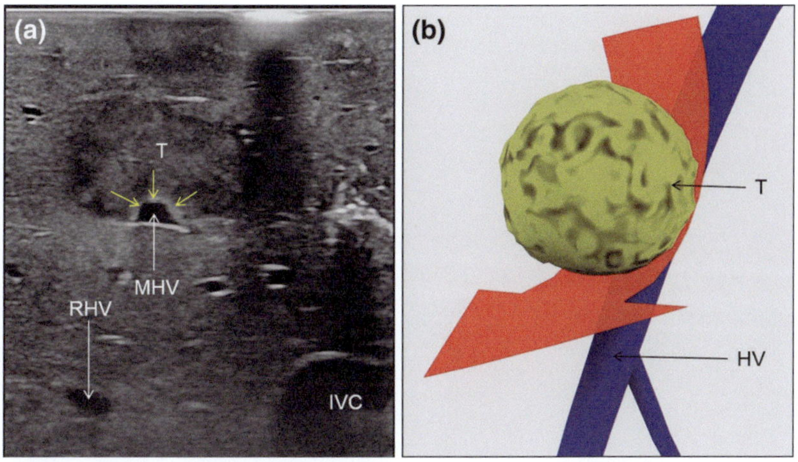

Fig. 7.15 **a** Colorectal liver metastasis (*T*) in contact with the middle hepatic vein (*MHV*) for an extension lower or equal than 2/3; **b** schematically this lesion can be classified as shown and in consequence a detachment of the tumor from the hepatic veins (*HV*) may be feasible, and the drawn dissection line (*red arrow*) is planned; inferior vena cava (*IVC*); right hepatic vein (*RHV*)

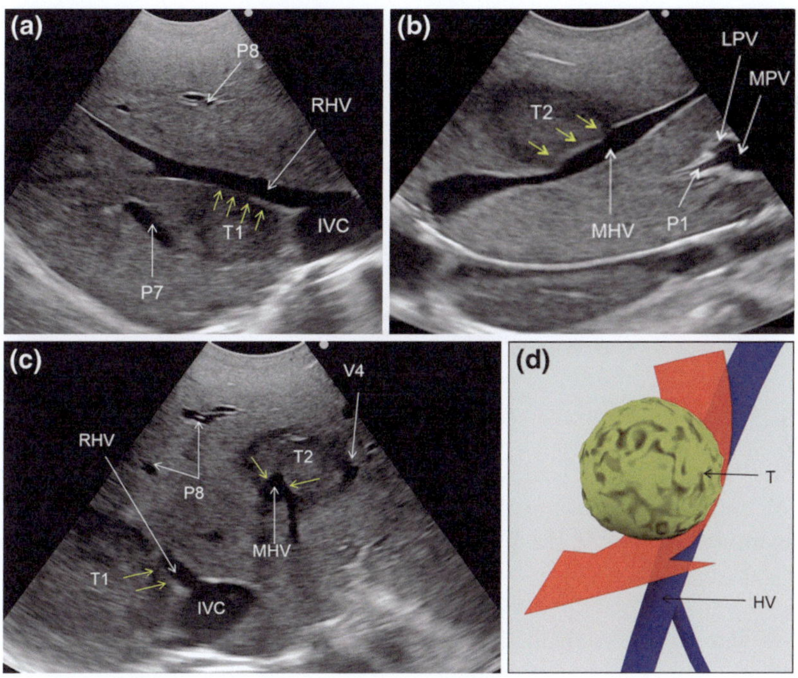

Fig. 7.16 **a** IOUS image of a colorectal liver metastasis in segment 7 (*T1*) in contact (*yellow arrows*) with the right hepatic vein (*RHV*); **b** IOUS image of a colorectal liver metastasis in segments 4 superior and 8 (*T2*) in contact (*yellow arrows*) with the middle hepatic vein (*MHV*); **c** transverse scan at IOUS of *T1*, *T2* in contact (*yellow arrows*) respectively with the RHV and MHV; **d** dissection (*red arrow*) followed for removing these two lesions; **e** IOUS image of a colorectal liver metastasis (*T3*) in contact (*yellow arrows*) with the left hepatic vein (*LHV*) at the caval confluence and another (*T4*) which infiltrates (*yellow arrows*) the LHV just peripherally in respect to T3; **f** dissection (*red arrow*) followed for removing these two lesions which is motivated by the type of relationship between T4 and LHV; **g**, **h** cut surface for removing those lesions depicted in the previous pictures: in particular, MHV was detached from T2 (**g**) and RHV from T1 (**h**); hepatic vein (*HV*); inferior vena cava (*IVC*); left portal vein (*LPV*); main portal vein (*MPV*); portal branch to segment 1 (*P1*); portal branch to segment 7 (*P7*); portal branch to segment 8 (*P8*); hepatic vein draining segment 4 (*V4*)

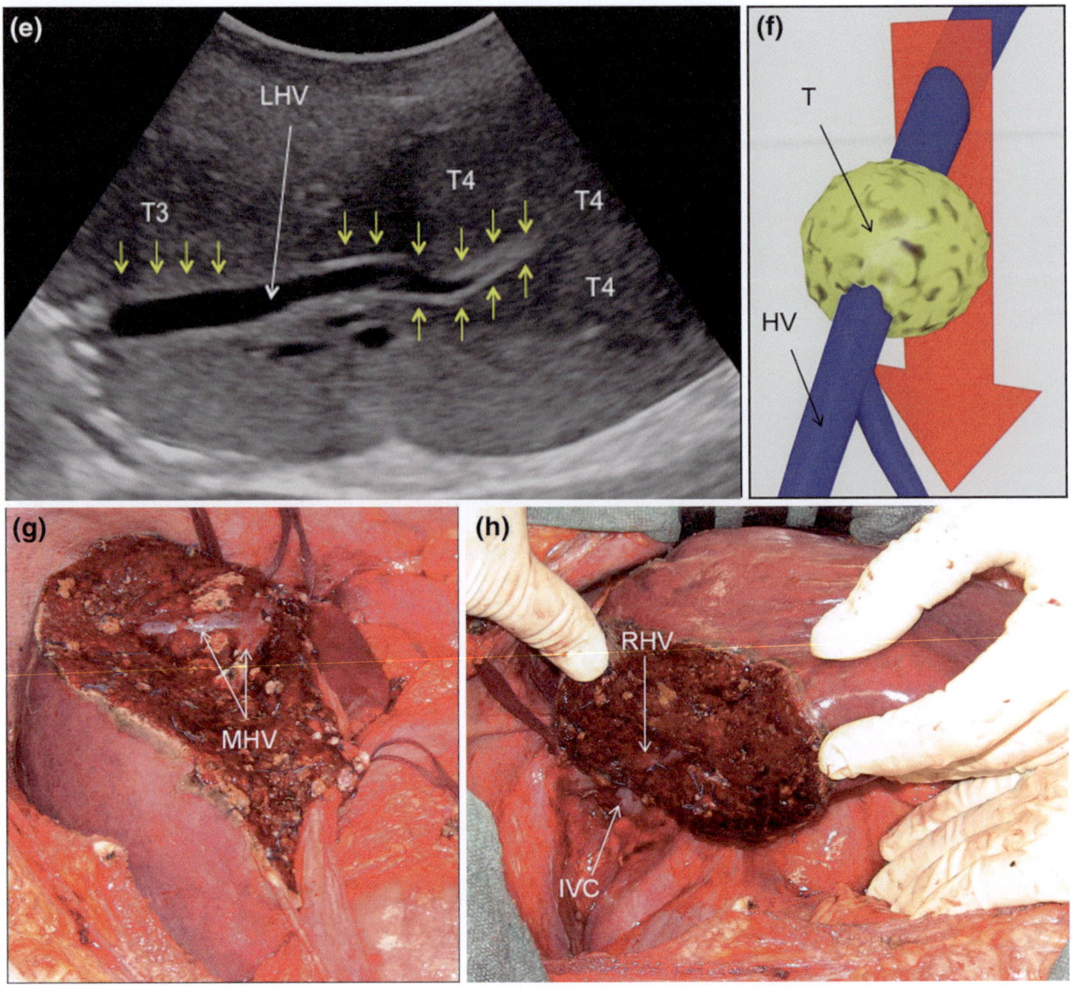

right posterior section, vessel wall invasion, or, for CLM, contact wider than two-third of pedicle circumference (Fig. 7.31a–k).

Procedure

In conditions A and B, extension to the right anterior section is tailored just to warrant the complete removal of the tumor, and the dissection line is drawn on the left side of the RHV which is also resected: flow direction in right anterior portal branch at CFIOUS is estimated as previously described once RHV is clamped if not occluded (Fig. 7.29d). In condition C, the extension of the resection into the right anterior section is tailored preserving most of the parenchyma of segment 8, the tract of the RHV at the hepatocaval confluence, and the left portion of segment 5 without division of the right anterior pedicle. In all the conditions suitable for SERPS the right anterior pedicle can remain exposed on the cut surface (Fig. 7.28f, g) or not (Figs. 7.29g and 7.31g).

7.1.2.2 Mini-Mesohepatectomy

This is an alternative to the conventional mesohepatectomy applied in case of tumors invading the MHV at its caval confluence, and consists of a limited resection including the tract of the invaded vein without its reconstruction sparing part of segment 4 and/or of the right anterior

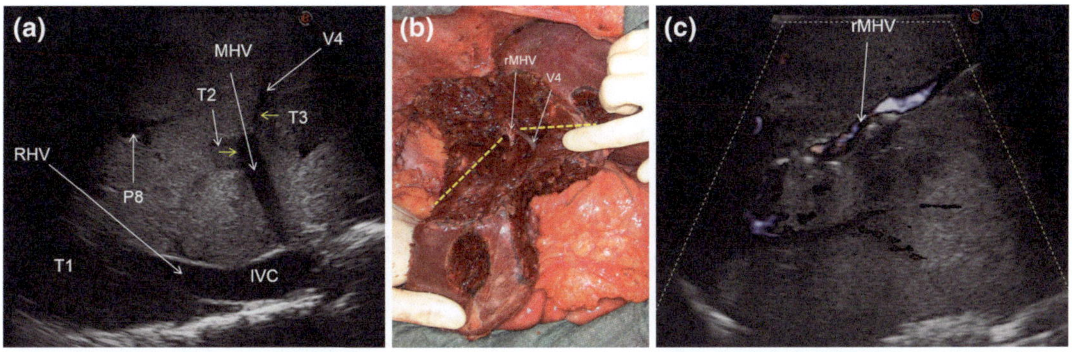

Fig. 7.17 **a** IOUS image of 3 out of 15 colorectal liver metastases (*T1*, *T2*, *T3*): two of them (*T2*, *T3*) have a contact (*yellow arrows*) with the mid-portion of the middle hepatic vein (*MHV*) and the branch draining segment 4 (*V4*); **b** the association of the two lesions close to each others and surrounding MHV and V4 at their junction made unfeasible their detachment without resection of a portion of vessel wall; the absence of communicating veins lead to vein reconstruction performed with a patch of bovine pericardium (*rMHV*) to allow proper drainage of a relevant part of remnant liver (the portion of liver located inferiorly to the two *yellow dashes lines*) considering the sacrificed parenchyma for having removed the other lesions distributed on both lobes; **c** CFIOUS image confirming the patency of the reconstructed vein: inferior vena cava (*IVC*); portal branch to segment 8 (*P8*)

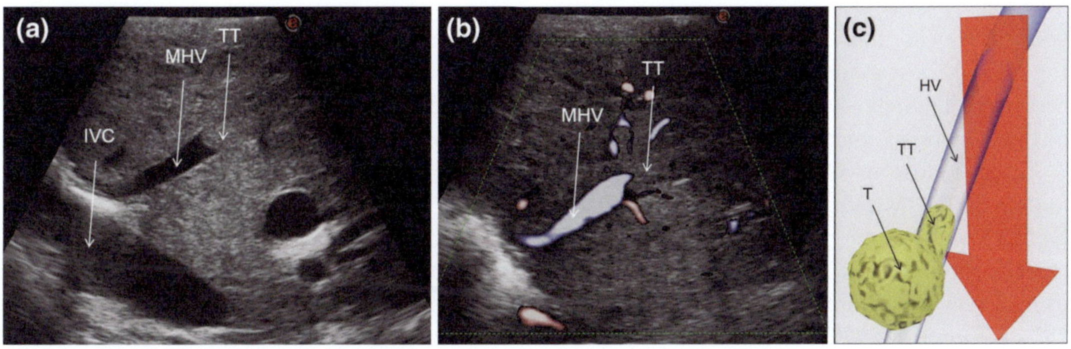

Fig. 7.18 **a** IOUS of an HCC having invaded with a tumor thrombus (*TT*) the middle hepatic vein (*MHV*); **b** CFIOUS image of that previously shown in (**a**); **c** schematically this lesion can be classified as shown and in consequence the dissection line (*red arrow*) has to consider hepatic vein (*HV*) resection; inferior vena cava (*IVC*); tumor (*T*)

section as shown in Fig. 7.32a, b, as further elaborated in the following paragraph [7].

Eligibility Criteria

Patients suitable for mini-mesohepatectomy (MMH) are those with tumors bearing macroscopic signs of vascular invasion (preoperative imaging and IOUS) of the MHV close to the hepatocaval confluence (within 4 cm) (Fig. 7.33a).

Procedure

The steps of MMH are represented here in detail in three cases (Figs. 7.33a–j, 7.34a–j, and 7.35a–k). If the tumor is large, and the relation with the MHV is just at the caval confluence, the MHV itself or more frequently the common trunk with the LHV is encircled and taped for eventual clamping (Figs. 7.34h and 7.35f). If not (small tumor and adjacent but not exactly at the caval confluence), the control of the MHV backflow bleeding could be done without preventive vein encirclement. The anterior surface of the hepatocaval confluence is exposed and a space between the RHV and MHV extrahepatic tracts prior to their caval confluence is obtained by dissection to accommodate the surgeon's fingertip (see Chap. 8). Finger compression is then applied to the MHV at its caval confluence

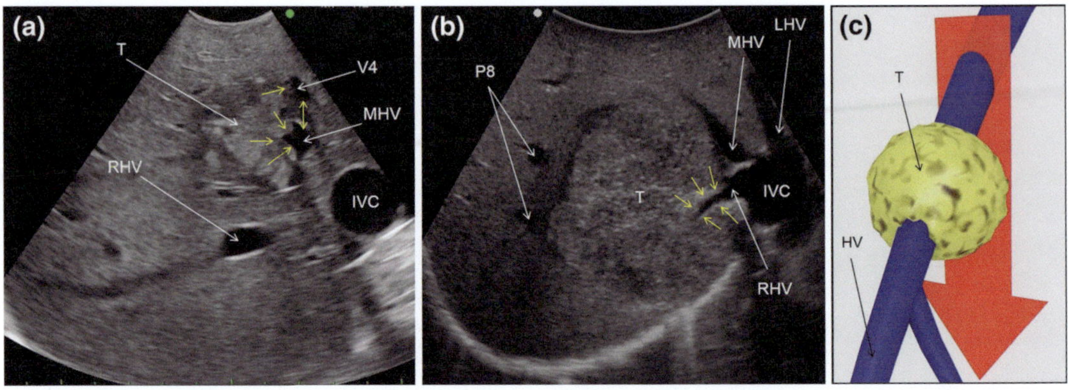

Fig. 7.19 **a** IOUS image of a colorectal liver metastasis (*T*) invading (*yellow arrows*) the middle hepatic vein (*MHV*), and the vein draining segment 4 (*V4* or scissural vein); **b** IOUS image of a colorectal liver metastasis (*T*) invading (*yellow arrows*) the right hepatic vein (*RHV*), and being in contact with the MHV; **c** schematically both lesions can be classified as shown and in consequence the dissection line (*red arrow*) has to consider resection of the MHV and RHV, respectively; hepatic vein (*HV*); inferior vena cava (*IVC*); left hepatic vein (*LHV*); portal branches to segment 8 (*P8*)

verifying by CFIOUS the disappearance of the blood flow in the MHV or its inversion (Fig. 7.36). For planning an MMH at least one of these three findings should be confirmed during the finger compression clamping test of the MHV: 1. Reversal flow in CFIOUS in the peripheral portion of the MHV, which suggests drainage through collateral circulation in the RHV/LHV depending on the side of the MHV branch with reversal flow (Fig. 7.33f). 2. Detectable shunting CV at CFIOUS with RHV, LHV, or IVC (Figs. 7.33c, d, e, 7.34d, and 7.35c, d).

3. Hepatopetal flow in P5-8 and/or P4inf portal branches (Figs. 7.33f and 7.34j). If none of these finding is confirmed and, in particular, hepatofugal flow direction in P5-8 and/or P4 inf is detected, hepatectomy has to be extended to the area fed by those portal branches.

The posterior wall of the MHV (Fig. 7.37a, b) or of the tumor once it is involving the paracaval portion (Fig. 7.33h), together with the surgeon's left-hand fingertip positioned between the IVC and the palpable cranial edge of the tumor (Figs. 7.33g, h; 7.34f, g; and 7.35b) are used as landmarks for delimiting the resection area. A crucial point for proper accomplishment of the MMH in presence of CV is to delineate a dissection plane, which does not interrupt the CV itself. This is generally obtained by dividing the MHV closest to its point of infiltration then allowing the vascular arches of the branches flowing into the main trunk to remain open: in this way, the latter will keep the respective drained areas connected with the CVs and thus also the adjacent hepatic vein (Figs. 7.33i and 7.34i).

7.1.2.3 Upper Transversal Hepatectomy

For tumors involving from more than one to nearly all of the hepatic veins at the hepatocaval confluence, major hepatectomy or vascular reconstruction or even unresectabilty are claimed. In 1987, Makuuchi et al. [14] reported that in case of a thick IRHV at preoperative imaging or in IOUS, resection of the tumor together with the RHV may have been feasible without carrying out a formal right hepatectomy rather limiting the liver tissue removal to that of segments 7 and 8. This was the first report showing how just the disclosure of an anatomical feature makes feasible surgical procedures that otherwise would have been unfeasible: the latter paper, apart of the mentioned procedure, also reports on three other new operations. After SERPS and MMH, profiting from the pioneering experience of Makuuchi, which opened new perspectives in the planning of surgical strategies, we continued by developing the procedure of upper transversal hepatectomy (UTH) [8].

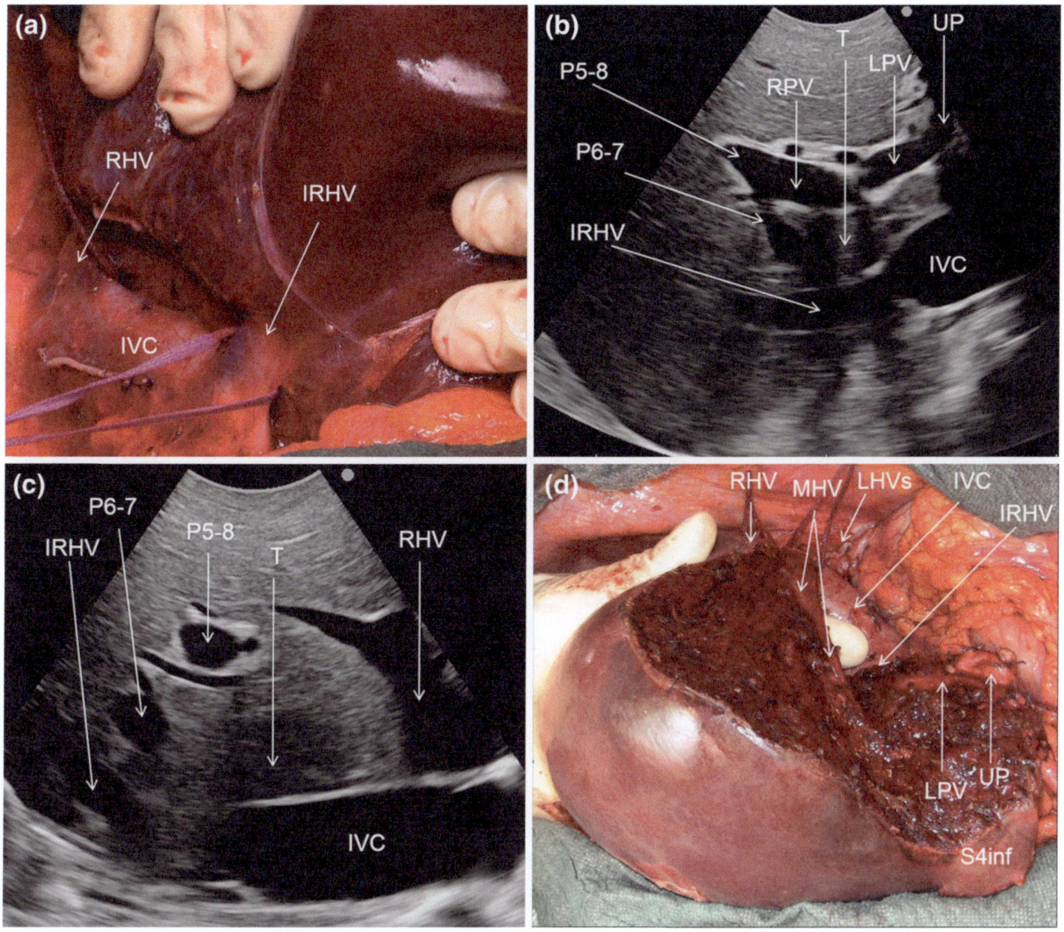

Fig. 7.20 **a** Surgical image of the inferior right hepatic vein (*IRHV*) flowing into the inferior vena cava (*IVC*) and its topographic relation with the right hepatic vein (*RHV*); **b** in IOUS the IRHV runs behind the right portal vein (*RPV*) and the branch to the right posterior section (*P6-7*); **c** on a sagittal IOUS scan the relation between the RHV and the IRHV is well disclosed: here, a colorectal liver metastasis is also evident located in between these two veins and in contact with the inferior vena cava (*IVC*); **d** at surgery the exposure, mobilization, and IOUS guidance made feasible the selective removal of the tumor between the two veins together with the removal of a large lesion in contact with the middle hepatic vein (*MHV*), and invading the left hepatic vein, which was resected (*LHVs*) anyway keeping the inferior portion of segment 4 (*S4inf*), then avoiding a formal left hepatectomy; left portal vein (*LPV*); portal branch to the right anterior section (*P5-8*); umbilical portion (*UP*)

Eligibility Criteria

The tumor at the caval confluence should have invaded two of the hepatic veins in the presence of IRHV and CVs (Fig. 7.38) or just CVs (Fig. 7.39a–p). The tumor could lie over the hilar plate with contact but not invading the right and left portal branches (Fig. 7.39d–g), and the segmental portal branches to segments 4 inferior, 5, and 6.

Procedure

UTH involves the total or partial resection of the superior liver segments (2,4sup,7,8) including partially or completely segment 1 together with two of the three hepatic veins but preserving the inferior portion of the liver which is possible through the natural by-passes represented by the CV with (Fig. 7.38) or without (Fig. 7.39a–p) accessory veins guaranteeing the outflow of the

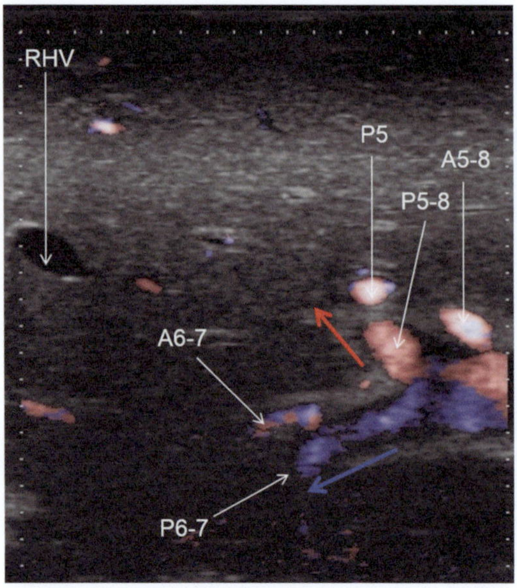

Fig. 7.21 CFIOUS image of the right portal vein (*RPV*) branching into the right anterior branch (*P5-8*) and the right posterior one (*P6-7*); the arteries to the same liver sections are also evident (*A5-8* and *A6-7*): the colors show the flow direction (*colored arrows*) which is hepatopetal both in the portal and arterial branches; portal branch to segment 5 (*P5*); right hepatic vein (*RHV*)

inferior portion of the liver theoretically drained by the resected hepatic veins. The ultrasound study in these patients should precisely map the accessory veins, IRHV included, and the CVs to determine whether their pattern merely connects two adjacent HVs (Fig. 7.39h, i) or an HV and the IVC: in the latter case the short hepatic vein connected to the obstructed HV through the CV has to be preserved, while in the absence of accessory veins flowing into the IVC, even in a similar tumor presentation, the caval plane can fully be freed (Fig. 7.39j). Also, adequate exposure and mobilization should allow positioning the left hand at the posterior aspect of the defined dissection plane (Fig. 7.39j). For all these reasons, a J-shaped thoracophrenolapatotomic access is frequently applied in such cases. The direct view afforded by this incision to the hepatocaval plane allows tailoring an adequate mobilization of the liver from the caval plane (Fig. 7.39j); in the case of an IRHV, this approach facilitates liver mobilization without sectioning this vein root. The access, the mobilization, the in- and outflow mapping, and the IOUS guidance lead to the removal of a relatively small and almost completely diseased part of the liver keeping the vast majority of the

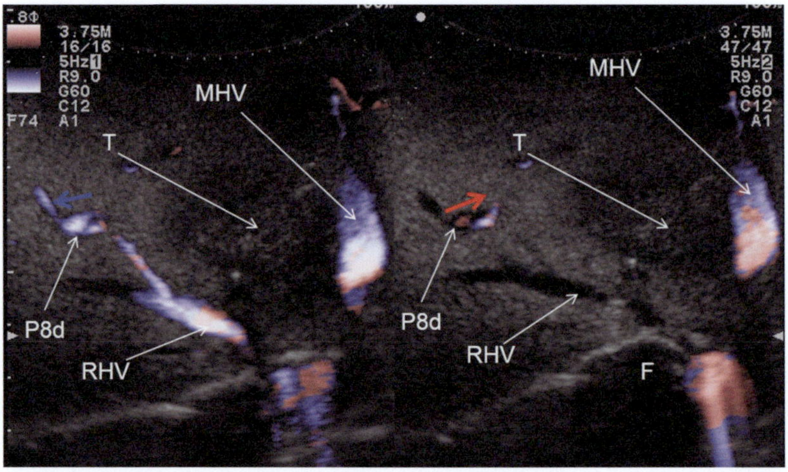

Fig. 7.22 CFIOUS images on the modifications of the portal flow directions induced by the occlusion of the hepatic vein outflow: on the left, the right hepatic vein (*RHV*) is patent, and the flow in the dorsal branch of the portal vein for segment 8 (*P8d*) shows an hepatopetal blood flow (*blue arrow*). On the right, once having occluded the RHV by finger compression (*F*) the blood flow in P8d is inverted (*red arrow*) becoming hepatofugal, which means that for this particular subsegment the liver is exclusively drained by the RHV, without communicating veins shunting the blood to another outflow route; middle hepatic vein (*MHV*); tumor (*T*)

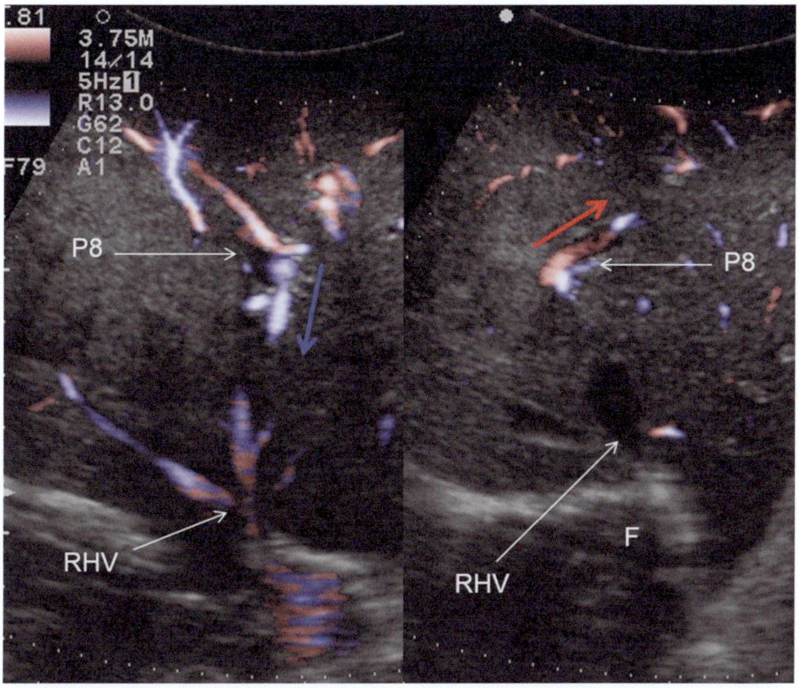

Fig. 7.23 CFIOUS images (as in Fig. 7.22) on the modifications of the portal flow directions induced by the occlusion of the hepatic vein outflow: on the left, the right hepatic vein (*RHV*) is patent, and the flow in the portal vein for segment 8 (*P8*) shows an hepatopetal blood flow (*blue arrow*). On the right, once having occluded the RHV by finger compression (*F*) the blood flow in P8 is inverted (*red arrow*) becoming hepatofugal, which means that for this particular subsegment the liver is exclusively drained by the RHV, without communicating veins shunting the blood to another outflow route

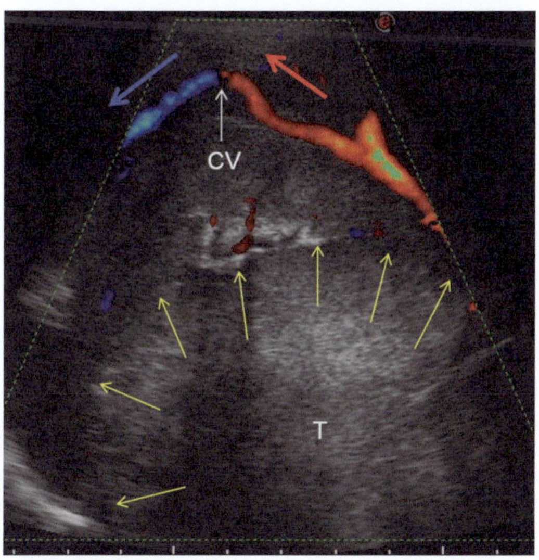

Fig. 7.24 CFIOUS image of a communicating vein (*CV*) shunting the blood flow from two adjacent hepatic veins in the presence of a large tumor (*T*) of which the *yellow arrows* indicate the margins and which compresses one of the two veins at its caval confluence provoking a sort of secondary Budd-Chiari Syndrome

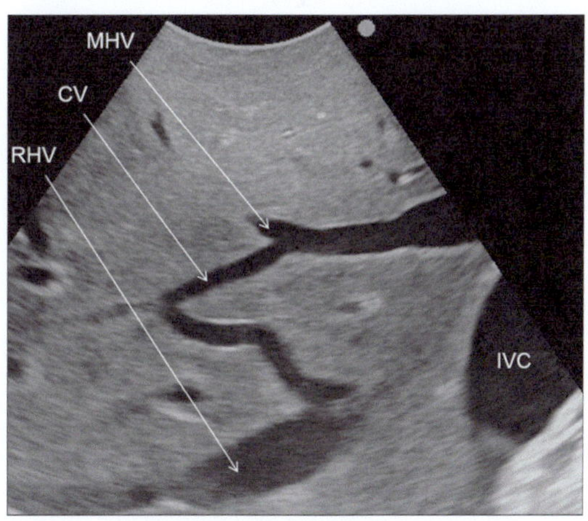

Fig. 7.25 IOUS image of a communicating vein (*CV*) shunting the blood flow between the middle (*MHV*) and the right hepatic vein (*RHV*), in absence of a tumor compressing one of them at the caval confluence; inferior vena cava (*IVC*)

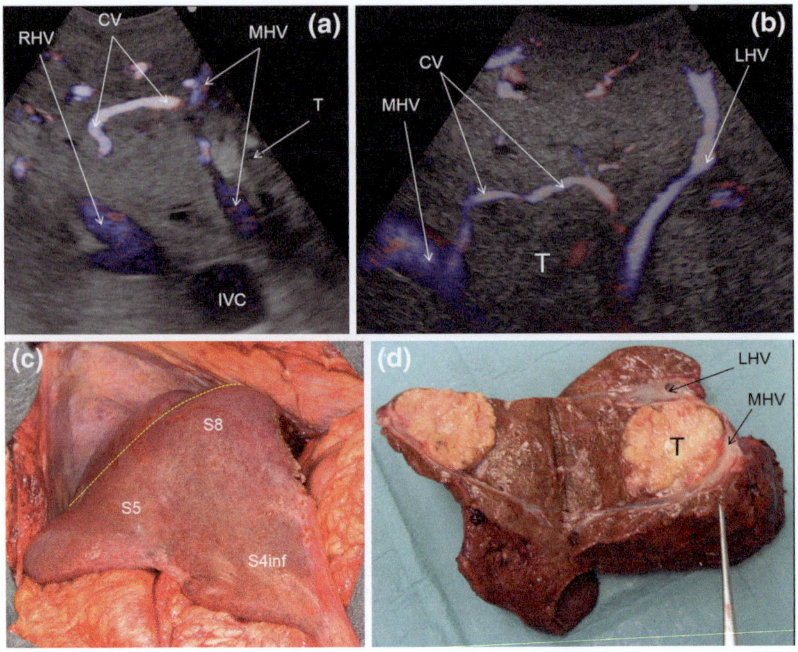

Fig. 7.26 **a** CFIOUS image of a communicating vein (*CV*) shunting the blood flow between the middle (*MHV*) and the right hepatic vein (*RHV*); **b** in the same patient, a further CV connecting the left hepatic vein (*LHV*) and the MHV by surrounding the tumor (*T*) which compresses both of them; **c** this feature allows instead of performing an extended left hepatectomy (*yellow dashed line*), just a left lobectomy (segments 2 and 3) extended to segment 4 superior; **d** the specimen shows T surrounded by LHV and MHV; segment 4 inferior (*S4inf*); segment 5 (*S5*); segment 8 (*S8*); inferior vena cava (*IVC*)

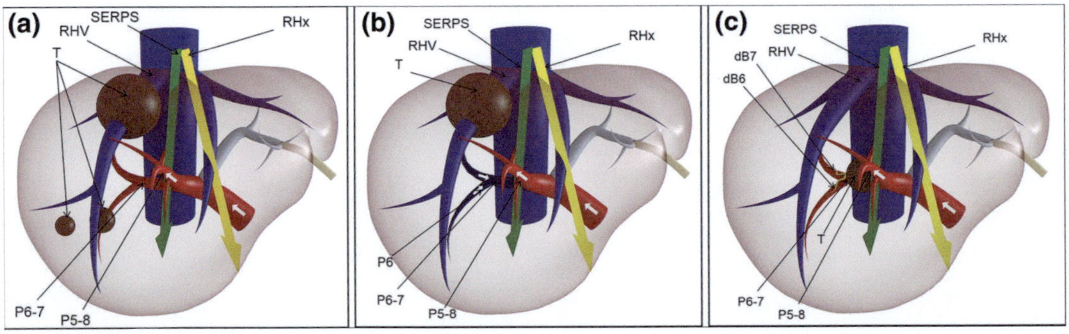

Fig. 7.27 Eligibility criteria for systematic extended right posterior sectionectomy (*SERPS*) featured by a dissection line passing between the portal branch to the right anterior section (*P5-8*), and the right hepatic vein (RHV) (*green arrow*) rather than that for a conventional right hepatectomy (RHx) (*yellow arrow*): in all cases, in CFIOUS the hepatopetal portal blood flow (*red colored* branch with *arrows* indicating the flow direction) must be evident in *P5-8* once the *RHV* is clamped if not already occluded. **a** Presence of vascular invasion of the RHV at the hepatocaval confluence (within 4 cm), with tumors (*T*) also in segment 6; **b** Presence of vascular invasion of the RHV at the hepatocaval confluence, without any tumor in segment 6, but without accessory veins and/or with hepatofugal portal blood flow (*blue colored* branch with *arrows* indicating the flow direction) in the portal branch to segment 6 (*P6*) with RHV clamped if not already occluded; **c** Presence of vascular invasion of the right posterior portal branch (*P6-7*) or anyway biliary dilation of the bile ducts draining segment 6 (*dB6*), and segment 7 (*dB7*), with T in contact with P5-8 without signs of biliary dilation in the right anterior section

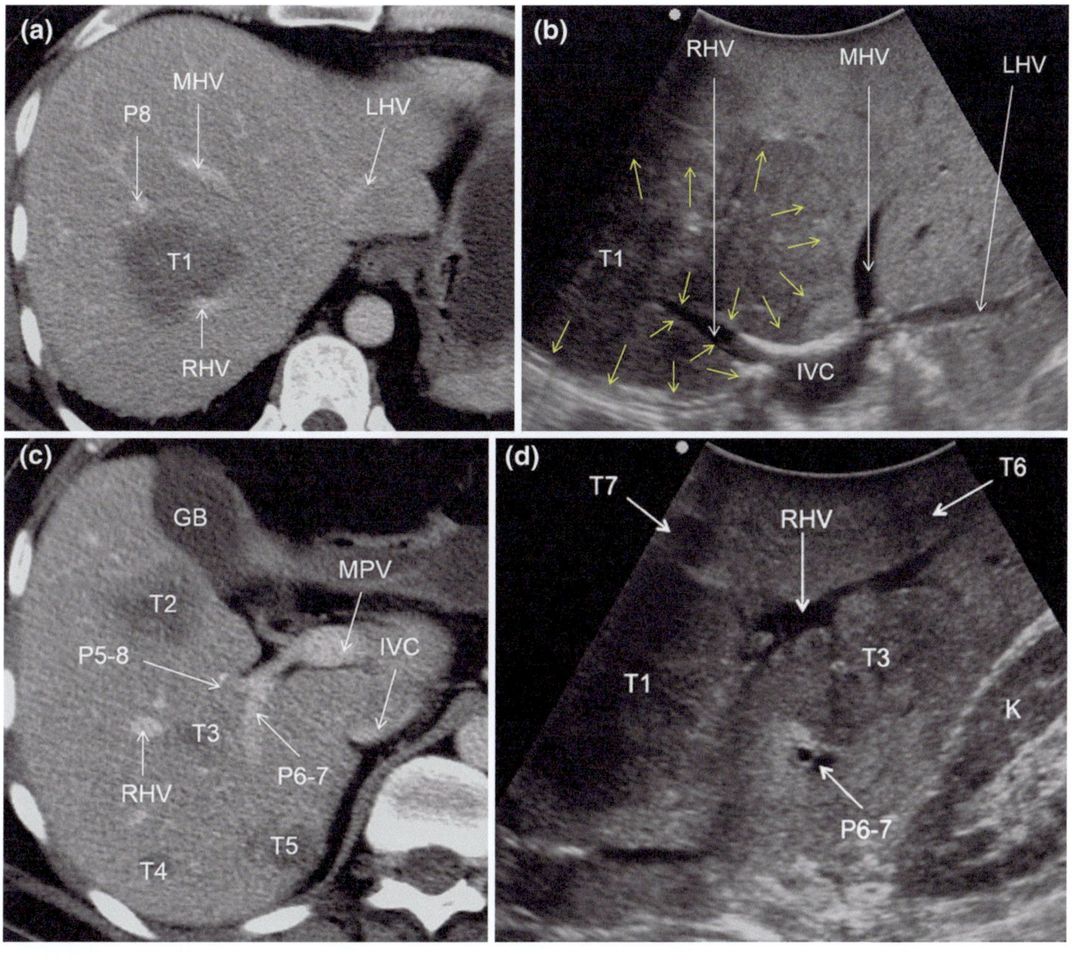

Fig. 7.28 **a** Computed tomography (*CT*) image of a colorectal liver metastasis (*T1*) invading the right hepatic vein (*RHV*); **b** IOUS image of the same pattern with T1 (*yellow arrows*) surrounding the RHV; **c** CT image of the lesions occupying the inferior portion of the right hemiliver (*T2-5*); **d** IOUS image of the pattern just shown in CT while disclosing further lesions (*T6,7*) using compulsorily a slightly different scan; **e** dissection line, which should be used for a formal right hepatectomy (*yellow arrows*) and inversely that built accordingly along the SERPS criteria for type (**a**) pattern (*green arrows*); **f** the cut surface after the resection with the portal branch to the right anterior section (*P5-8*) exposed; **g** CFIOUS showing the hepatopetal direction (*red arrow*) of blood flow in P5-8; cut surface (*CS*); gallbladder (*GB*); kidney (*K*); inferior vena cava (*IVC*); left hepatic vein (*LHV*); middle hepatic vein (*MHV*); main portal vein (*MPV*); portal branch to segment 8 (*P8*); portal branch to the right posterior section (*P6-7*)

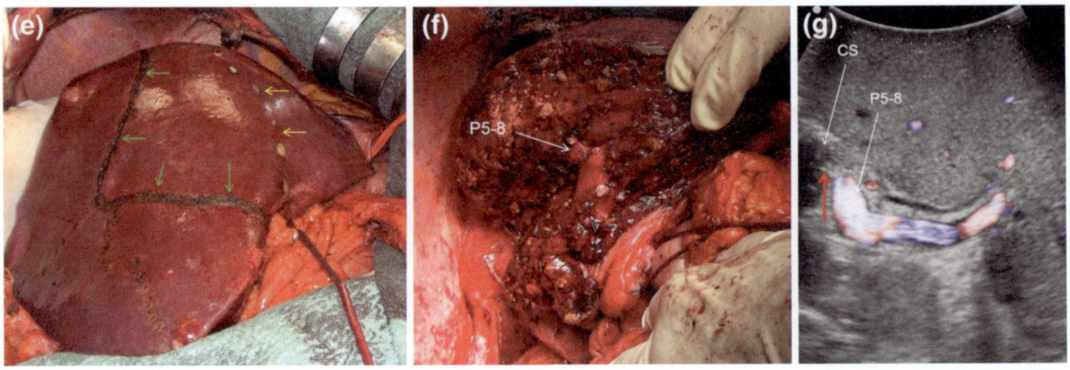

Fig. 7.28 (Continued)

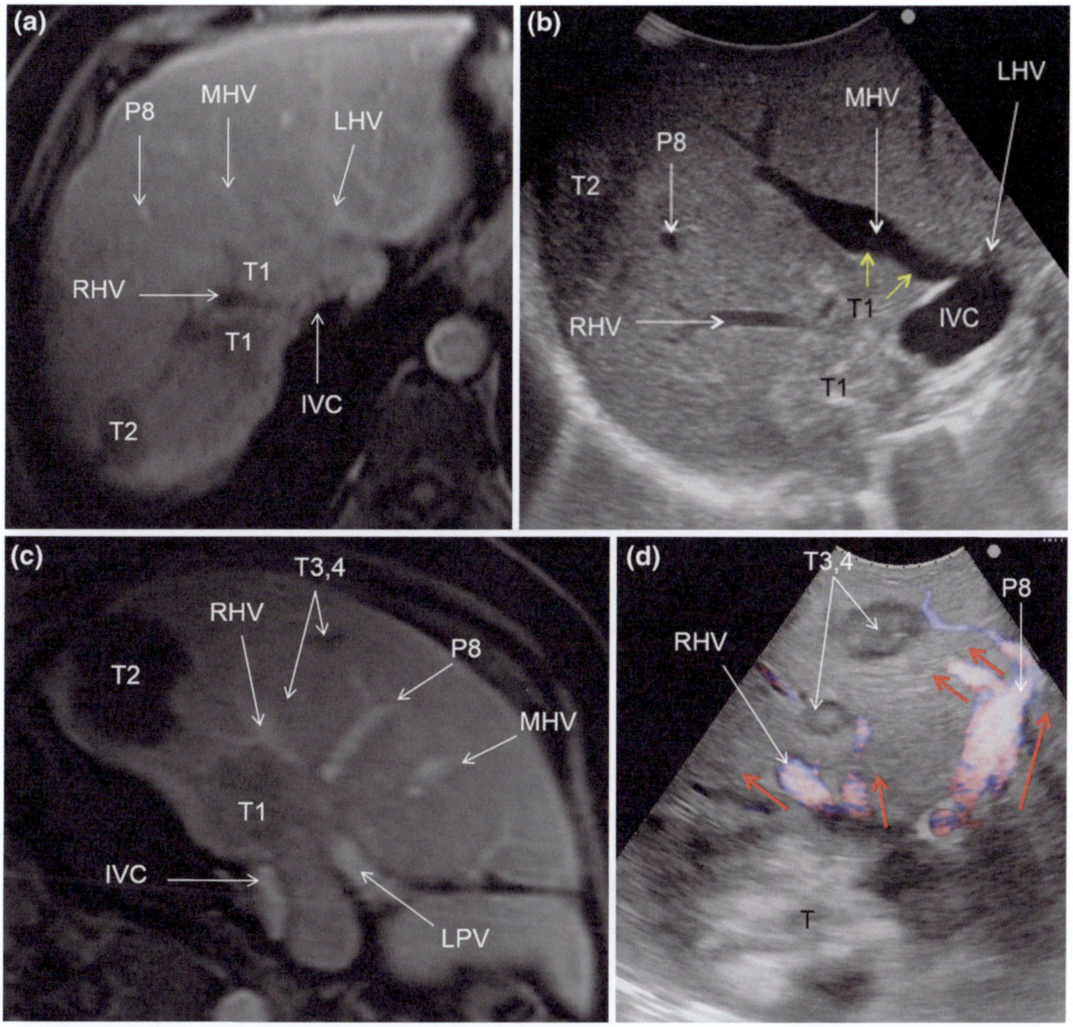

Fig. 7.29 **a** Magnetic resonance (*MRI*) image of a colorectal liver metastasis (*T1*) invading the right hepatic vein (*RHV*); **b** IOUS image of T1 invading the RHV as previously shown, but better disclosing the contact (*yellow arrows*) between T1 itself and the middle hepatic vein (*MHV*); **c** MRI image of T1 invading the RHV, contacting the branch to the right anterior section in proximity of the origin of the branch to segment 8 (*P8*), and with the inferior vena cava (*IVC*) by occupying segment 1. Also, this shows the existence of other lesions surrounding the tumor; T2, an hemangioma; T3 and T4, other metastases; **d** CFIOUS image demonstrating the hepatopetal blood flow in P8 (*red arrows*), and the reverse flow in the RHV (*red arrows*); **e** dissection line which should be used for a formal right hepatectomy (*yellow dashed line*), and inversely that built following the SERPS criteria for type (**b**) pattern (*green arrows*); **f** the liver observed frontally resembles the entire apart from the small areas in which local resections have been done (*arrows*); **g** the cut surface after SERPS extended to segment 1 with the stumps for the portal pedicles for the dorsal part of segment 8 dorsal (*P8d*) for segment 7 (*P7*) and for segment 6 (*P6*), and exposure of the MHV; **h** IOUS image of a further lesion (*T5*) located between the branches to segments 2 (*P2*) and 3 (*P3*); **i** the cut surface (*arrow*) after removal also of this lesion; hepatic pedicle (*HP*); left hepatic vein (*LHV*); left portal vein (*LPV*); portal branch to segment 4 (*P4*); stump of the RHV (*RHVs*); round ligament (*RL*); umbilical portion (*UP*)

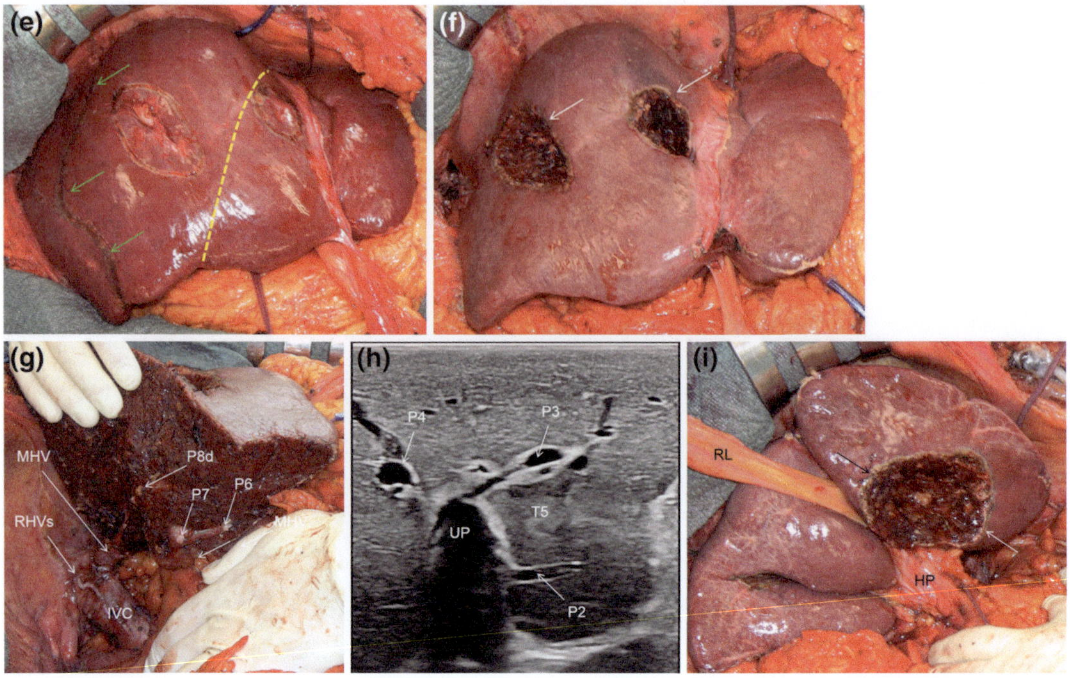

Fig. 7.29 (Continued)

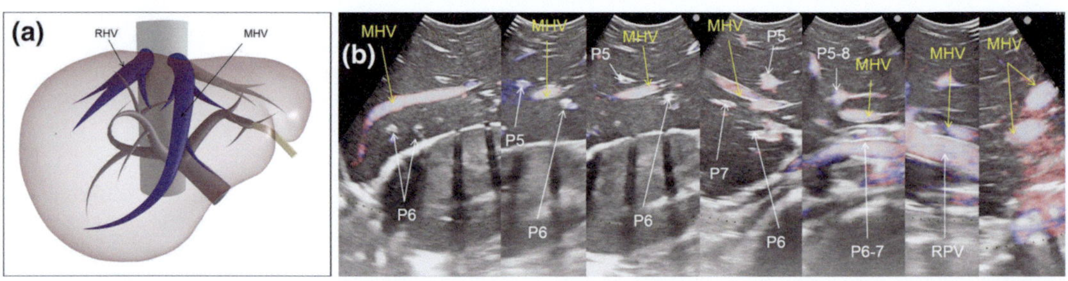

Fig. 7.30 **a** Pattern arising once a dominant middle hepatic vein (*MHV*) exists that drains the right inferior hemiliver including segment 6; **b** CFIOUS serial images of the entire route of the branch of the MHV draining segment 6; portal branch to segment 5 (*P5*); portal branch to segment 6 (*P6*); portal branch to the right anterior section (*P5-8*); portal branch to the right posterior section (*P6-7*); right hepatic vein (*RHV*); right portal vein (*RPV*)

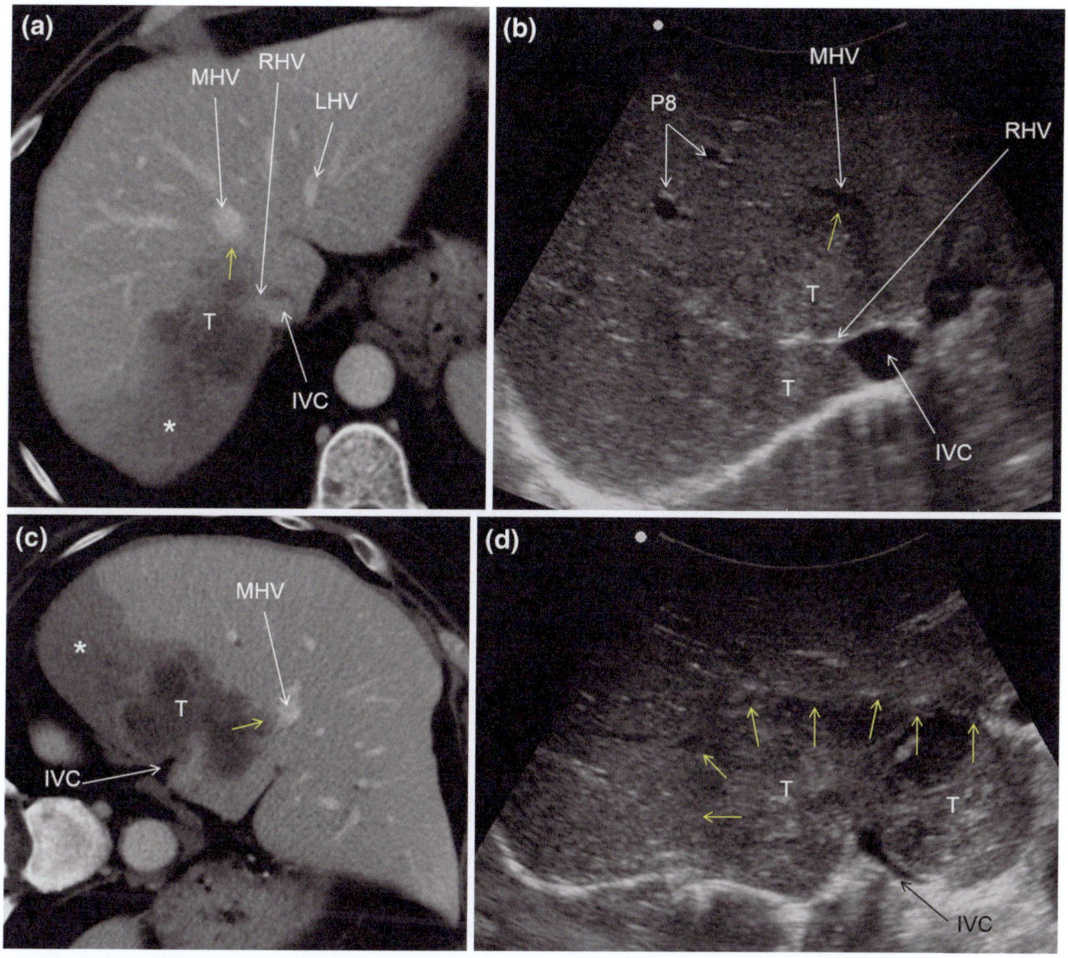

Fig. 7.31 **a** Computed tomography (*CT*) image of a colorectal liver metastasis (*T*) invading the right hepatic vein (*RHV*), close to (*yellow arrow*) the middle hepatic vein (*MHV*), and in close contact with the inferior vena cava (*IVC*); **b** the corresponding IOUS image with T invading the RHV, in close proximity (*yellow arrows*) to the MHV, and extensive contact with the IVC; **c** CT image of T deforming the profile of the IVC, again getting close (*yellow arrow*) to the MHV; **d** IOUS image of T occupying the entire segment 1 and surrounding and deforming the IVC; **e** CT image of T distally as it invades the portal branch to the posterior section of which the biliary tract is visible (*B6-7*) (*yellow arrows*); **f** similar IOUS image of T showing its relation (*yellow arrows*) with the portal branch to the posterior section (*P6-7*); **g** SERPS was carried out according to the procedure for (**b**)-(**c**) pattern extending the resection to segment 1: the cut surface (*CS*) showing the portion of the MHV exposed since in contact with T, the RHV stump (*RHVs*), the IVC, and its portion in which a wall resection was carried out reconstructing the vein by direct suture (*sIVC*); **h** the liver observed frontally appears to be entire as compared to that which should have been removed performing a formal right hepatectomy (*yellow dashed line*); **i** CFIOUS confirming the hepatopetal direction (*red arrows*) of the blood flow into the portal branch to the right anterior section (*P5-8*), and more peripherally to segment 8 (*P8*), and the hepatofugal blood flow into the MHV (*blue arrow*); **j** specimen including essentially segments 1 (*S1*), 6 (*S6*), and 7 (*S7*), and partially segments 5 (*S5*), and 8 (*S8*); **k** detail of the tumor showing that part which was markedly hypodense in CT (**e**), and anechoic in IOUS (**f**) as necrotic (*Tn*), and also disclosing the liver bed surrounding the retrohepatic IVC (*IVCb*), which was entirely occupied by T. *: liver parenchyma with different density at CT due to the lack of vascular supply by tumoral infiltration of P6-7; cut surface (*CS*); left hepatic vein (*LHV*); left portal vein (*LPV*)

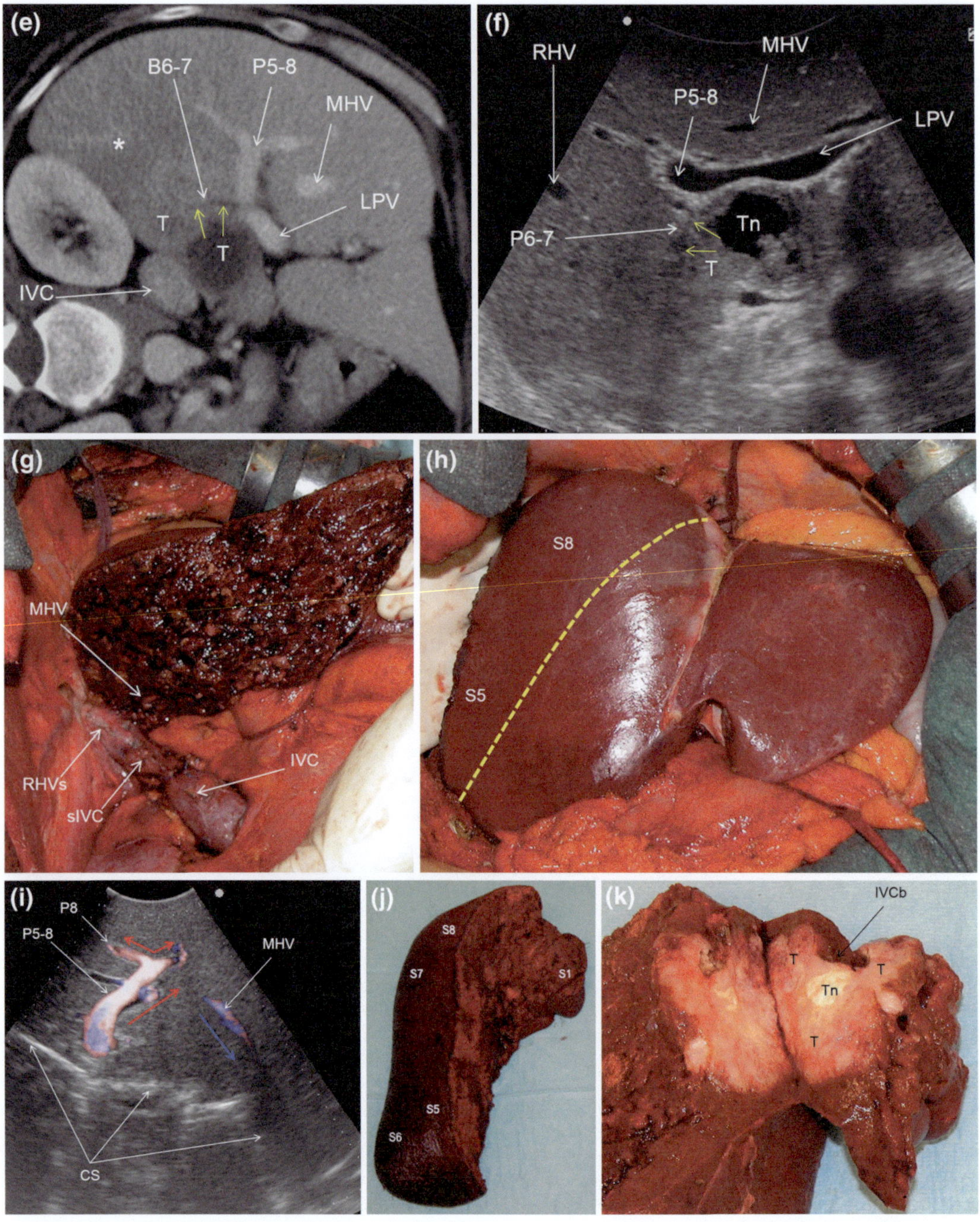

Fig. 7.31 (Continued)

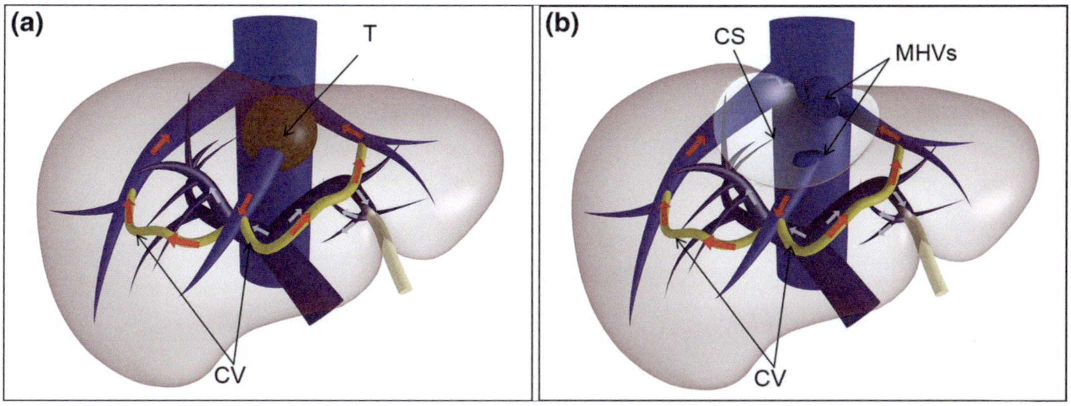

Fig. 7.32 Pattern of presentation of a tumor (*T*) invading the middle hepatic vein (*MHV*) at the hepatocaval confluence with communicating veins (*CV*) between the MHV itself and one or both of the adjacent hepatic veins allowing the blood to be drained by those veins (*red arrows*) (**a**), then enabling a limited resection referred to as mini-mesohepatectomy (**b**); cut surface (*CS*); middle hepatic vein stump (*MHVs*)

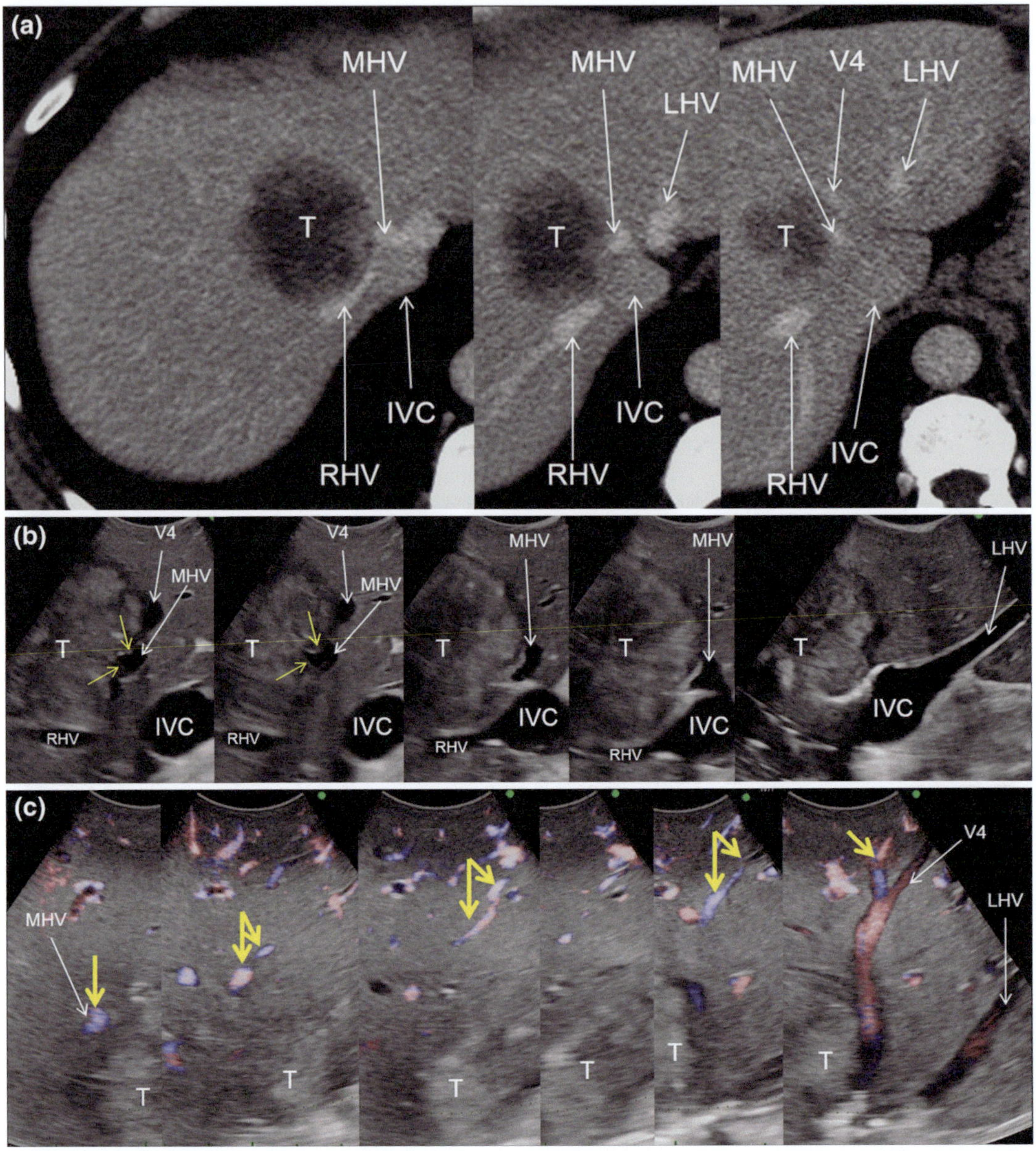

Fig. 7.33 **a** Computed tomography (*CT*) image of a colorectal liver metastasis (*T*) invading the middle hepatic vein (*MHV*), in contact with the scissural vein (*V4*), and in contact with the right hepatic vein (*RHV*), at caval confluence; **b** the correspondent IOUS serial images with T invading the MHV (*yellow arrows*), in contact with V4 and the RHV, and getting in touch with the inferior vena cava (*IVC*); **c** CFIOUS serial showing the complex but detectable route of a communicating vein (*yellow arrows*) flowing from the distal portion of the MHV to V4; **d** CFIOUS image of another communicating vein between the MHV and V4 (*yellow arrows*); **e** CFIOUS serial pictures showing another complex but detectable route of a communicating vein (*yellow arrows*) flowing from the distal portion of the MHV to the RHV; **f** CFIOUS showing that once the MHV has a reversal flow (*red arrow*), anyway the portal branch to the right anterior section (*P5-8*) maintains an hepatopetal blood flow direction (*red arrow*); **g** the virtual dissection line (*yellow dashed line*) connecting the electrocautery (*EC*) and the surgeon's fingertip (*F*) passes through the axis of the MHV (*red dashed line*); **h** the virtual dissection line (*yellow dashed line*) connecting EC and F is shown in relation to the posterior tumoral (*T*) edge which bulges into the paracaval portion of the liver behind the MHV (*yellow arrows*); **i** the cut surface at the end of the resection showing the intrahepatic side of the stump of the MHV (*MHVs2*) with the preserved venous arch (*yellow dashed arrow*) which retains the possibility for the blood to flow into both the RHV and V4; **j** specimen including the tumor and the resected tract of the MHV; left hepatic vein (*LHV*); caval side of the MHV stump (*MHVs1*)

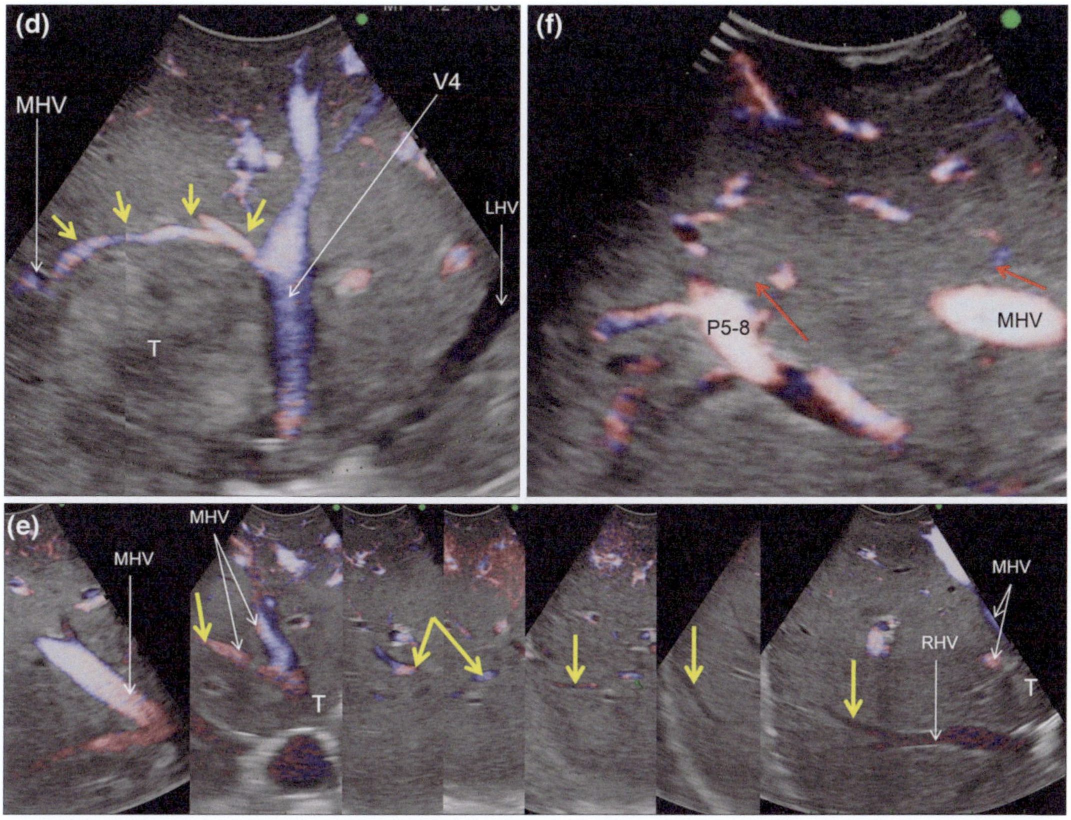

Fig. 7.33 (Continued)

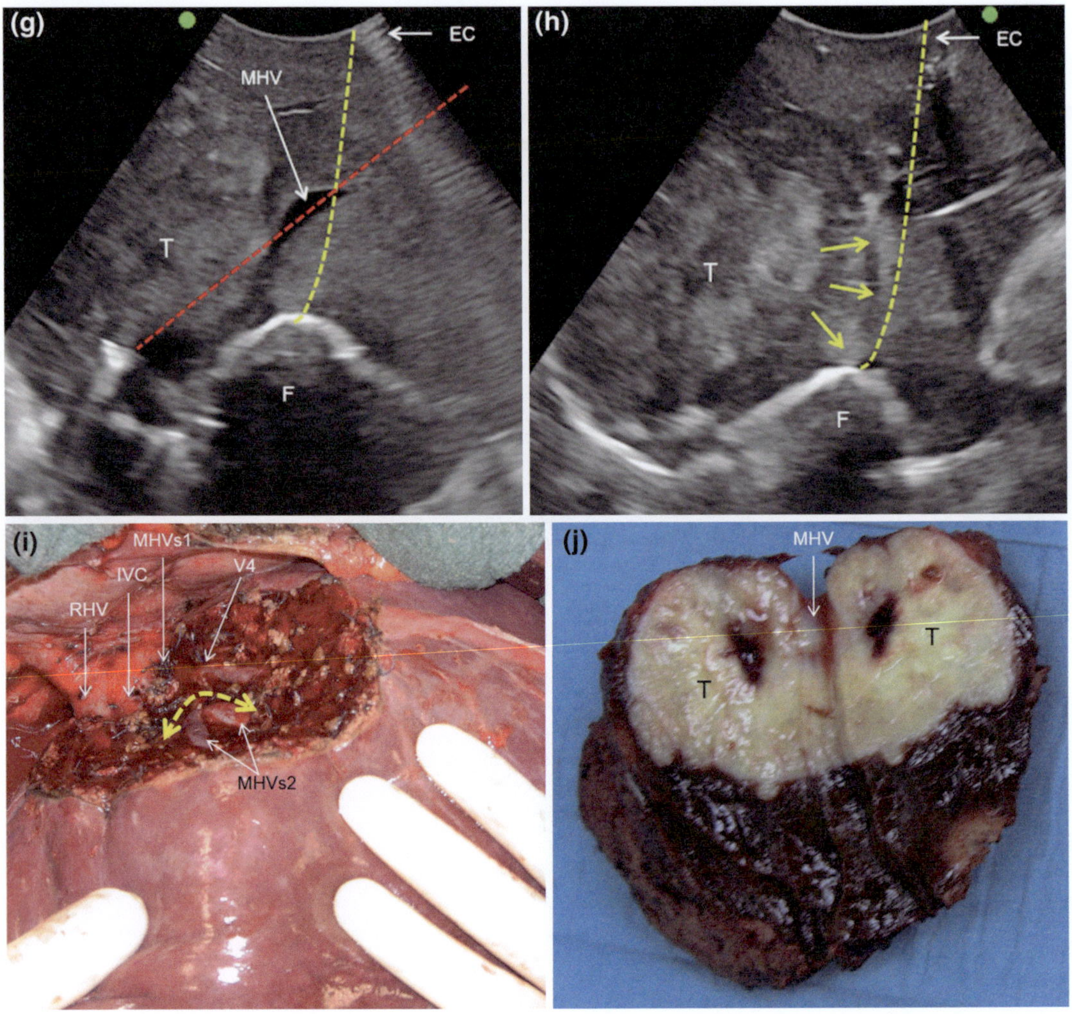

Fig. 7.33 (Continued)

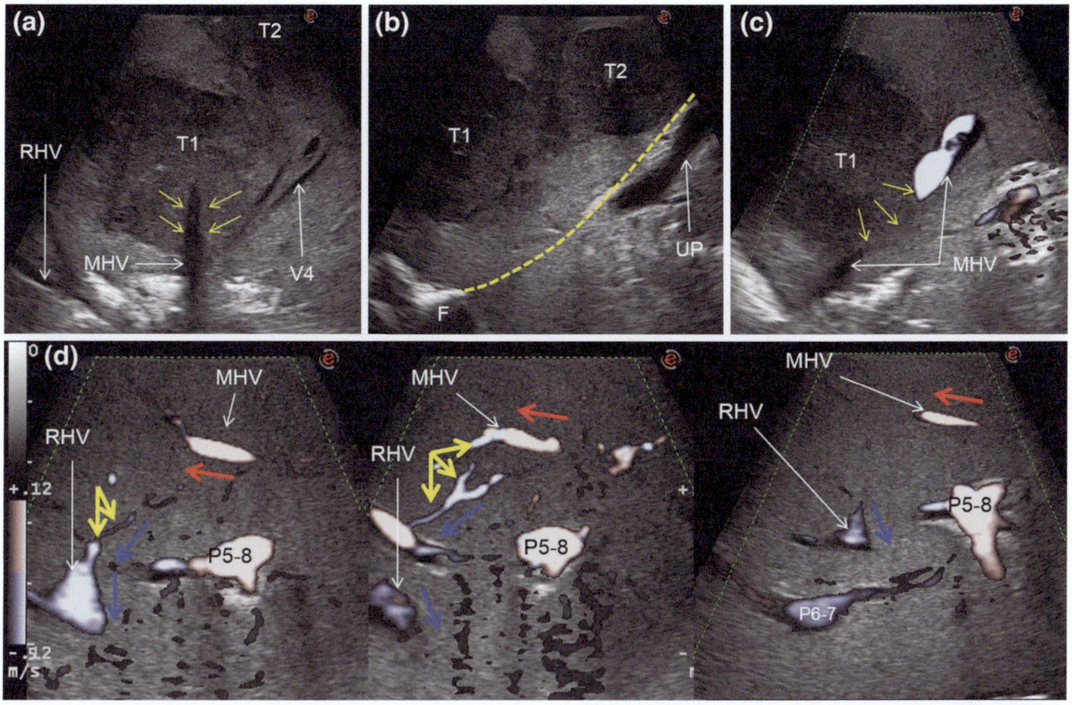

Fig. 7.34 **a** IOUS image of a colorectal liver metastasis (*T1*) invading (*yellow arrows*) the middle hepatic vein (*MHV*), contacting the scissural vein (*V4*), at the caval confluence; **b** another IOUS scan showing the relations of close adjacency between T2 and the umbilical portion (UP); the virtual dissection plan to detach T2 and UP is also shown (*yellow dashed line*); **c** IOUS image showing the degree of invasion (*yellow arrows*) of the MHV by T1; **d** CFIOUS serial images of a communicating vein between the right hepatic vein (RHV) and the MHV (*yellow arrows*) with the hepatic vein's blood flow direction represented by the *red* and *blue arrows*; **e** combined maneuver using the probe and the surgeon's left hand to disclose the resection area and determining the dissection plane to be followed (please also refer to Chap. 8); **f** based on the latter maneuver, this IOUS image shows the virtual dissection plan (*yellow dashed line*) connecting the electrocautery (*EC*) and the surgeon's fingertip (*F*) in relation to the MHV; **g** IOUS image showing the virtual dissection plan (*yellow dashed line*) connecting the electrocautery (*EC*) and the surgeon's fingertip (*F*) in relation to the UP; **h** the resection area is then drawn on the liver surface (*green arrows*); **i** the cut surface at the end of the resection showing the intrahepatic stump of the MHV (*MHVs2*) preserving the arch (*yellow dashed arrow*) which retains the possibility for the blood to flow into both the RHV and V4; **j** CFIOUS confirms the hepatopetal blood flow (*red arrows*) in the portal branch to the right anterior section (*P5-8*), and to segment 5 (*P5*); inferior vena cava (*IVC*); caval stump of the MHV (*MHVs1*); portal branch to segment 2 (*P2*); portal branch to segment 3 (*P3*); portal branch to segment 4 superior (*P4s*); portal branch to the right posterior section (*P6-7*); tourniquets (*Tp*) containing the tapes which are encircling the RHV and the common trunk of LHV and MHV

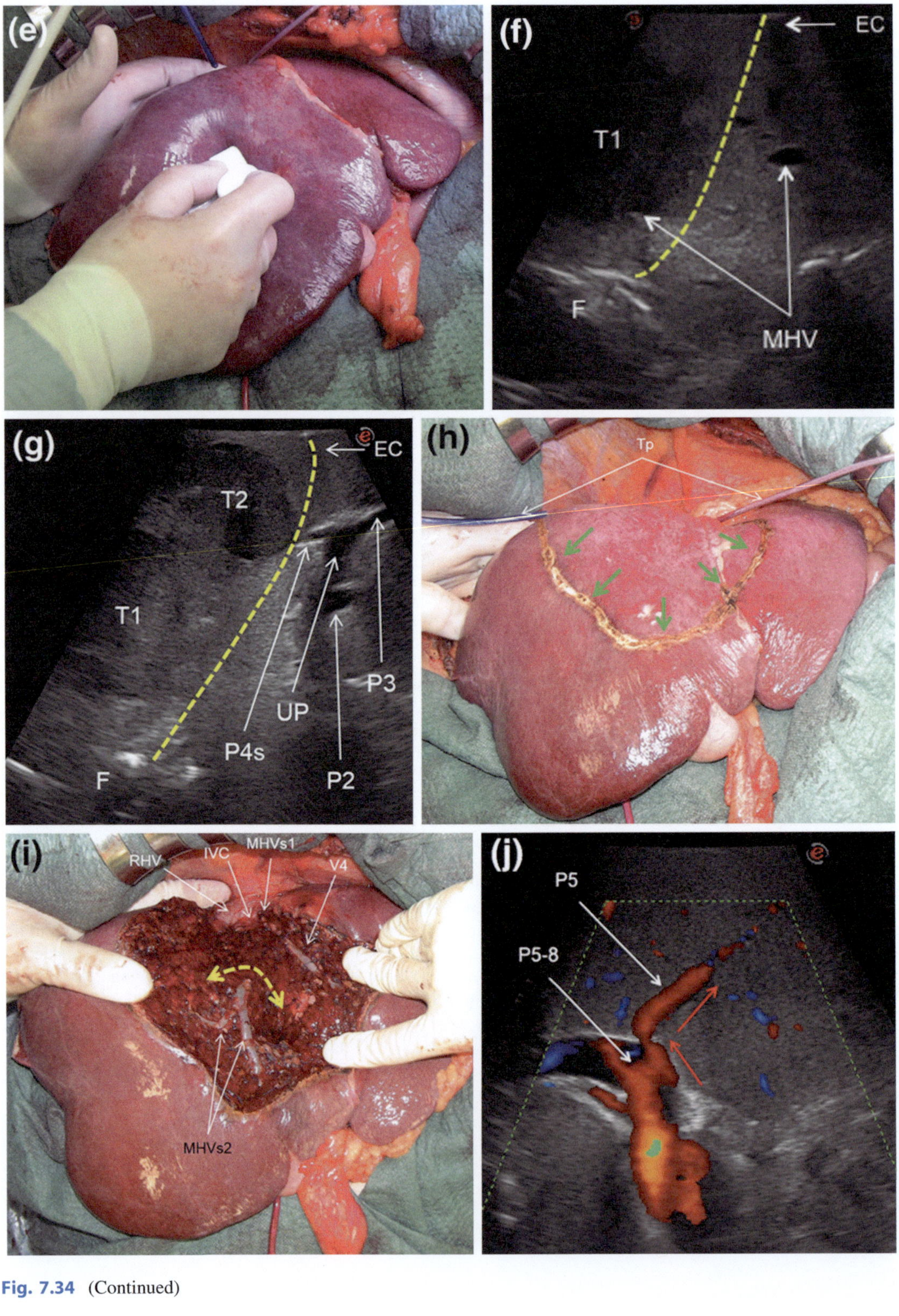

Fig. 7.34 (Continued)

Fig. 7.35 **a** IOUS image of a large (*yellow arrows* disclosing the edges) colorectal liver metastasis (*T*) invading the middle hepatic vein (*MHV*), dislodging the right (*RHV*) and the left hepatic vein (*LHV*), at the caval confluence; **b** serial IOUS images better disclosing for each hepatic vein the type of relation (*yellow arrows*), which is in contact and compression with the RHV (*left side*) and the LHV (*right side*), while it is clearly infiltrating the MHV (*center*); **c** CFIOUS disclosing a communicating vein (*CV*) between the RHV and the MHV: *red* and *blue colored arrows* indicate blood flow direction; **d** CFIOUS serial images of another communicating vein between the RHV and the MHV (*yellow arrows*), which in reality is composed by two branches (*yellow* and *green arrows*) originating from two different tracts of the RHV, then flowing together into a single branch connected with the MHV; **e** the main dissection plane for this resection (*red arrow*): as in Fig. 7.13, for this large CLM a parenchyma-sparing procedure, so-called "liver tunnel", is indicated, combined with, for this particular condition, mini-mesohepatectomy; **f** from left to right: the resection areas (*green arrows*) for removing the main lesion and those associated (totally 12 lesions): on the right the main lesion (*T*) is visible just below the Arantius ligament (*AL*); **g** the cut surface in segment 4inf-5 with exposure of the right (*RPV*) and the left portal branch (*LPV*); **h** the liver tunnel at the end of the removal of T exposing on the cut surface the portal branch to segment 8 (*P8*), the root of the right posterior branch (*P6-7*), the RPV and LPV (both exposed also on the opposite cut surface), the umbilical portion (*UP*), the LHV and the RHV: the inferior vena cava (*IVC*) is fully exposed and the stump of the MHV is visible too (*MHVs*). The *dashed yellow lines* more or less represent the edges of the spared parenchyma for the presence of the communicating veins which vicariate the MHV in draining the blood from segments 4 inferior and 5; **i** from left to right: the main specimen which occupied segments 4 superior, segment 8 (*S8-4s*), and the entire segment 1; on the right the intratumoral fossa in which the MHV was fully included is shown; **j** the schema is representing the condition which has allowed the operation herein shown: the existence, recognition, and respect of the communicating veins (*CV*); **k** the schematic of the cut surface (*CS*) at the end of the resection; caudate lobe (*CL*); surgeon's fingertip (*F*); hepatic pedicle (*HP*); portal branch to the right anterior section (*P5-8*); round ligament (*RL*); tourniquet (*Tp*) containing the tape encircling the common trunk of LHV and MHV

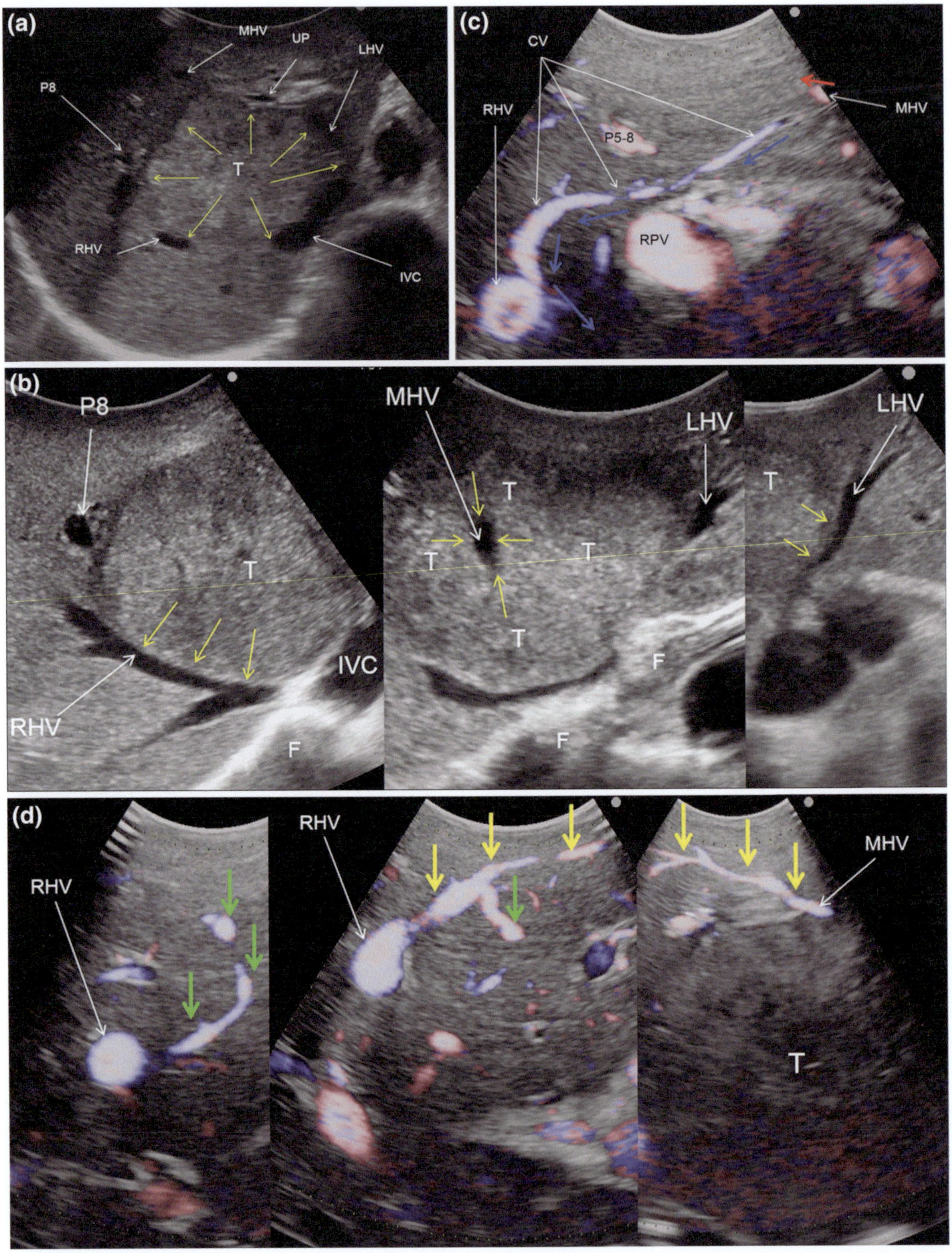

Fig. 7.35 (Continued)

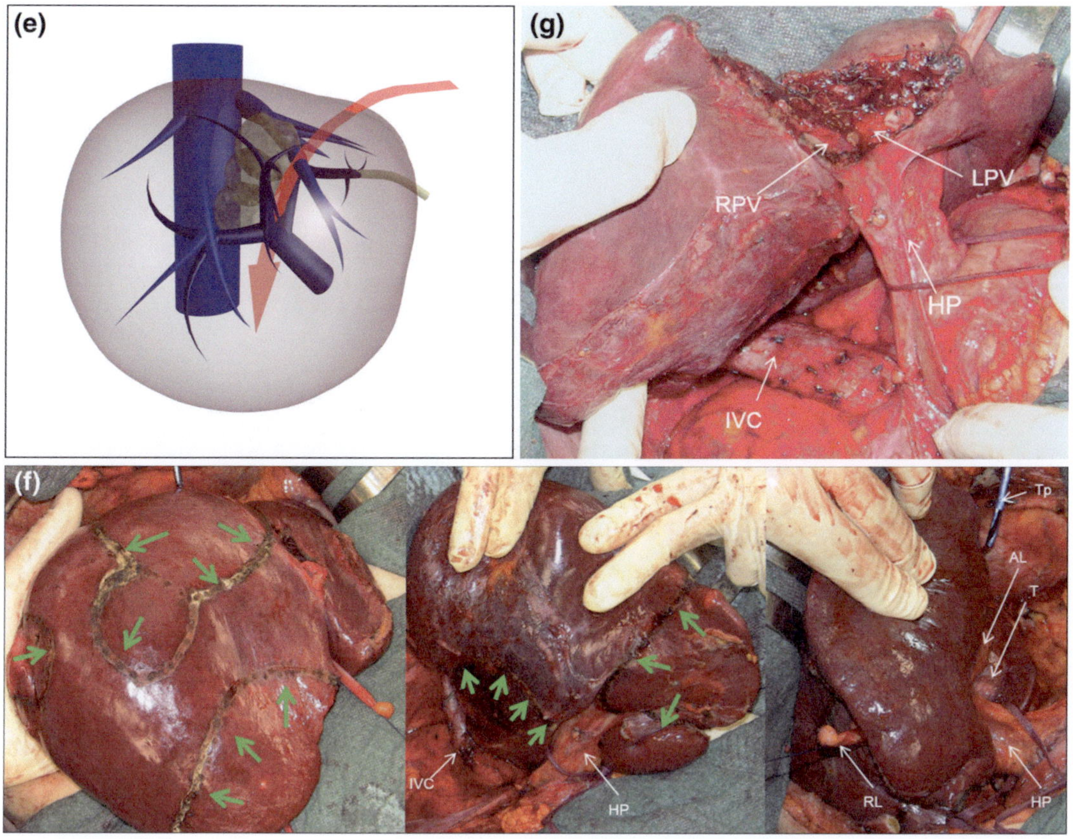

Fig. 7.35 (Continued)

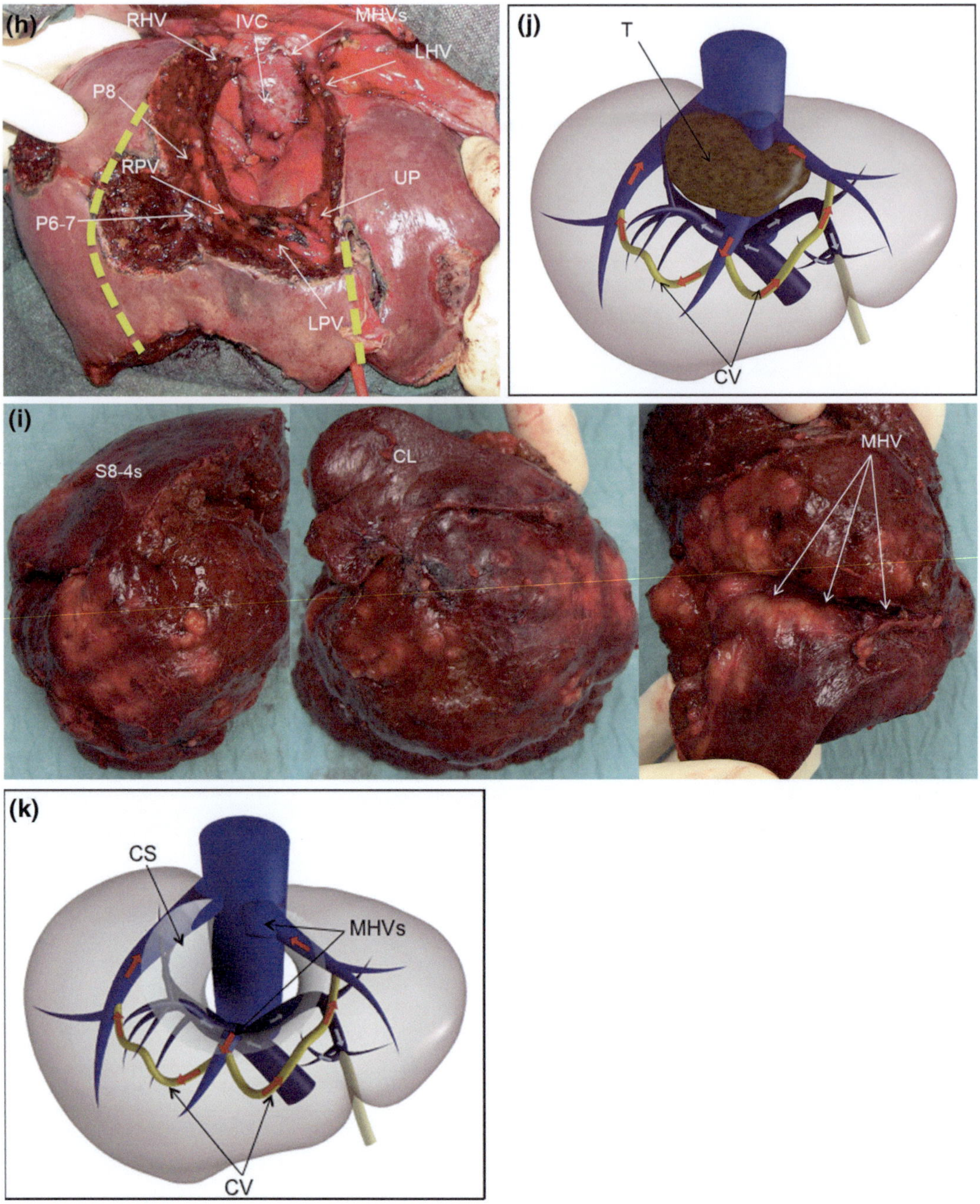

Fig. 7.35 (Continued)

functioning liver parenchyma intact with adequate in and outflow (Fig. 7.39k–p). The existence and preservation of an IRHV and the CV could make feasible the removal of all the superior segments and of the three HVs (Fig. 7.40a–e), extending to segment 4 inferior and 5 and even segment 3 the preservation of just segment 6, as initially described by Makuuchi in 1987 [14].

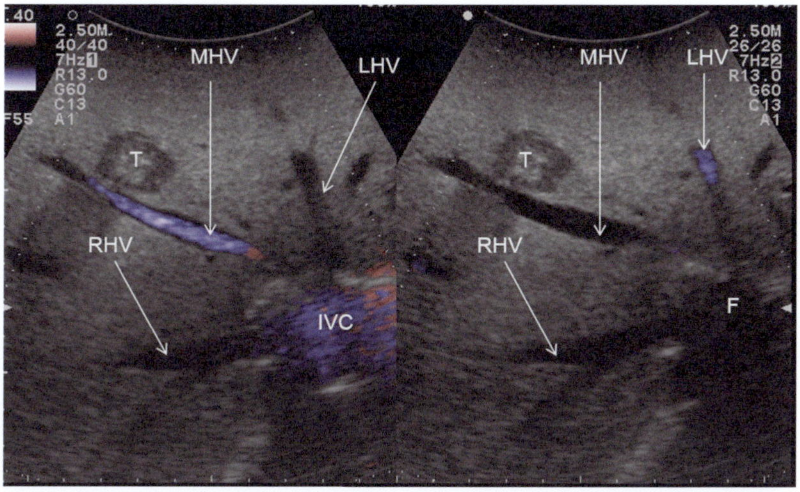

Fig. 7.36 Maneuver for controlling the backflow bleeding from the hepatic veins by means of finger compression: on the left in CFIOUS, the middle hepatic vein (*MHV*) has a color signal inside, which means blood flow, while, on the right, once finger (*F*) compression is applied to its confluence into the inferior vena cava (*IVC*), the color disappears which indicates the drastic reduction or absence of blood flow inside the vein; left hepatic vein (*LHV*); right hepatic vein (*RHV*); tumor (*T*)

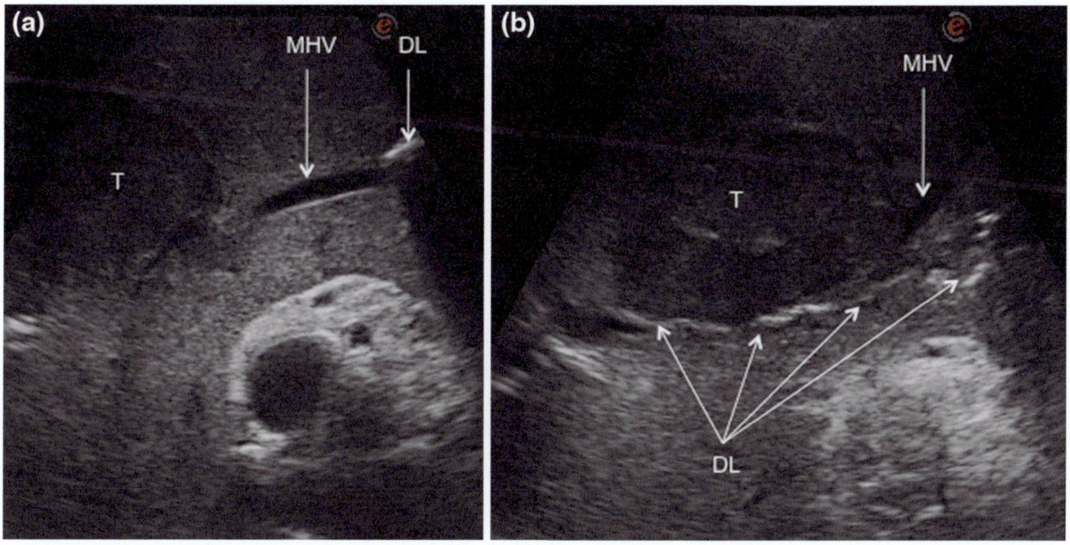

Fig. 7.37 **a** Dissection line (*DL*) approaching the middle hepatic vein (*MHV*); **b** once dividing the MHV, its posterior wall is followed for accomplishing the DL to complete removal of the tumor (*T*)

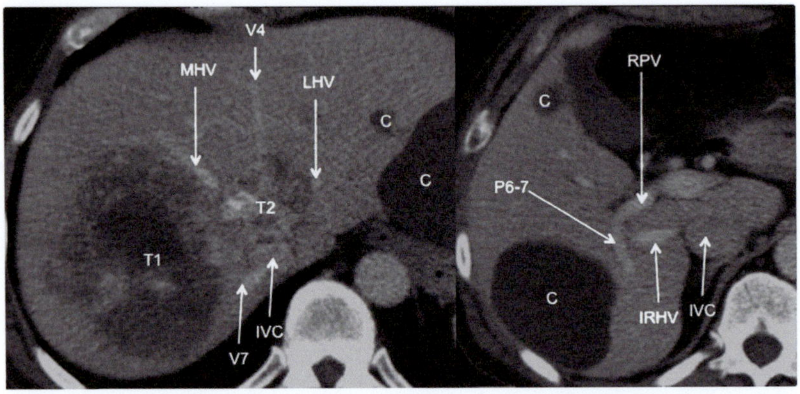

Fig. 7.38 Justification of the so-called "upper transversal hepatectomy": the right (*RHV*) and middle hepatic veins (*MHV*) are affected by two large tumors (*T1* and *T2*), the left hepatic vein (*LHV*) is also in contact with T2, and a thick inferior right hepatic vein (*IRHV*) is evident: in the case of communicating veins connecting the involved hepatic veins with the IRHV it would be possible to remove the segment 4 superior, 8, and 7 together with MHV and RHV leaving the inferior portion of the liver drained by the communicating veins and the IRHV; cyst (*C*); inferior vena cava (*IVC*); right portal vein (*RPV*); portal branch to the right posterior section (*P6-7*); scissural vein (*V4*)

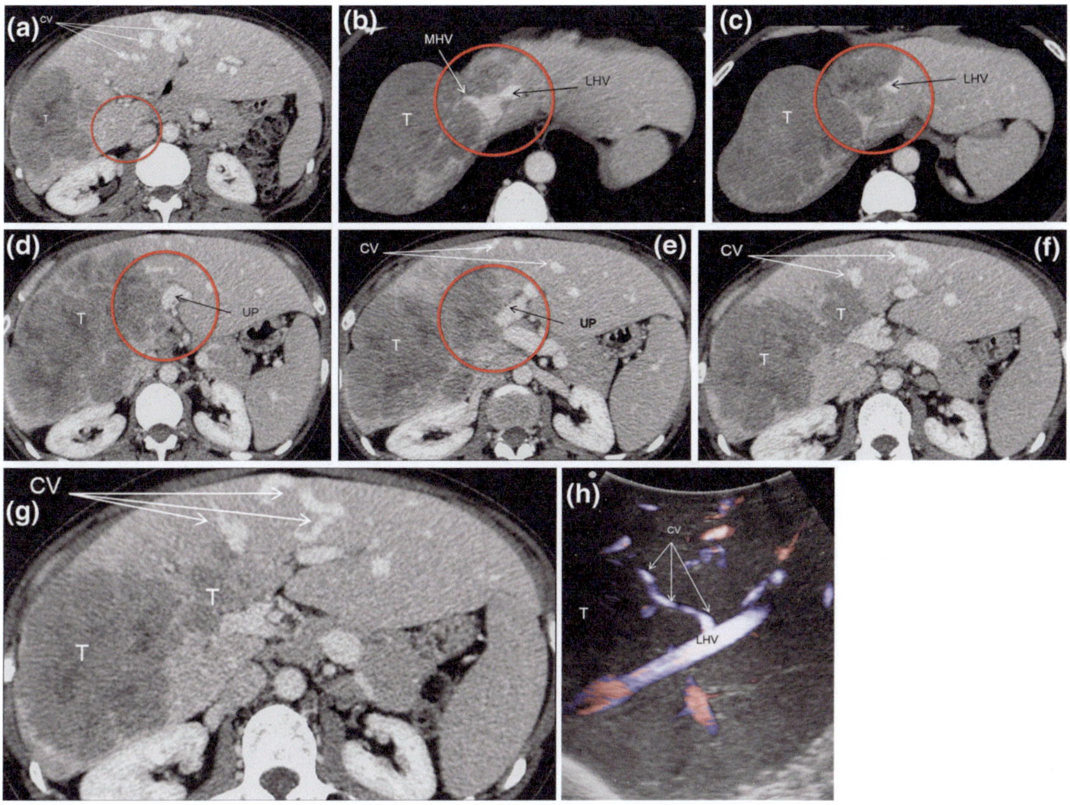

Fig. 7.39 **a–g** Computer tomography (*CT*) of patient having another condition suitable for "upper transversal hepatectomy": the right (*RHV*) and middle hepatic veins (*MHV*) are involved by a large colorectal liver metastasis (*T*), which has a wide contact (*red circle* in **b** and **c**) with the left hepatic vein (*LHV*), without the existence (*red circle* in **a**) of an inferior right hepatic vein (*IRHV*), but with clearly visible thick communicating veins (*CV*) (**a**, **e–g**). The tumor bulges over the hilar plate (**d–g**) having a wide contact up to the umbilical portion (*UP*) (*red circles* in **d** and **e**); **h**, **i** the CVs are recognized in CFIOUS; **j** the resection area is devised accordingly (*green arrows*) having had the foresight of preparing an adequate exposure by means of a J-shaped thoracophrenolaparotomy with a caudal extension of the midline incision for performing the removal of the primary tumor in the sigmoid colon by means of a Hartmann procedure. The latter was selected to avoid the coexistence of an intestinal anastomosis with this complex hepatectomy; **k** after upper transversal hepatectomy the cut surface shows the left (*LPV*) and the right portal branches (*RPV*), the LHV which was detached from the tumor removing part of its wall and reconstructing the vein by direct suture (*LHVr*); the RHV and MHV stumps (*RHVs*/*MHVs*) are also shown; **l** this view makes more evident also the full removal of segment 1 with full exposure of the inferior vena cava (*IVC*); **m** frontal view at the end of the resection; well visible (*black circle*) the respected CVs appearing on the glissonian surface of the liver; **n** representing the condition which has allowed the operation herein shown as the existence, recognition, and respect of the communicating veins (*CV*); **o** the cut surface (*CS*) at the end of the resection; **p** postoperational control at two years: in the meanwhile the patients had the closure of the colostomy: the absence of tumor recurrence and the patency of numerous CVs are evident; portal branch to segment 2 (P2)

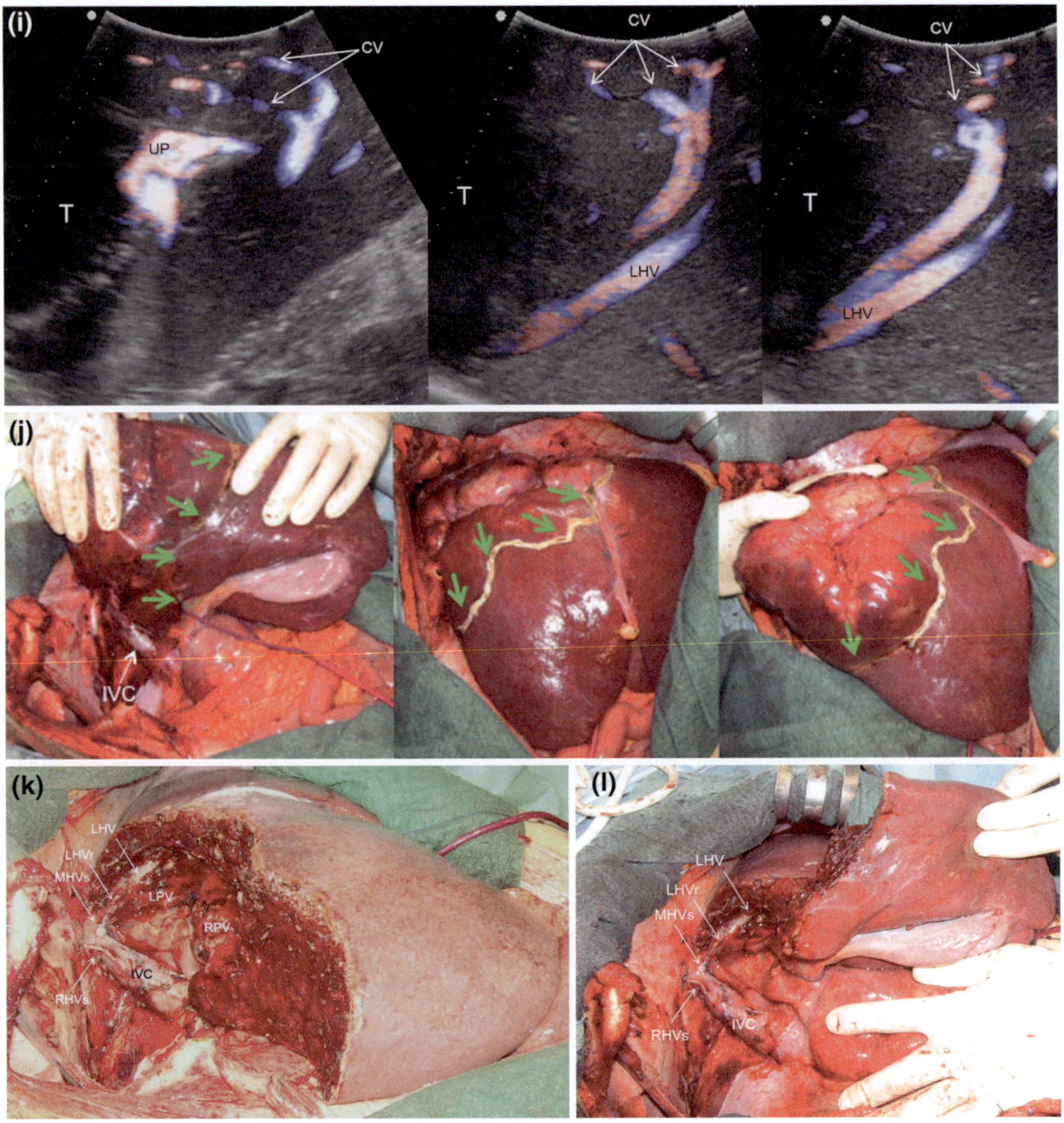

Fig. 7.39 (Continued)

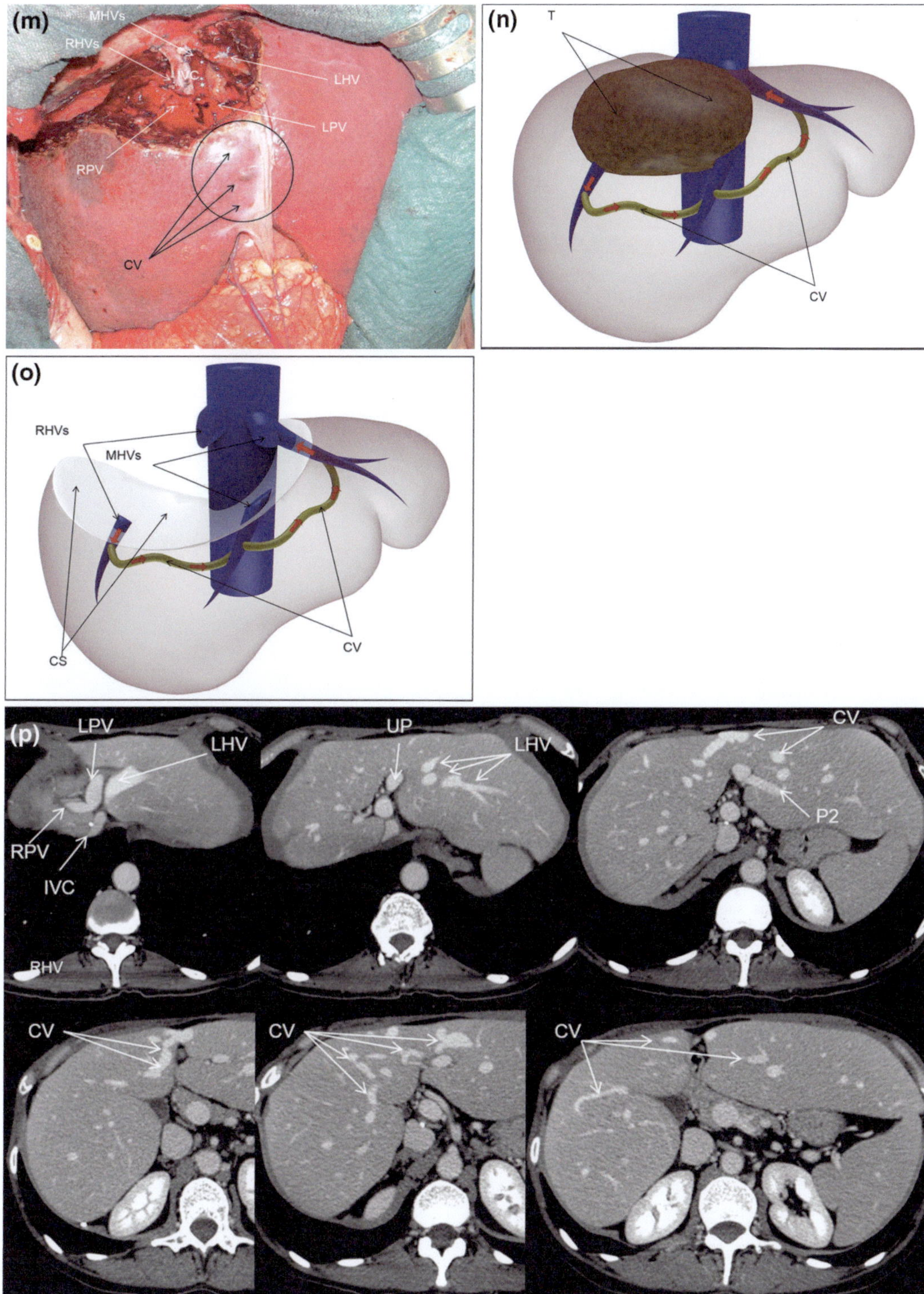

Fig. 7.39 (Continued)

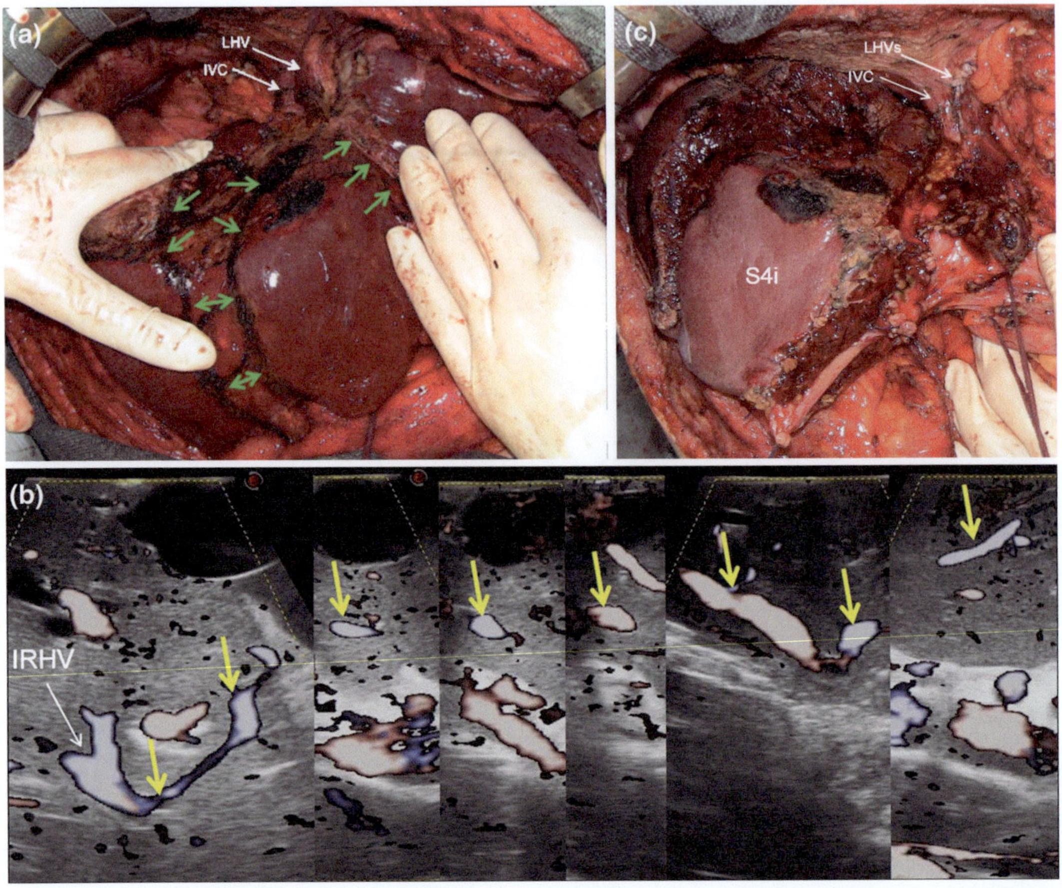

Fig. 7.40 **a** the surgical field of a reoperation for disease recurrence after "upper transversal hepatectomy" for colorectal liver metastases (original presentation shown in Fig. 7.38): the *green arrows* indicate the resection areas which include the sacrifice of the left hepatic vein (*LHV*); **b** this is feasible because of the presence of an inferior right hepatic vein (*IRHV*) and the communicating veins (*CV*), which both allowed the previous operation and were all confirmed and respected by CFIOUS (*yellow arrows*); **c** the resection was accomplished preserving the segment 4 inferior (*S4i*); **d** a congested area (*arrows*) was left; **e** the congested area was retained to leave functioning the thickest (*CV2*) of the two CVs for ensuring adequate drainage through the CV and the IRHV of the S4i; **f** schematically the operation can be figured as shown; cut surface 1 (*CS1*); cut surface 2 (*CS2*); inferior vena cava (*IVC*); left hepatic vein stump (*LHVs*); middle hepatic vein stump (*MHVs*); right hepatic vein stump (*RHVs*); segment 5 (*S5*); segment 6 (*S6*)

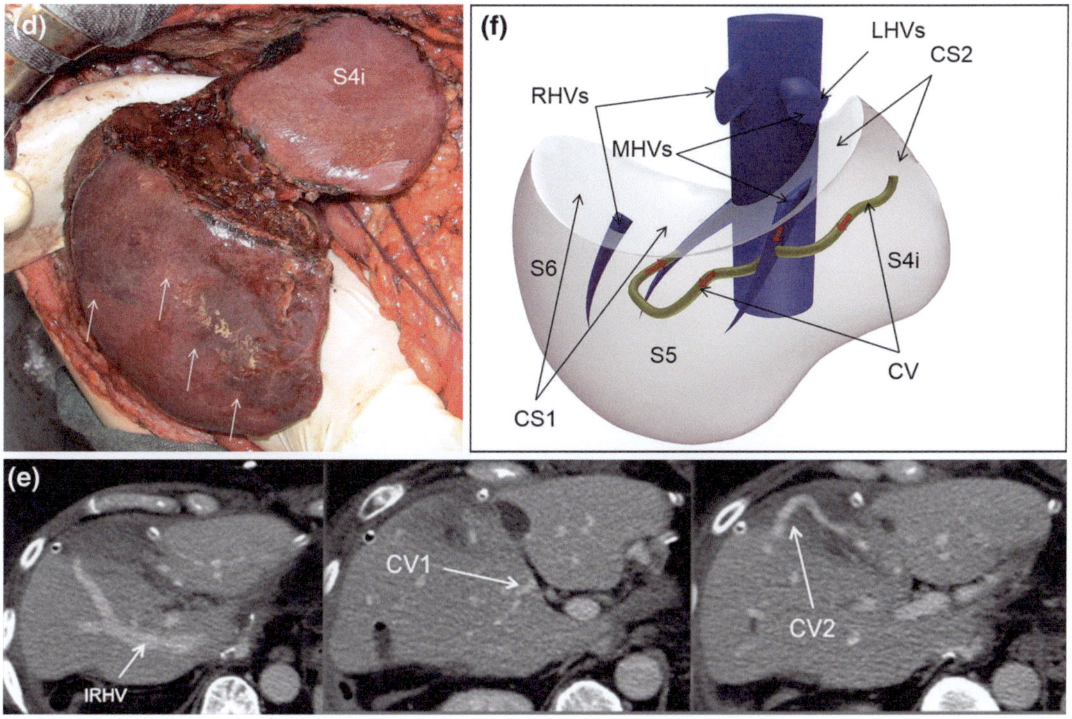

Fig. 7.40 (Continued)

References

1. Jarnagin WR, Bach AM, Winston CB (2001) What is the yield of intraoperative ultrasonography during partial hepatectomy for malignant disease? J Am Coll Surg 192:577–583
2. Cerwenka H, Raith J, Bacher H et al (2003) Is intraoperative ultrasonography during partial hepatectomy still necessary in the age of magnetic resonance imaging? Hepatogastroenterology 50:1539–1541
3. Torzilli G, Procopio F, Botea F et al (2009) One-stage ultrasonographically guided hepatectomy for multiple bilobar colorectal metastases: a feasible and effective alternative to the 2-stage approach. Surgery 146:60–71
4. Narita M, Oussoultzoglou E, Jaeck D et al (2011) Two-stage hepatectomy for multiple bilobar colorectal liver metastases. Br J Surg 98(10):1463–1475
5. Schnitzbauer AA, Lang SA, Goessmann H et al (2012) Right portal vein ligation combined with 433 in situ splitting induces rapid left lateral liver lobe hypertrophy enabling 2-staged extended right hepatic resection in small-for-size settings. Ann Surg 255(3):405–414
6. Torzilli G, Donadon M, Marconi M et al (2008) Systematic extended right posterior sectionectomy: a safe and effective alternative to right hepatectomy. Ann Surg 247:603–611
7. Torzilli G, Palmisano A, Procopio F et al (2010) A new systematic small for size resection for liver tumors invading the middle hepatic vein at its caval confluence: mini-mesohepatectomy. Ann Surg 251(1):33–39
8. Torzilli G, Procopio F, Donadon M et al (2012) Upper transversal hepatectomy. Ann Surg Oncol 19(11):3566
9. Torzilli G, Montorsi M, Donadon M et al (2005) "Radical but conservative" is the main goal for ultrasonography-guided liver resection: prospective validation of this approach. J Am Coll Surg 201:517–528
10. Torzilli G, Montorsi M, Del Fabbro D et al (2006) Ultrasonographically guided surgical approach to liver tumours involving the hepatic veins close to the caval confluence. Br J Surg 93:1238–1246
11. Torzilli G, Donadon M, Palmisano A et al (2007) Back-flow bleeding control during resection of right-sided liver tumors by means of ultrasound-guided finger compression of the right hepatic vein at its caval confluence. Hepatogastroenterology 54:1364–1367

12. Sano K, Makuuchi M, Miki K et al (2002) Evaluation of hepatic venous congestion: proposed indication criteria for hepatic vein reconstruction. Ann Surg 236:241–247
13. Torzilli G, Garancini M, Donadon M et al (2010) Intraoperative ultrasonographic detection of communicating veins between adjacent hepatic veins during hepatectomy for tumours at the hepatocaval confluence. Br J Surg 97:1867–1873
14. Makuuchi M, Hasegawa H, Yamazaki S et al (1987) Four new hepatectomy procedures for resection of the right hepatic vein and preservation of the inferior right hepatic vein. Surg Gynecol Obstet 164:68–72

8 Resection Guidance

Guido Torzilli, Fabio Procopio, and Guido Costa

The Chap. 7 described how IOUS with the information provided can lead to otherwise unsuitable approaches. Here, we will show how new strategies require IOUS assistance not only for checking their suitability but also for being realized in practice.

IOUS-guided liver dissections do not only require an ultrasound system equipped with adequate probes and an adequate background in ultrasound imaging interpretation. A targeted surgical maneuver thus also needs to be aimed at facilitating the IOUS-guided maneuver. Two main steps need to be considered in accomplishing ultrasound-guided resections:

- Achievement of adequate exposure of the surgical field implying adequate abdominal incision and liver mobilization for allowing proper maneuver both with the probe and the surgeon's left hand. The latter is used other than for sustaining or literally hanging the organ, and limiting blood loss, also as a landmark for maintaining, together with the information provided by the real-time IOUS, the correct trajectory of the liver parenchyma dissection.
- Proper IOUS-guided demarcation of the resection area.

Once these two steps are achieved, all the conditions to be able to perform a real IOUS-guided dissection of the liver parenchyma are in the surgeon's hands.

This chapter elaborates on insights into the preparation and execution of a fully IOUS-guided liver resection.

8.1 Abdominal Incision and Mobilization of the Liver

As a general principle, mobilization should allow the surgeon to have his left hand passing over the resection area established by means of IOUS: in this perspective the incision is selected, with J-shaped laparotomy as the standard incision (Fig. 8.1a, b). The latter, which includes the removal of the xiphoid process, other than being propaedeutic for handling the liver with the left hand (Fig. 8.1c), also allows a vertical view of the hepatocaval confluence both from above with the surgeon standing (Fig. 8.1d), and from the right side with the surgeon seated while approaching the hepatocaval plane (Fig. 8.1e).

When the tumor is located in the paracaval portion of segment 1 or anywhere at the hepatocaval confluence, and the control of the hepatic veins at this level seems not fully achievable with the abdominal incision only due

G. Torzilli (✉) · F. Procopio · G. Costa
Department of Hepatobiliary Surgery,
University of Milan-School of Medicine,
Humanitas Research Hospital-IRCCS,
Via A. Manzoni 56, 20089 Rozzano, MI, Italy
e-mail: guido.torzilli@humanitas.it;
guido.torzilli@unimi.it

G. Torzilli (ed.), *Ultrasound-Guided Liver Surgery*,
DOI: 10.1007/978-88-470-5510-0_8, © Springer-Verlag Italia 2014

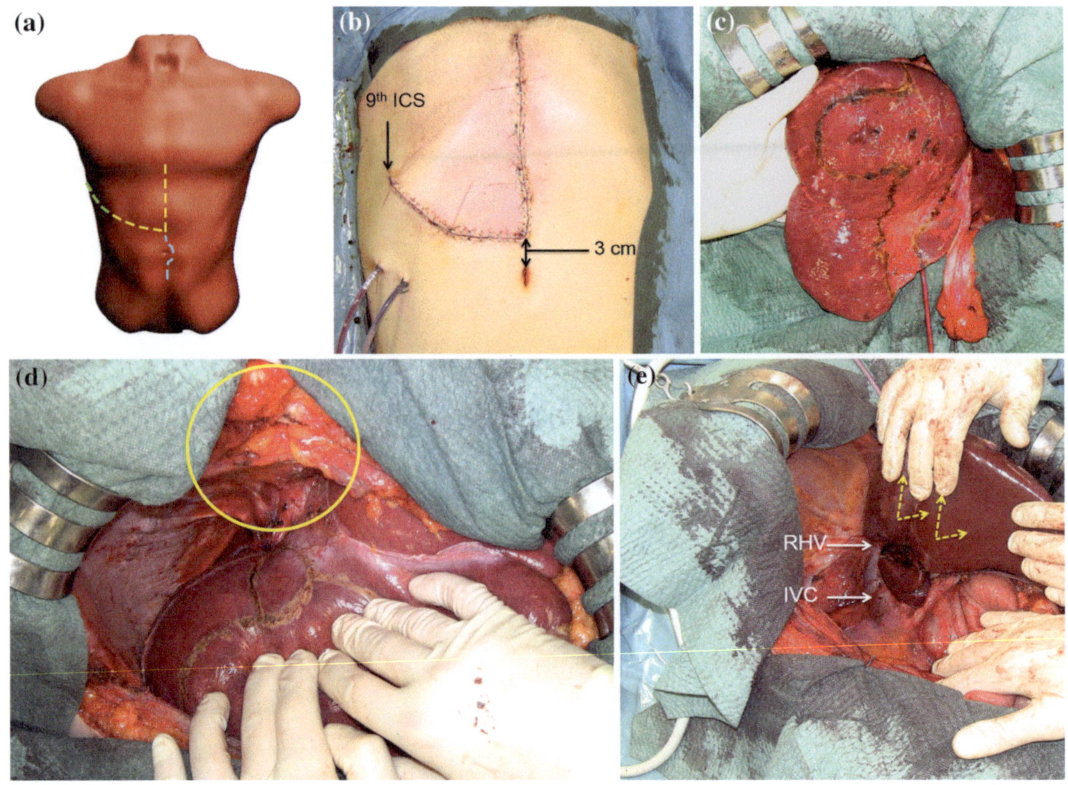

Fig. 8.1 **a** The J-shaped laparotomy is represented by the *dashed yellow line*: the midline starts at the root of the xiphoid process (which is always removed to open a better view over the anterior aspect of the hepatocaval confluence), and proceeds on the midline up to 3 cm above the umbilicus. At this point the transverse portion starts dividing the rectus muscle and approaching the costal arch at the level of the 9th intercostal space (*ICS*); **b** appearance of the J-shaped laparotomy after suturing; **c** the incision has to allow placement of the surgeon's left-hand which sustains the liver aiding in controlling bleeding during dissection, and moreover, representing the backside landmark for guiding resection; **d** the hepatocaval confluence is perpendicularly visualized by means of removal of the xiphoid process: the *yellow circle* highlights the area; **e** this incision enables an adequate view of the retrohepatic area, allowing the liver to be retracted to the left but moreover pulled up from the inferior vena cava (*IVC*), rather than crushed against it as in the case of a subcostal access: *dashed yellow arrows* indicate the traction lines (upward and laterally to the left); right hepatic vein (*RHV*)

Fig. 8.2 **a** The J-shaped thoracophrenolaparotomy is represented by the *dashed yellow line* together with the *green line*. As for the previous incision, the midline starts at the root of the xiphoid process and proceeds on the midline up to 3 cm above the umbilicus. At this point the transverse portion starts dividing the rectus muscle and approaching the costal arch at the level of the 9th intercostal space (*ICS*) which is opened up to the posterior axillary line (the skin is divided up to the mid-axillary line); **b** appearance of the J-shaped thoraco-phreno-laparotomy after suturing; **c**, **d** this incision allows better placement of the surgeon's left-hand compared to the abdominal approach only. This is particularly useful in case of lesions to be removed at the caval confluence especially if in a parenchyma-sparing modality: indeed, just after mobilization through an abdominal incision only, the surgeon may feel confident to handle the organ adequately. However, the difficulties raised by the lack of a thoraco-abdominal approach generally start in the late phases of the resections once the specimen has to be divided from the caval confluence and the left-hand handling would benefit from its placement through the opened intercostal space as shown in these pictures; **e** the surgeon's perspective being seated while dissection of the liver from the inferior vena cava is performed; chest tube (*CT*) ▶

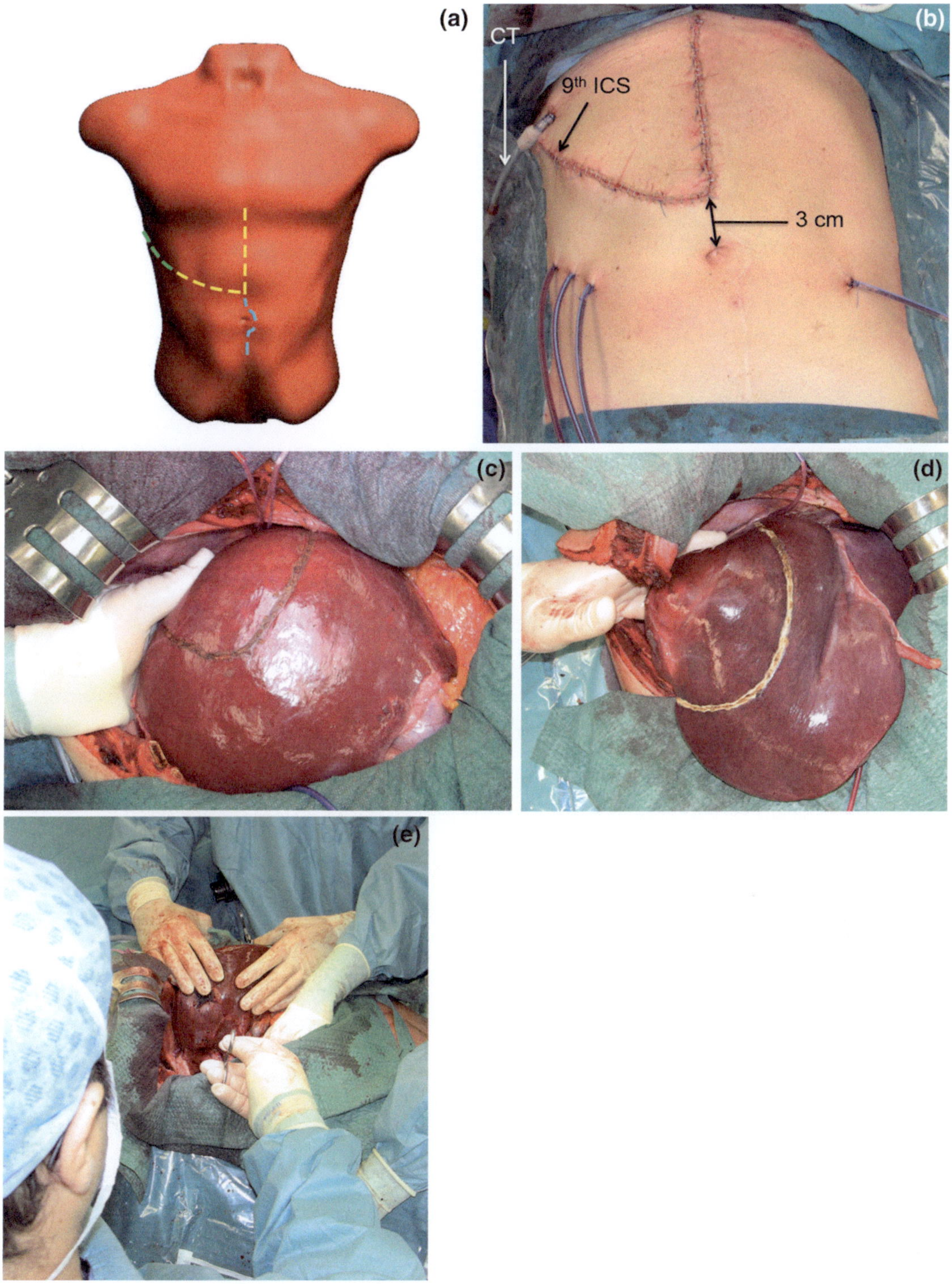
(a)
(b)
CT
9th ICS
3 cm
(c)
(d)
(e)

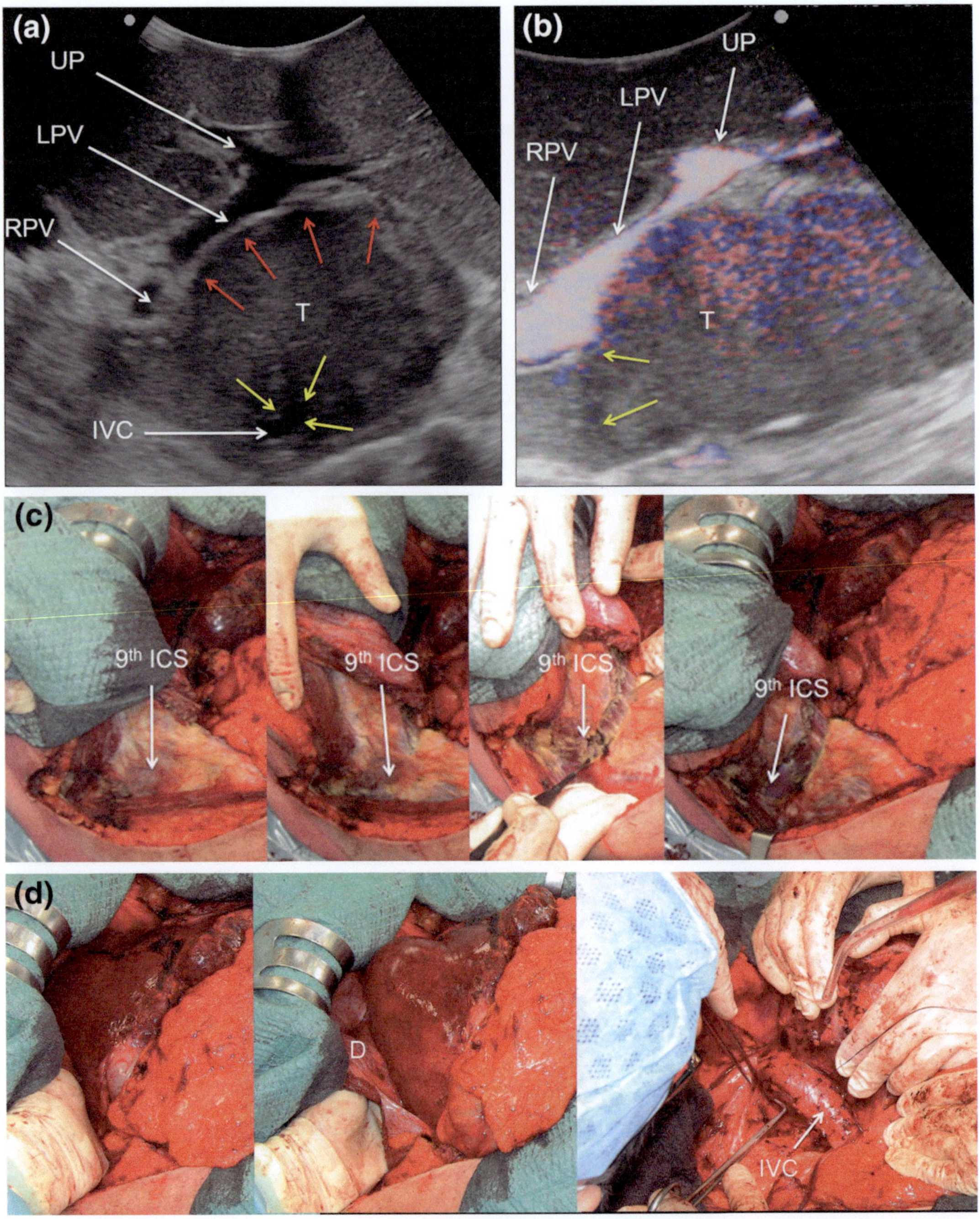

Fig. 8.3 **a** IOUS of a large tumor (*T*) in segment 1 dislodging anteriorly and compressing (*red arrows*) the left portal vein (*LPV*) and surrounding and deforming (*yellow arrows*) the inferior vena cava (*IVC*); **b** CFIOUS image better showing the right-sided extension of the tumor (*yellow arrows*) to the caudate process; **c** from left to right, the progressive opening of the 9th intercostal space (*ICS*); **d** from left to right, the surgeon's left hand positioned in the chest through the divided diaphragm (*D*) is pulling upward the liver; in this way the dissection of the retrohepatic plane is proceeded meticulously and progressively detaching the tumor from the inferior vena cava (*IVC*); **e** in this way dissection of the IVC from the tumoral fossa (*IVCfossa*) in which it was lying is completed without performing any resection of the vessel wall or proceeding to the total vascular exclusion although the tapes (*Tp*) were previously positioned for caution; **f** the specimen removed with the *arrows* indicating the IVC fossa; the right posterior section was also removed for the presence of two other lesions; right hepatic vein (*RHV*); right portal vein (*RPV*); umbilical portion (*UP*)

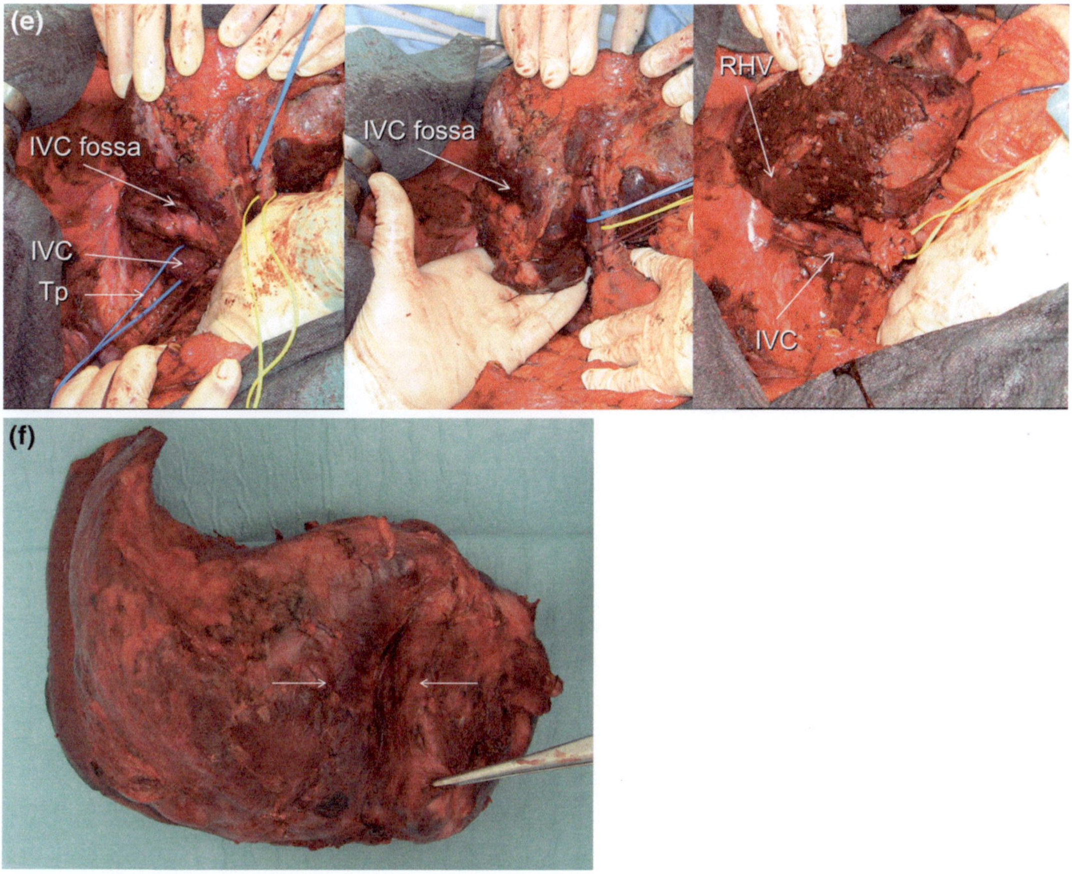

Fig. 8.3 (continued)

to patient characteristics and/or the tumor features (position, relations, and size), two solutions are possible. Both represent an extension of the J-shaped laparotomy and both aim to extend the working space for the surgeon especially at the mid-to-late phases of the dissection and in general when the major veins are approached. A J-shaped thoracophrenolaparotomy is shown in Fig. 8.2a, b: this incision allows the operator himself to have more space for positioning the left hand and for related liver handling (Fig. 8.2c, d), and moreover, allows a better view of the hepatocaval plane, which falls in line with the visual plane of the operator (Fig. 8.2e), being particularly useful for affording conservative resection of large tumors located in segment 1 (Fig. 8.3a–f). It is important to note that opening the chest may not be necessary for mobilization of the liver, but generally may be crucial during dissection and particularly towards the end when the specimen is detached from the hepatic veins and more space for handling particularly with the left hand could be needed. Therefore, paradoxically, chest opening is a maneuver more frequently carried out by expert surgeons rather than young fellows, since it is a decision derived from background experience that leads the operator to foresee the potential difficulties of the resection, and to shift to a thoracophrenolaparotomic approach without hesitation.

A median extension to the lower abdomen is selected (Fig. 8.4), particularly in case of an existing median incision: this access facilitates

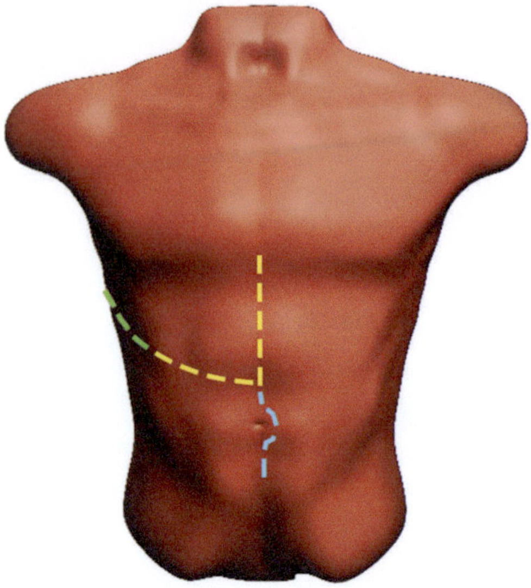

Fig. 8.4 The J-shaped laparotomy is extended distally on the midline (*dashed blue line*), particularly when associated procedures have to be performed in the mid-lower abdomen

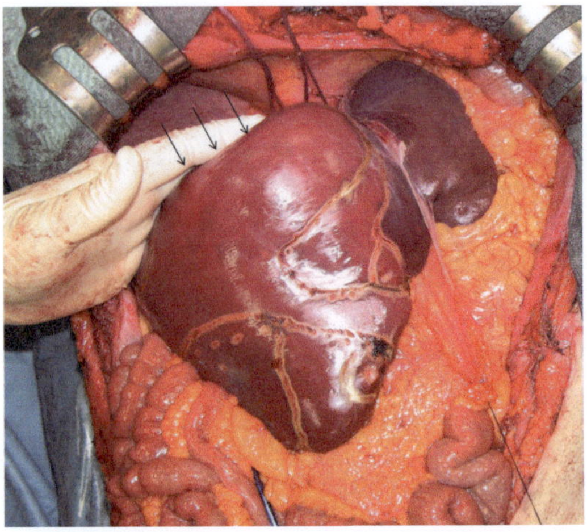

Fig. 8.6 The midline extension also allows easier placement of the left hand with respect to the J-shaped incision if just laparotomic, and enables opening of the angle between the dome of the liver and the caval confluence of the hepatic veins by pulling the liver downward (*arrows*)

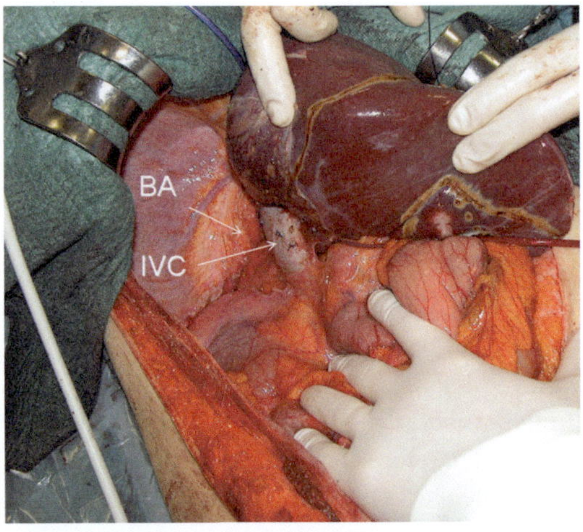

Fig. 8.5 The midline extension allows adequate exposure of the bare area (*BA*) and the inferior vena cava (*IVC*)

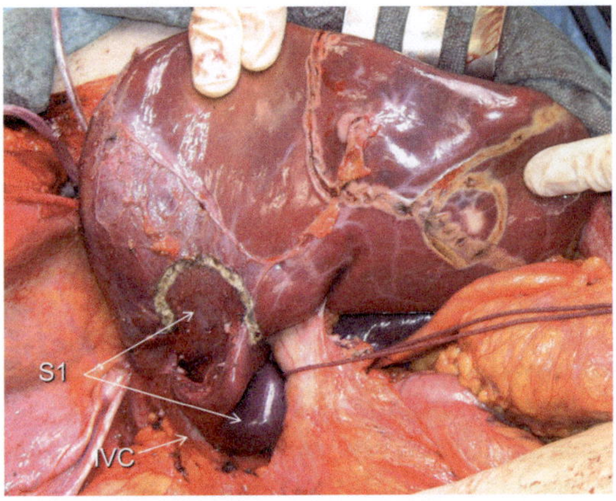

Fig. 8.7 The midline extension, although allowing easier placement of the left hand with respect to the J-shaped incision if just laparotomic, and permitting a complete hepatocaval dissection, as compared to the thoracophrenolaparotomic one, does not enable a perpendicular visual plane of the retrohepatic area; inferior vena cava (*IVC*); segment 1 (*S1*)

caudal tilting of the liver once mobilized (Fig. 8.5), and provides a larger space for positioning the left hand, then for handling the liver (Fig. 8.6). However, this access is not featured by a surgeon's visual plane perpendicular to the hepatocaval space (Fig. 8.7), and is probably linked to a higher risk of wound hernias.

For right-sided segmentectomies or subsegmentectomies or sectionectomies the bare area is dissected and the right hemiliver is mobilized till the surgeon's left hand is positioned behind the

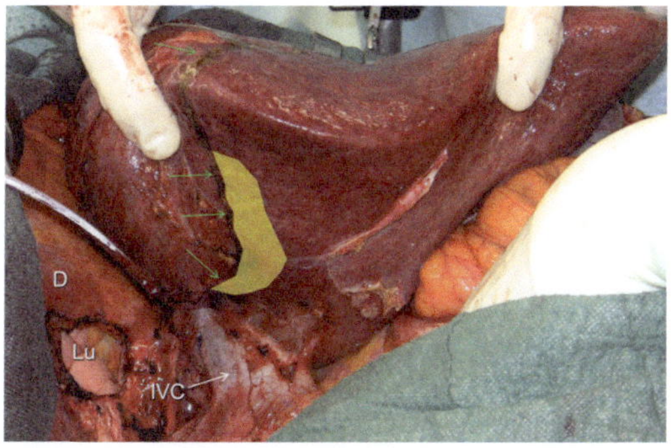

Fig. 8.8 The *yellow* area just at the edge of the dissection area drawn with the electrocautery (*green arrows*) shows the position of the left-hand's fingertips during liver dissection to aid in driving the proper trajectory for liver division; diaphragm (*D*); inferior vena cava (*IVC*); lung (*Lu*)

hemiliver, sustaining it, and as mentioned is comfortably positioned over the posterior aspect of the dissection plane drawn during the definition of the surgical strategy (Fig. 8.8). This mobilization should be extensive enough to allow allocation of the surgeon's hand, and to avoid damaging of the adjacent structures, and particularly not to injure any short hepatic vein eventually left at the edge of the dissection area. Such an injury can be the source of conspicuous bleeding from the IVC, and can be massive as generally recognized late and potentially extended to the caval wall.

Therefore, a slight mobilization of the right hemiliver just dividing the triangular ligament and partially or completely the bare area will be accomplished for lesions located in segments 5, 6, 7 inferior, and 8 ventral (Fig. 8.9a, b). Conversely, the right side of the retrohepatic IVC is reached for lesions located in segments 7 and 8 dorsal. If the lesion is located in segment 7 superior or 8 dorsal, close to the hepatocaval confluence (last 4 cm), but is not in contact with the hepatic veins, the hepatocaval ligament is not divided (Fig. 8.10a, b), and only the space between the RHV and the MHV is dissected for allowing fingertip insertion and eventual compression (Fig. 8.11a, b). The caval confluence of the RHV is recognized following the trajectory of the right inferior phrenic vein (RIPV), which flows into the IVC adjacent to the RHV, and for that a reliable landmark (Figs. 8.10b and 8.12) [1].

If the lesion is still right-sided but in contact with a hepatic vein at its caval confluence (Fig. 8.13a–g), or involves the paracaval portion of segment 1 (Fig. 8.14a–e), liver mobilization includes division of the hepatocaval ligament and exposure of the retrohepatic IVC till the area to be resected is under control of the surgeon's left hand (surgeon's fingertip getting over the most distal portion of the planned dissection plane) (Figs. 8.13b, and 8.14c). This detachment proceeds unless the control is obtained even

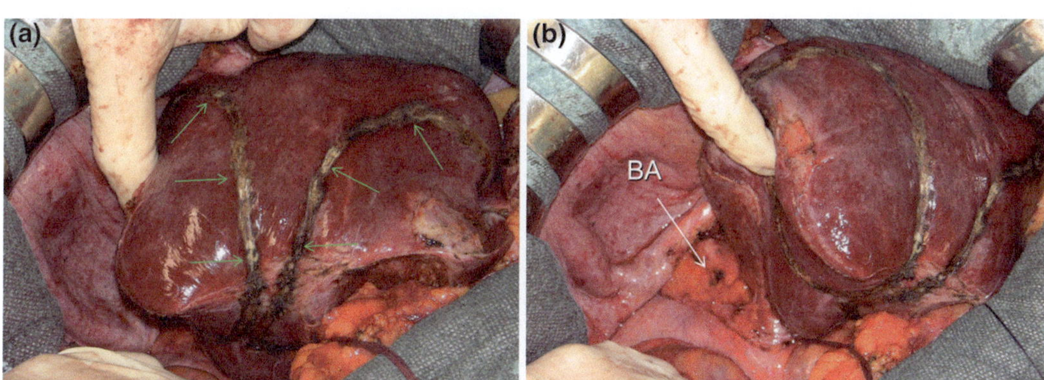

Fig. 8.9 For lesions located in the right inferior portion of the liver, for which limited resections (*green arrows*) could be enough (**a**), liver mobilization may be limited to the partial division of the bare area (*BA*) (**b**)

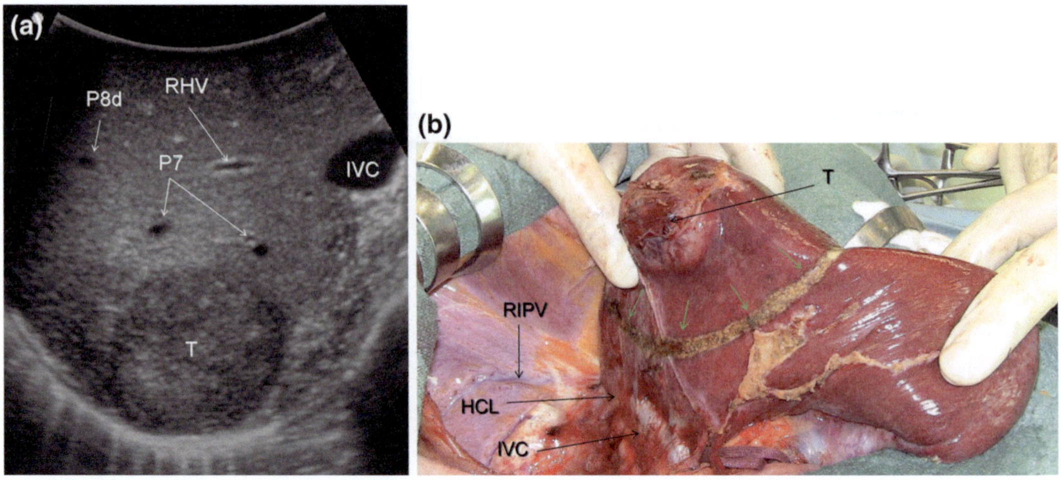

Fig. 8.10 For lesions (*T*) located close to the caval confluence, but without having close vascular relations (**a**), the dissection line (*green arrows*) is drawn relatively far from the caval confluence (**b**), and mobilization proceeds unless the inferior vena cava (*IVC*) is exposed but the hepatocaval ligament (*HCL*) may not be necessarily divided; right inferior phrenic vein (*RIPV*); right hepatic vein (*RHV*), portal branches to segment 7 (*P7*); portal branch to subsegment 8 dorsal (*P8d*)

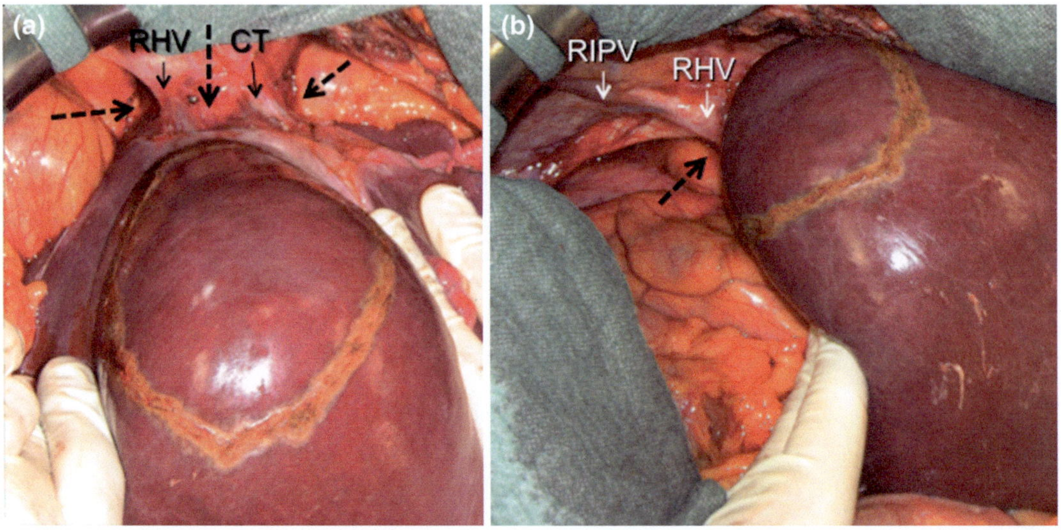

Fig. 8.11 For lesions located close to the caval confluence, but without having close vascular relations, the hepatocaval confluence is prepared just for fingertip positioning enabling compression of the hepatic veins for reducing backflow bleeding: in (**a**) the dissection for finger positioning is shown, with the *dashed black arrows* indicating the place where the fingertip should be placed; in (**b**) a right-sided perspective indicating the posterior aspect of the right hepatic vein (*RHV*) is shown; common trunk (*CT*) of left and middle hepatic vein; right inferior phrenic vein (*RIPV*)

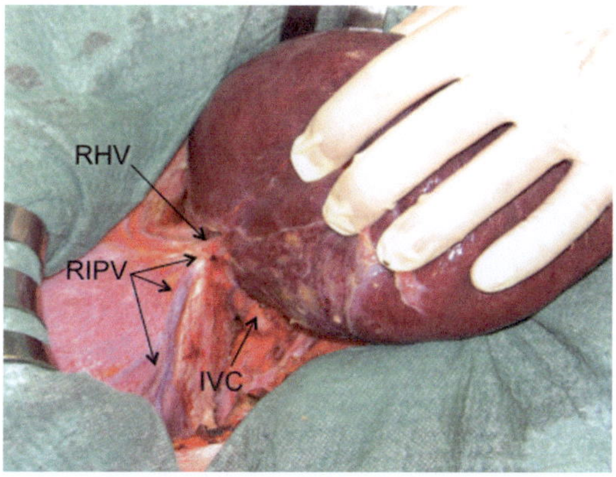

Fig. 8.12 The right inferior phrenic vein (*RIPV*) indicates the confluence of the right hepatic vein (*RHV*). This is particularly useful during dissections approaching the hepatocaval confluence in presence of adhesions between the diaphragm and the liver or in concurrence with tumoral invasion of the diaphragm itself

though this means achieving complete detachment from the IVC (Fig. 8.15a–c). In this case, once the mobilization of segment 1 is complete and carried out through a right-sided approach, the left-hand fingertips are positioned at the edge between segments 2 and 1 where the Arantius' ligament runs, somehow hooking the caudate lobe (Fig. 8.16).

For segment 2 and 3 segmentectomies or subsegmentectomies, the left triangular ligament and the left coronary ligament are divided and with the surgeon's left hand the left lobe is handled.

For lesions located at segment 4 superior at the hepatocaval junction, the mobilization combines the one described for lesions at segments 7 inferior and 8 ventral and for those in the left lobe. For these lesions once there is a relationship with the main trunk of the MHV, particular attention should be given to the fact that this vein is generally featured by a vertical confluence into the IVC (Fig. 8.17), which makes its length shorter than the others and its central position makes its compression more difficult. For these reasons, injury of this vein during dissection could be a source of massive bleeding and therefore preventive check of the control of the vein flow by finger compression (Fig. 8.18), or vein encirclement itself is always to be considered (Fig. 8.19).

A particular trick that deserves to be mentioned is the use of IOUS to help mobilization when there are adhesions that may mask important structures to be recognized and preserved as the hepatic hilum, the IVC, and the hepatic veins. Just positioning the probe to localize these structures in relation to the dissection area and the distance between the latter and the structures themselves helps to avoid their damage and the severe consequences related to it (Fig. 8.20).

8.2 IOUS-Guided Demarcation of the Resection Area

Demarcation of the resection area can be accomplished in an anatomical or nonanatomical fashion according to the type of the tumor, and the background liver. For anatomical demarcation the edges between adjacent portions of the liver having different inflow are outlined using various methods. However, before discussing these modalities, a brief comment on one of the most misleading uses of IOUS is required. The person with sufficient skills in IOUS within a surgical team usually is asked to disclose the plane containing the MHV by just contacting the probe with the liver surface. It is clear that any transverse or longitudinal scan merely viewing the MHV does not disclose the actual plane dividing the right and left liver in which the MHV itself is contained, since to define such a plane two landmarks are needed. Therefore, even for this purpose making apparent the demarcation line between the right and left liver on the hepatic surface is indispensable for identifying the only anatomical plane passing through the MHV (Fig. 8.21a, b).

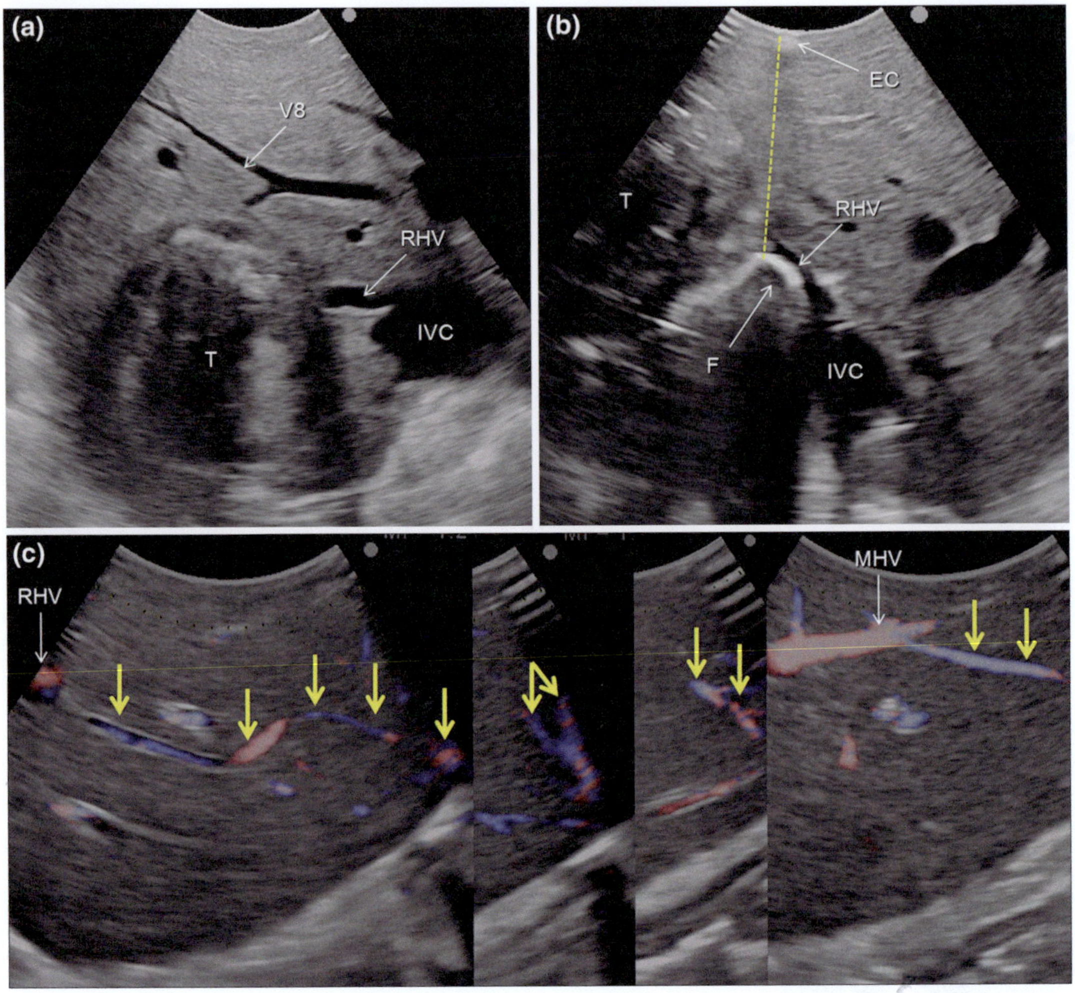

Fig. 8.13 **a** IOUS of a colorectal liver metastasis (*T*) previously treated and relapsed after thermal ablation and now invading the right hepatic vein (*RHV*) in proximity of its caval confluence; **b** upon adequate mobilization the surgeon's fingertip (*F*) is placed between the tumor and the inferior vena cava (*IVC*) at the level of the RHV confluence, and together with the electrocautery (*EC*) being positioned on the opposite side, the virtual dissection plane is planned (*dashed yellow line*); **c** a communicating vein between the RHV and the middle hepatic vein (*MHV*) (*yellow arrows*); **d**, **e** the RHV is taped (*Tp*) and the resection area is drawn (*green arrows*); **f**, **g** the resection is carried out sparing segment 6 (*S6*) (**f**), which is drained by the communicating veins connecting the intrahepatic stump of the RHV (*RHVs1*) with the MHV (**g**); caval stump of the RHV (*RHVs2*); scar from previous thermal ablation (*S*); hepatic vein draining segment 8 and flowing into MHV (*V8*)

8.2.1 Anatomical Resection

Selection of an anatomical resection for CLM seems not to be oncologically relevant [2], while its use for HCC is still controversial [3–8]: for the latter there are no studies comparing in a reliably randomized fashion anatomical and nonanatomical resections. However, reports show long-term benefits of the anatomical approach over the nonanatomical [3–6, 9, 10] both in a large series contest [5] and by a statistical analysis weighted to rule out the possible significant effect of selection biases that may afflict the reliability of the results [9]. The rationale for anatomic resection for HCC is based on its pattern of intrahepatic dissemination

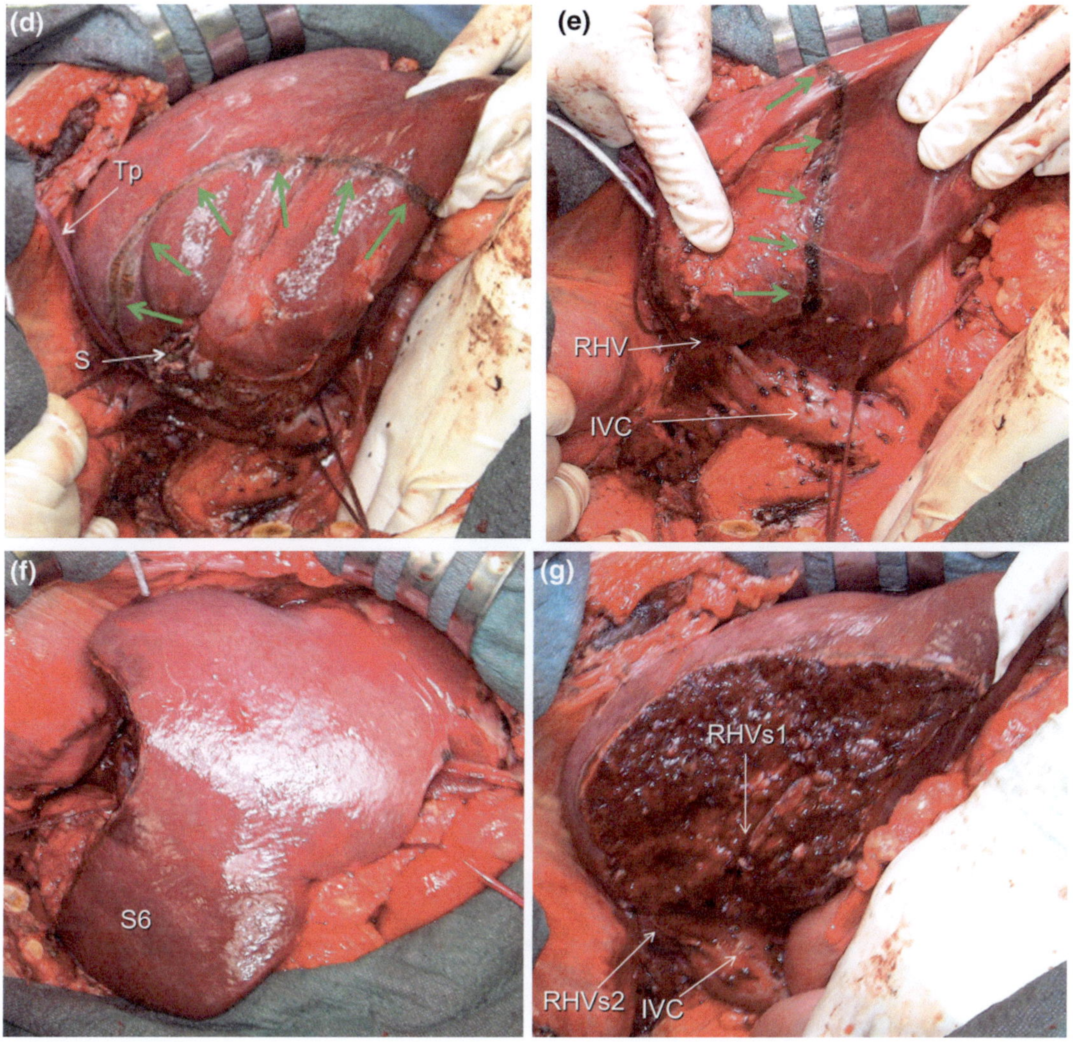

Fig. 8.13 (continued)

from the main lesion through the portal branches (Fig. 8.22). Thus, the resected specimen should include at least the portal area with the lesion (Fig. 8.23). On the other hand, the superiority of the anatomical resection seems more evident in those subgroups of patients with single HCCs larger than 2 cm in diameter [5] or with extranodular growth [10], which are usually those with higher risk of satellites and microvascular invasion.

However, no matter whether technical requirements for accomplishing truly anatomical sectionectomies and formal major hepatectomies are more uniformly accepted, the agreement on the requirements for defining a subsegmental resection as a real anatomical one is still vague, and thus a potential source of misunderstanding also in evaluating the data published in reports related to the topic. Indeed, recognition and demarcation of the segmental area to be removed in a fully anatomical way is still a matter of debate. The only certainty is that the segmental or subsegmental portal area feeding the tumor cannot be visualized on the liver surface without interventional techniques that allow their recognition. Almost all the proposed

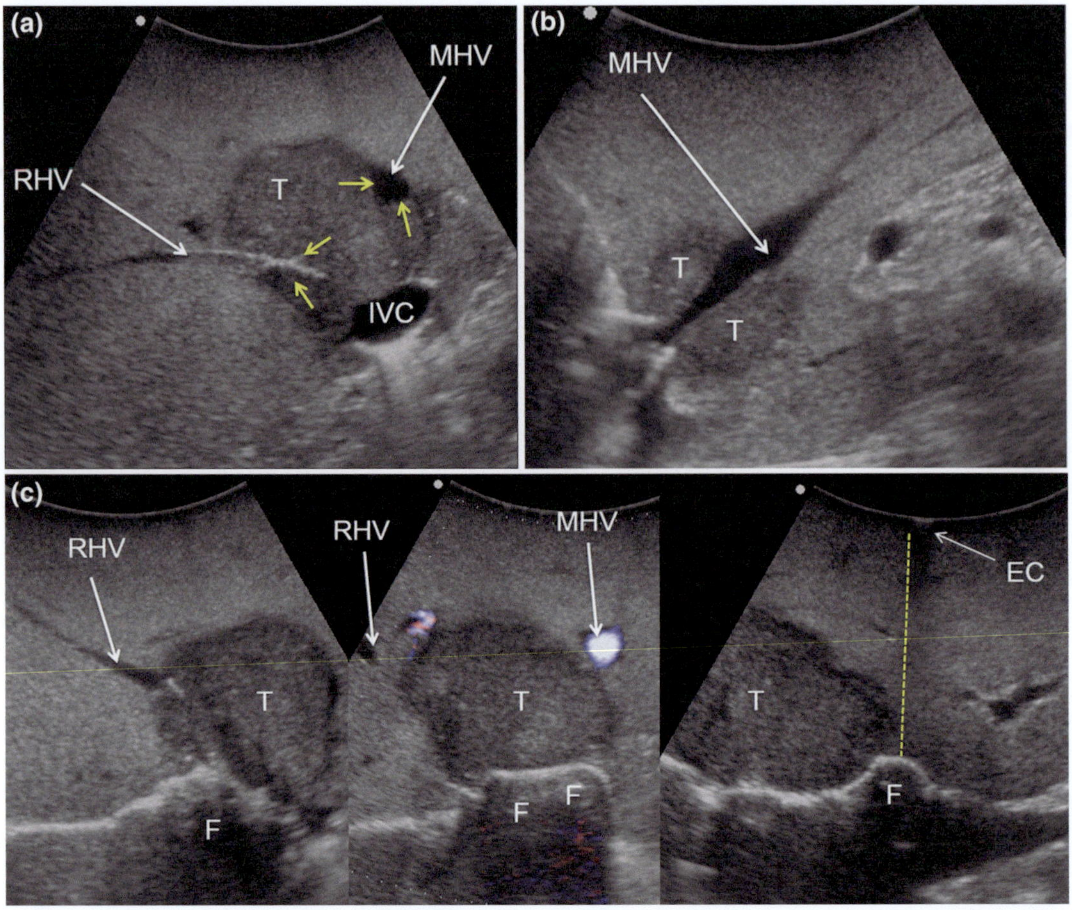

Fig. 8.14 **a** IOUS of a colorectal liver metastasis (*T*) invading the right hepatic vein (*RHV*) and in wide contact with the middle hepatic vein (*MHV*) (*yellow arrows*); **b** a sagittal scan showing the MHV in another plan; **c** from left to right, these serial images show mobilization proceeding unless the fingertip (*F*) can be positioned on the left side on the tumor margin and together with the electrocautery (*EC*) on the opposite side of the liver the virtual dissection plane is drawn (*dashed yellow line*); **d** late phase of liver mobilization in which the RHV is taped and then resected preserving the vein draining the caudate lobe (*HVS1*); **e** resection is carried out sparing segments 5 and 6, and preserving MHV; inferior vena cava (*IVC*); stump of the RHV (*RHVs*)

techniques are based on ultrasound guidance, especially in a cirrhotic liver where there are generally wide variations and abnormalities in the extension of the segmental areas. The first procedure described in this sense was the so-called *systematic segmentectomy* devised in the early 1980s [11]. The latter consists in the puncture of the portal branch feeding the tumor once the homolateral artery is clamped at the hepatic hilum: then the dye is injected into the punctured vein (Fig. 8.24a, b). More recently, alternatives to this approach have been devised.

The following paragraphs provide details concerning ultrasound-guided techniques for segmental and sectional resections.

8.2.1.1 Segmentectomies

Puncture of the Portal Branch

The portal branch feeding the tumor to be resected is punctured under IOUS-guidance through a free-hand technique or with a dedicated device, and then 3–5 ml of indigo carmine dye are injected into the vessel (Fig. 8.24a, b). The stained area becomes evident on the liver

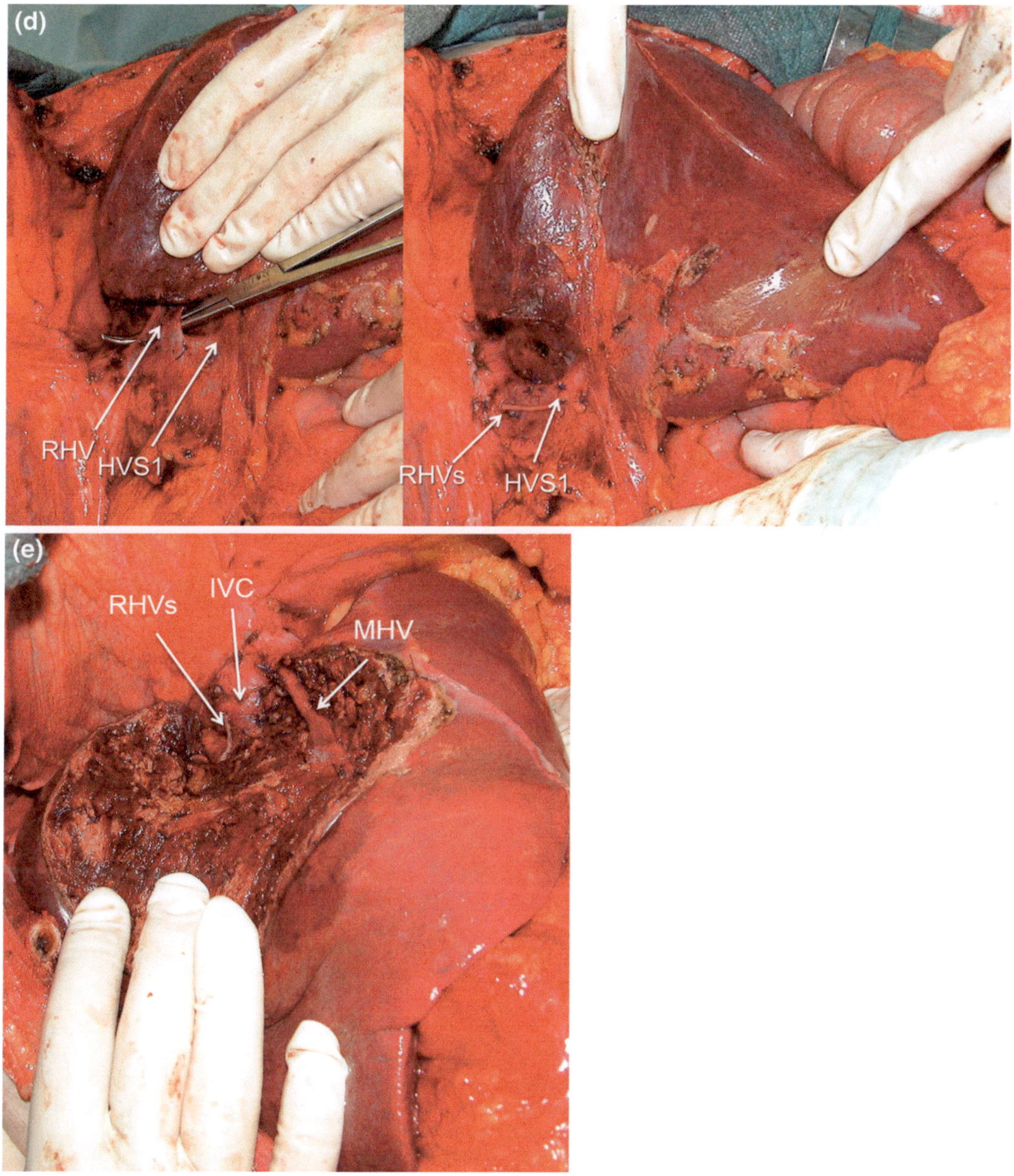

Fig. 8.14 (continued)

surface and is marked by electrocautery and the resection can be accomplished fully in an anatomical way. If the nodule is located between two adjacent segments, two portal branches afferent to the area should be punctured and injected. In this case, the deepest and most dorsal vessel must be punctured at first to avoid air bubbles contained in the dye from disturbing the ultrasonographic detection and puncture of the other branch. The portal branch is punctured 1–2 cm distally from its origin to avoid dye reflux and the direction and velocity of the

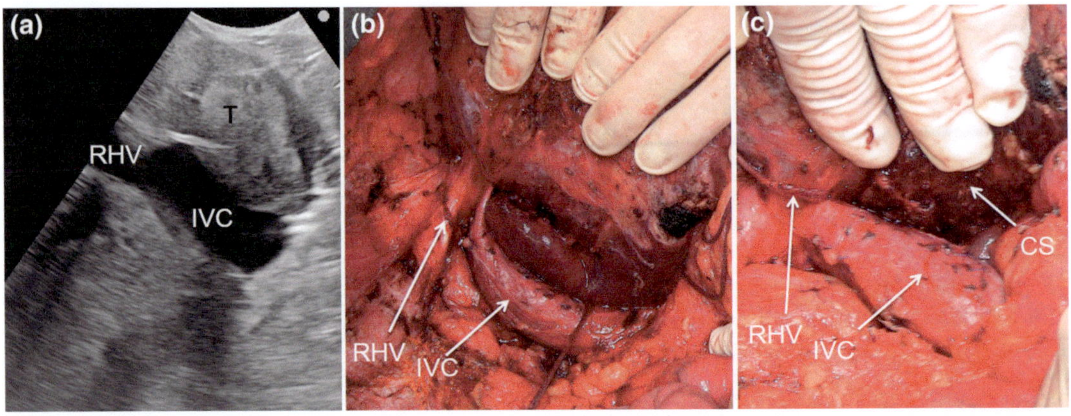

Fig. 8.15 **a** IOUS of a tumor (*T*) occupying segment 1 (caudate lobe) and compressing and dislodging on the right the inferior vena cava (*IVC*); **b** the liver is then mobilized approaching it from both sides but preferentially on the right completely freeing the IVC; **c** resection is then carried out; cut surface (*CS*); right hepatic vein (*RHV*)

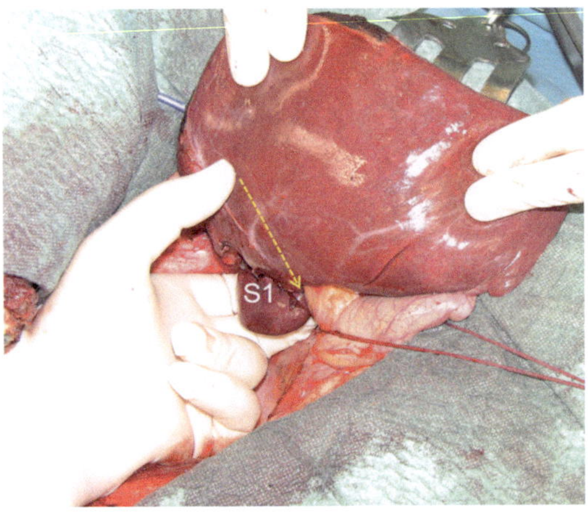

Fig. 8.16 Once the mobilization of segment 1 (*S1*) is completed by means of a right-sided approach, the left-hand fingertips are positioned at the edge between segments 2 and 1, where the Arantius' ligament runs, somehow hooking the caudate lobe and the virtual dissection plane can be determined (*dashed yellow arrow*)

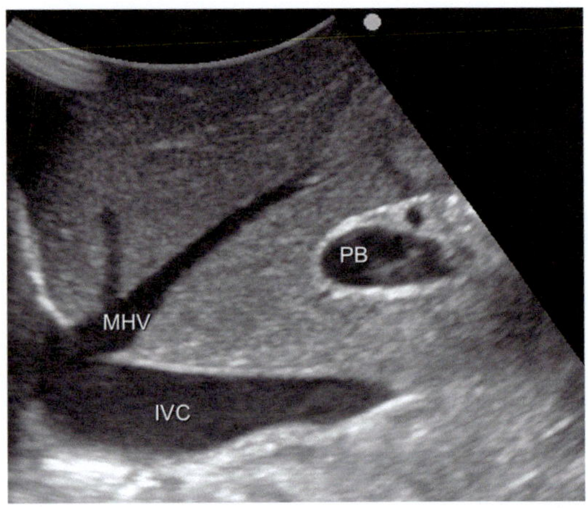

Fig. 8.17 IOUS shows the peculiarity of the middle hepatic vein (*MHV*) in most cases. It runs vertically toward its confluence into the inferior vena cava (*IVC*), and this has to be kept in mind during dissection in segments 4 and 5 seemingly far away from the hepato-caval confluence. Inversely, caval confluence is straight down a few centimeters, and consequently damaging the MHV may result in massive and usually unexpected bleeding, which may lead to panic unexperienced surgeons; portal bifurcation (*PB*)

infusion are controlled by IOUS. To prolong staining, the hepatic artery at the hilum is clamped before portal branch puncture. When there are numerous and thin vessels to be punctured or in the case of tumor thrombus in the segmental portal branch of the segment to be removed, the dye is injected in the portal branches afferent to the adjacent segments: this is the so-called *counterstaining technique* [12].

The above method remains the most precise way for segmental and subsegmental anatomical demarcation. Its main drawback, other than the required quite high skill of the surgeon in

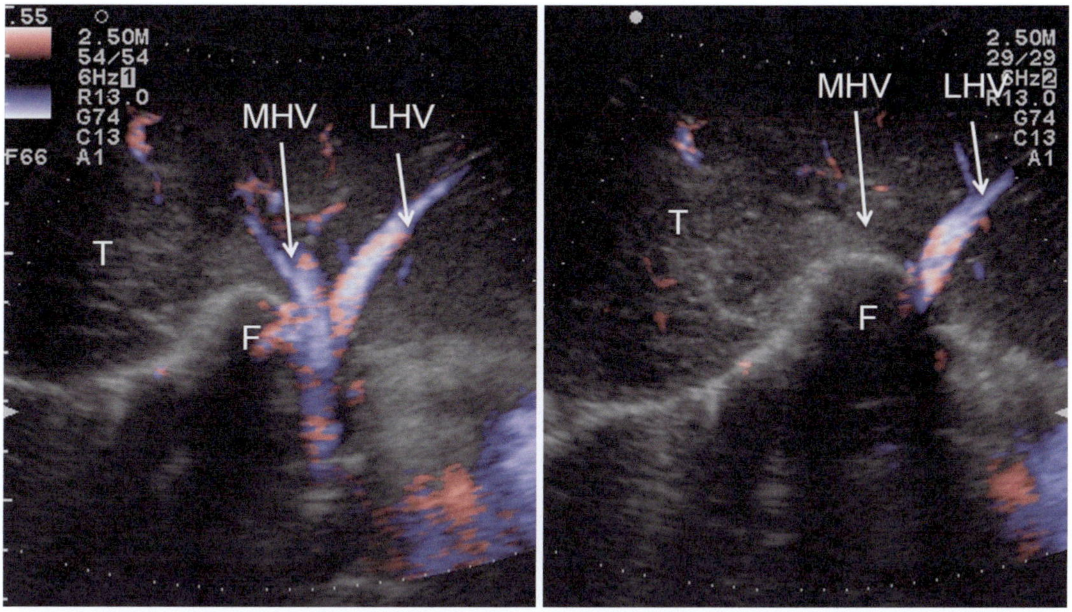

Fig. 8.18 CFIOUS showing the aforementioned technique (see Chap. 7 and herein) for controlling backflow bleeding in those conditions in which the hepatic veins have not been encircled. Just before starting dissection, once the hepatocaval confluence has been prepared (as in Fig. 8.11) it is possible to verify under CFIOUS guidance the adequacy of finger compression (*F*) just checking the disappearance of the color-flow once the compression has been applied (from *left* to *right*); left hepatic vein (*LHV*); middle hepatic vein (*MHV*)

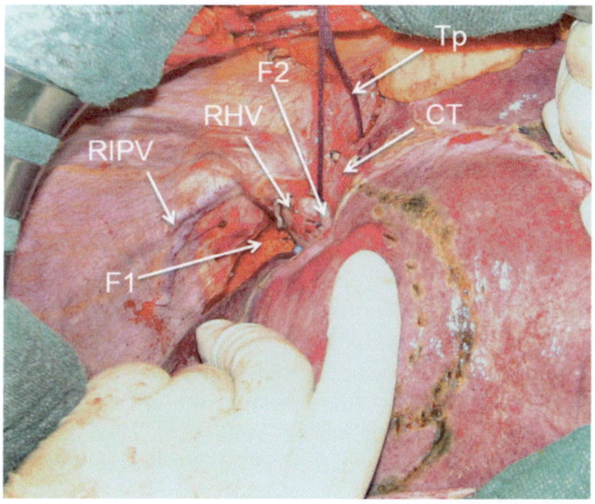

Fig. 8.19 Encirclement (*Tp*) of the common trunk (*CT*) and the sites for allocating the fingers for compressing the right hepatic vein (*RHV*) (*F1*) and the middle hepatic vein (*MHV*) (*F2*); right inferior phrenic vein (*RIPV*)

puncturing miniscule vessels, is the fact that if the ink regurgitates or is injected into the wrong portal branch, it could be then difficult to identify the proper area to be removed.

Compression of the Portal Branch

The procedure, as illustrated in Fig. 8.25a, b, initially was used for tumors located in the left hemiliver (see Fig. 1.10a in Chap. 1) [13], but more recently has been successfully extended to all segmental locations [14] and even to an entire sectional portion of the liver [15]. Once the feeding portal branch is identified by IOUS (Fig. 8.26a, e), it is compressed using the IOUS probe on one side of the liver and the finger on the opposite side (Fig. 8.26b, f), confirming the proper compression by IOUS real-time control (Fig. 8.26c, g). In this way it is possible to induce a transient ischemia of the portion of the liver distally to the compression site. This portion can be marked by electrocautery, the compression is released (Fig. 8.26d, h–j), and resection is carried out (Fig. 8.26k). This technique is simple, fast, noninvasive, and reversible. The possibility to modify the site of compression and then the resection volume allows tailoring the resection in function of the

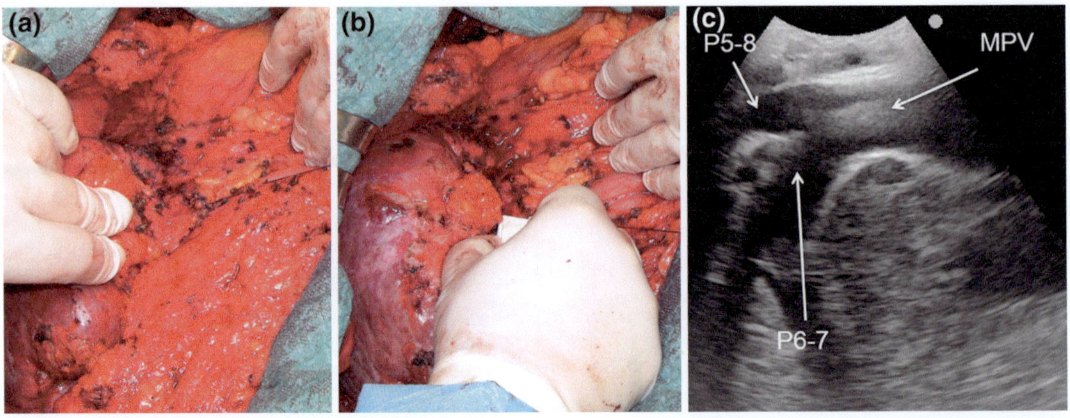

Fig. 8.20 **a** A surgical field with dense adhesions and an anatomy that, often due to previous operations and eventually previous resection too, has been modified; **b** the probe can be applied for better understanding the anatomy; **c** in this case it is useful to fix exactly the position of the hilar pedicle that has to be encircled avoiding its inadvertent damage; main portal vein (*MPV*); portal vein to the right anterior section (*P5-8*); portal vein to the right posterior section (*P6-7*)

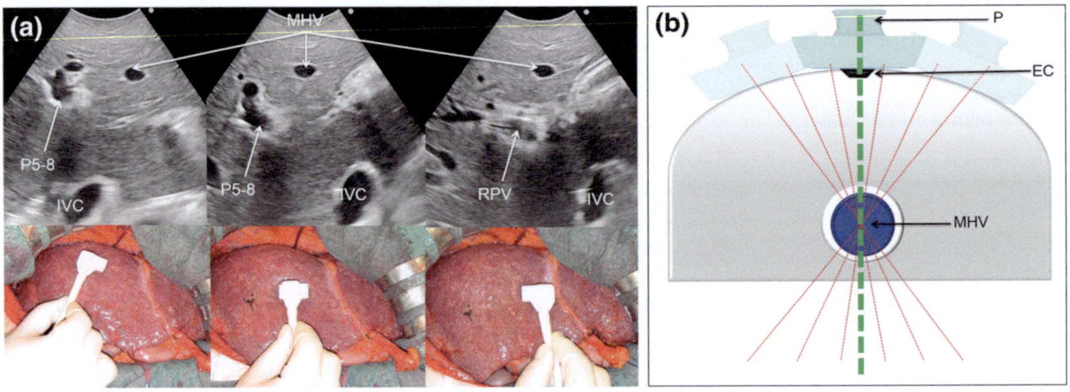

Fig. 8.21 **a** Comparison of different IOUS scans with related IOUS images, showing how it is misleading to consider the proper anatomical plan dividing the right and left liver anyone in which, by IOUS, the middle hepatic vein (*MHV*) is visualized. Here, three different scans are able to visualize the vein although other structures appear and disappear; **b** the elementary principle on which this finding is based: numerous plans (*dashed red lines*) pass through the single point represented by the MHV, but only one is adequate. To find the latter compulsorily requires another point as that represented by the demarcation line on the liver surface between the two hemilivers (*Cantlie's line*), which can be marked with electrocautery (*EC*) and then allowing to disclose the proper line passing through the MHV (*dashed green line*); inferior vena cava (*IVC*); portal vein to the right anterior section (*P5-8*); probe (*P*); right portal vein (*RPV*)

tumor features and the status of the background liver. Furthermore, the compression can be used in a *countercompression* perspective, alluding to the philosophy proposed by Takayama et al. of defining the adjacent segmental margins to disclose those of the targeted segment [12]. The latter was applied for complete and anatomical segment 1 resection using the aforementioned portal branches puncture technique. Indeed, for segments such as segment 8 and 4 superior for which direct compression of the feeding portal branch can be unfeasible, the compression of the adjacent segmental branch allows the definition of their segmental margins [14]. However,

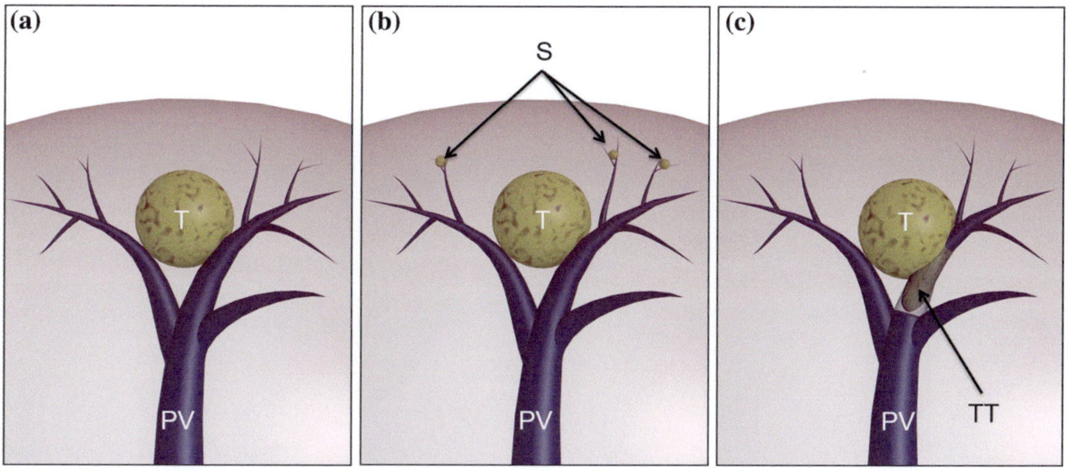

Fig. 8.22 **a** Relation between an HCC (*T*) and its feeding portal vein (*PV*); **b** the HCC tends to disseminate within its segment, developing satellites (*S*); **c** later its attitude is to spread through the liver by disseminating through the portal tree, and invading it with tumor thrombi (*TT*)

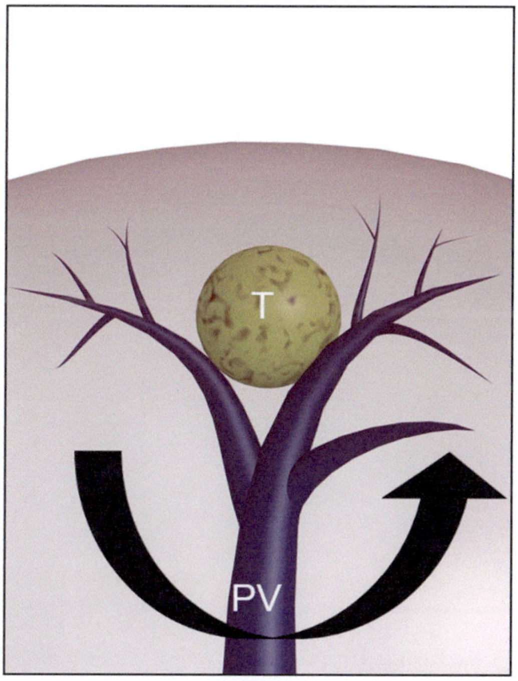

Fig. 8.23 According to Fig. 8.22, the best local treatment for HCC (*T*) should be the removal, in addition to the nodule, also of the segmental or subsegmental area fed by the portal tree (*PV*)

growing expertise has allowed to standardize the modality to perform a direct compression of segment 8 portal branch (P8) [16] (Fig. 8.27a–e), and even the selective compression of subsegmental branches feeding the ventral and dorsal portions of this segment (Fig. 8.28a–j), and that of the superior portion of segment 4 [17]. Briefly, the left hand of the surgeon together with the IOUS probe are positioned under IOUS guidance having P8 at the level selected for compression between them (Figs. 8.27a–e, 8.28a–j). A fundamental trick should be to select the compression site avoiding inadvertent compression of other vascular structures (Fig. 8.29a, b) that could mismatch the real segmental or subsegmental profile. Using the left fingertips and the IOUS probe itself, the surgeon compresses bilaterally the liver at the targeted position resulting in the compression of P8 (Fig. 8.27a–c) or its subsegmental ventral (P8v) (Fig. 8.28c–e) and dorsal (P8d) (Fig. 8.28f–h) branches; this maneuver is monitored constantly in real-time IOUS by means of the probe used for compression (Figs. 8.27a, 8.28c, e, f, h). For P8v, the probe compression sites are usually located on the superoanterior surface of the liver, and the finger compression sites are just in proximity and cranial with the hepatocaval junction (anterocranial approach). For the subsegmental dorsal area of segment 8, compression can be applied directly to its feeding portal branch (P8d) or on P7 as for a formal anatomical

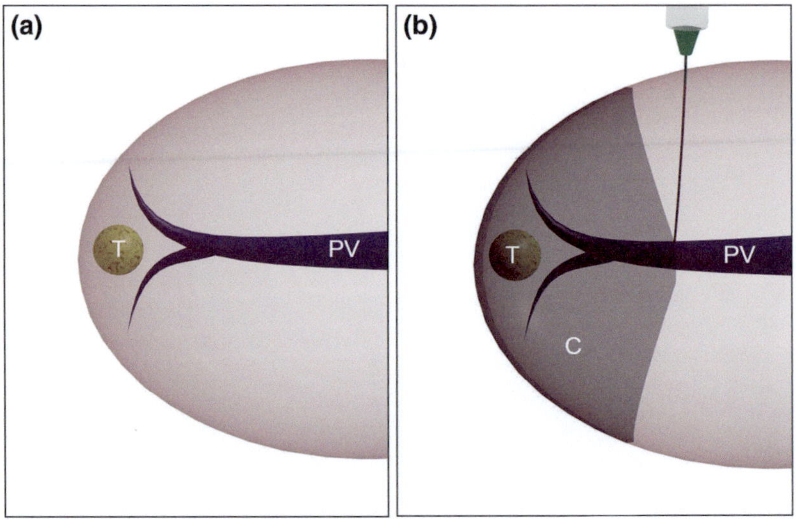

Fig. 8.24 Performance of a systematic segmentectomy for an HCC (*T*), by identifying the portal vein (*PV*) feeding the lesion (**a**), and by injecting dye (generally indigo carmine) into PV once the homolateral hepatic artery is clamped at the hepatic hilum, allowing the selective coloring of the part to be removed (*C*), which corresponds to the segment or subsegment with the tumor (**b**)

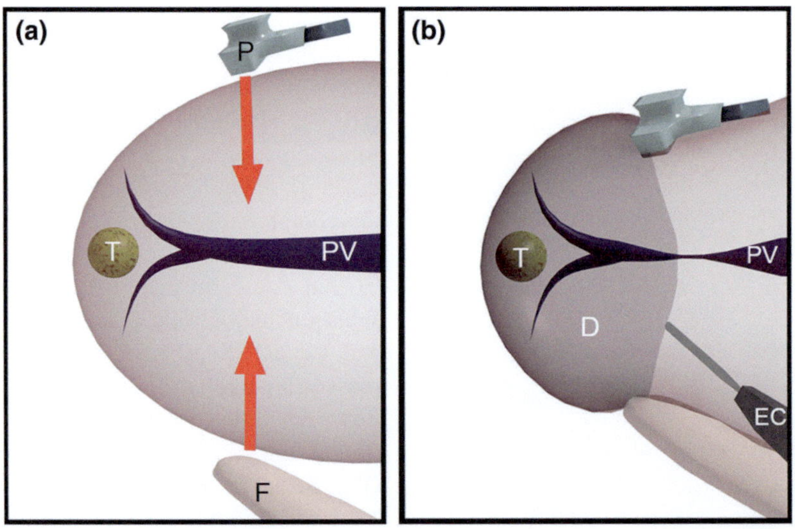

Fig. 8.25 Alternative approach for performing a systematic segmentectomy for an HCC (*T*) by identifying the portal vein (*PV*) feeding the lesion, and by compressing (*red arrows*) with the probe (*P*) and the finger (*F*) the feeding PV (**a**), determining a transient discoloring of the area (*D*), which can be marked with electrocautery (*EC*), and which corresponds to the segment or subsegment with the tumor (**b**)

segmentectomy of segment 7 (Fig. 8.30a–e), but only in a countercompression manner. In both cases, the compression window on the IOUS scan is obtained by positioning the finger compression site on the posterior surface of the liver, which was previously mobilized (antero-posterior approach). Compression is maintained until the surface of the liver distal to the

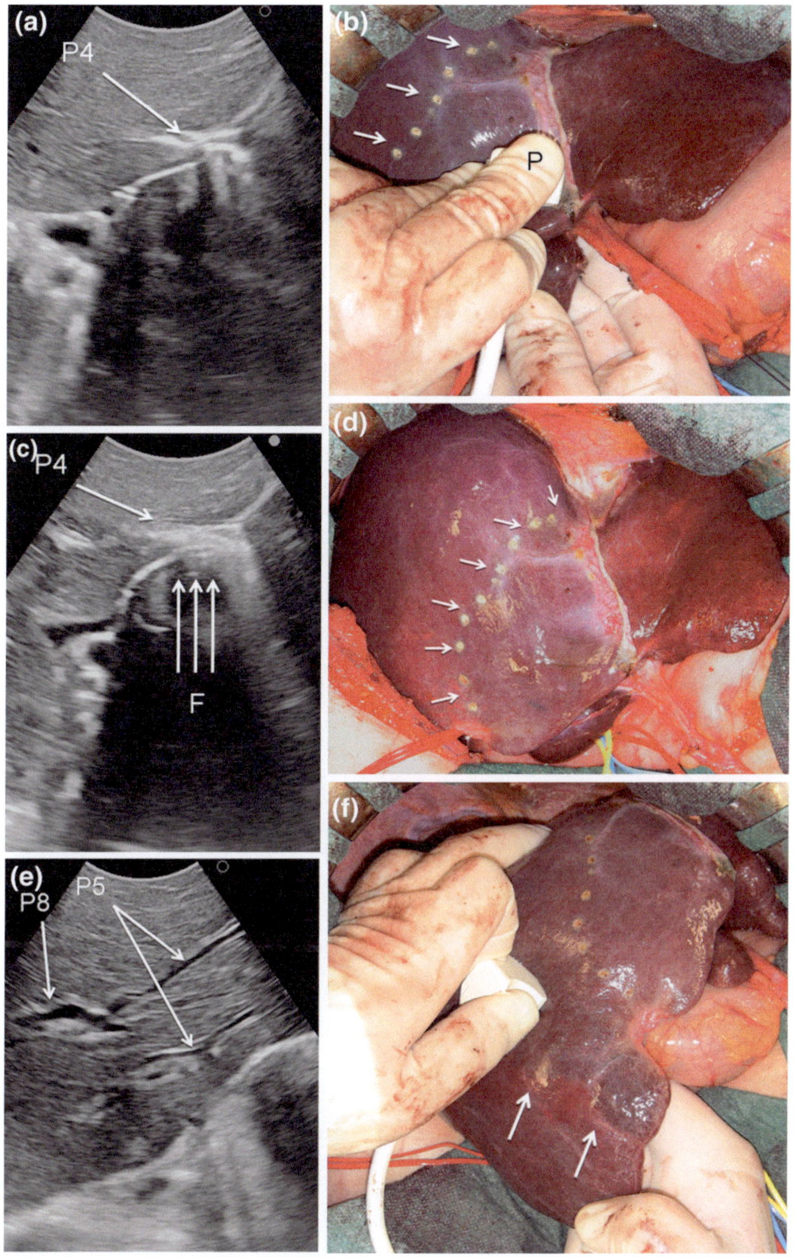

Fig. 8.26 **a** IOUS scan identifying the common portal branch for segment 4 (*P4*); **b** once identified under IOUS guidance P4 compression is carried out by means of the probe (*P*) and the surgeon's finger positioned on the opposite side, resulting in discoloring of the segmental portion to be removed (*arrows*); **c** the maneuver is monitored under continuous IOUS control; **d** the area is marked by electrocautery (*arrows*); **e–i** the same maneuver for the segment 5 portal branches (*P5*), which are identified in IOUS (**e**), then compressed revealing the discolored area (*arrows*) (**f**) under constant IOUS real-time control (**g**), and at the end the demarcation of the area (*arrows*) with electrocautery is performed (**h**, **i**); **j** the whole area including segments 4 (*S4*) and 5 (*S5*) is more clearly demarcated (*arrows*); **k** resection is carried out; finger (*F*); portal vein to segment 8 (*P8*)

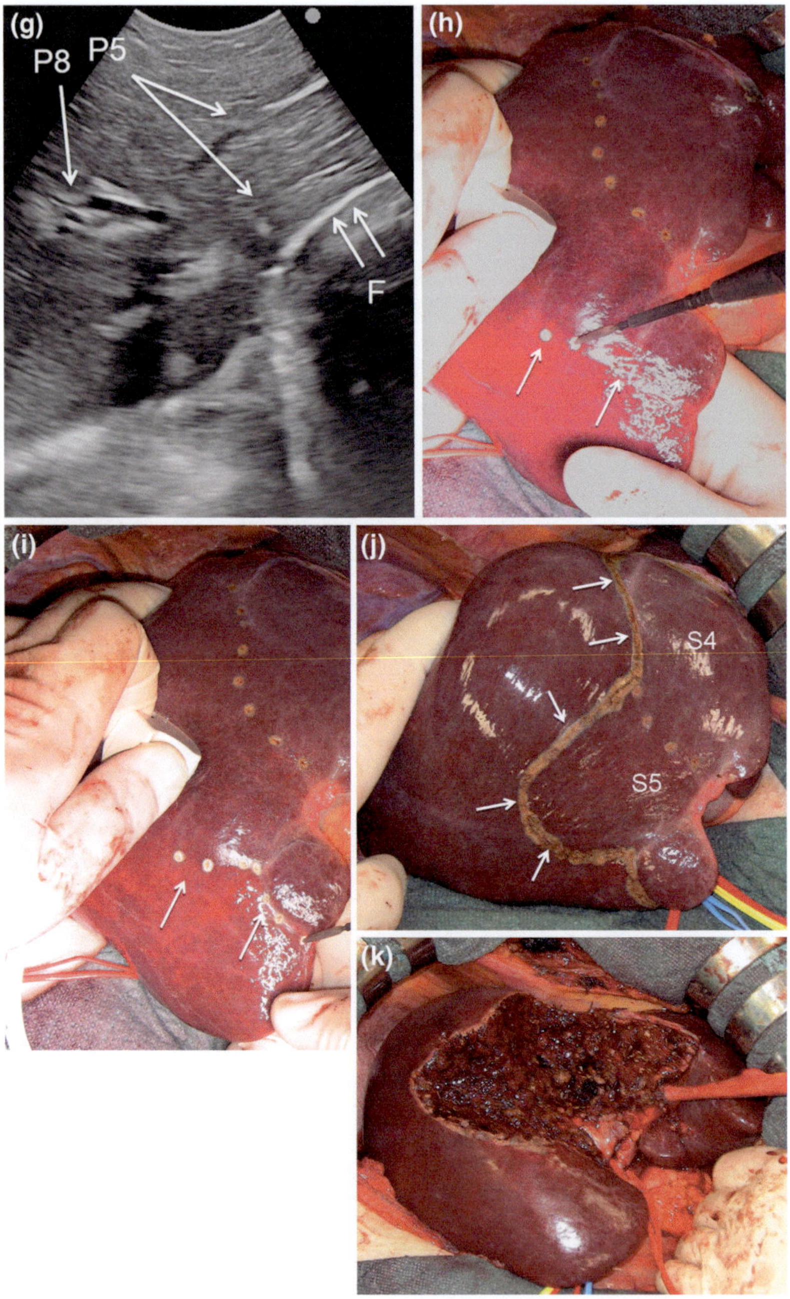

Fig. 8.26 (continued)

Fig. 8.27 **a** IOUS scan showing on the left the portal branch (*P8*) feeding the tumor (*T*) in segment 8, and on the right its compression by means of the probe and the surgeon's finger (*F*) positioned on the opposite side; **b** compression results in discoloring of the segmental portion to be removed (*arrows*); **c** the area is marked by electrocautery (*arrows*); **d** the liver at the end of the segmental resection showing on the cut surface the middle (*MHV*) and right hepatic veins (*RHV*), and the stump of P8, which are a marking proof of the full anatomicity of the segment removal; **e** the same cut surface visualized from above to show the perpendicular plane (when compared to the frontal body axis), which has to be followed once resection of segment 8 has to be done; inferior vena cava (*IVC*)

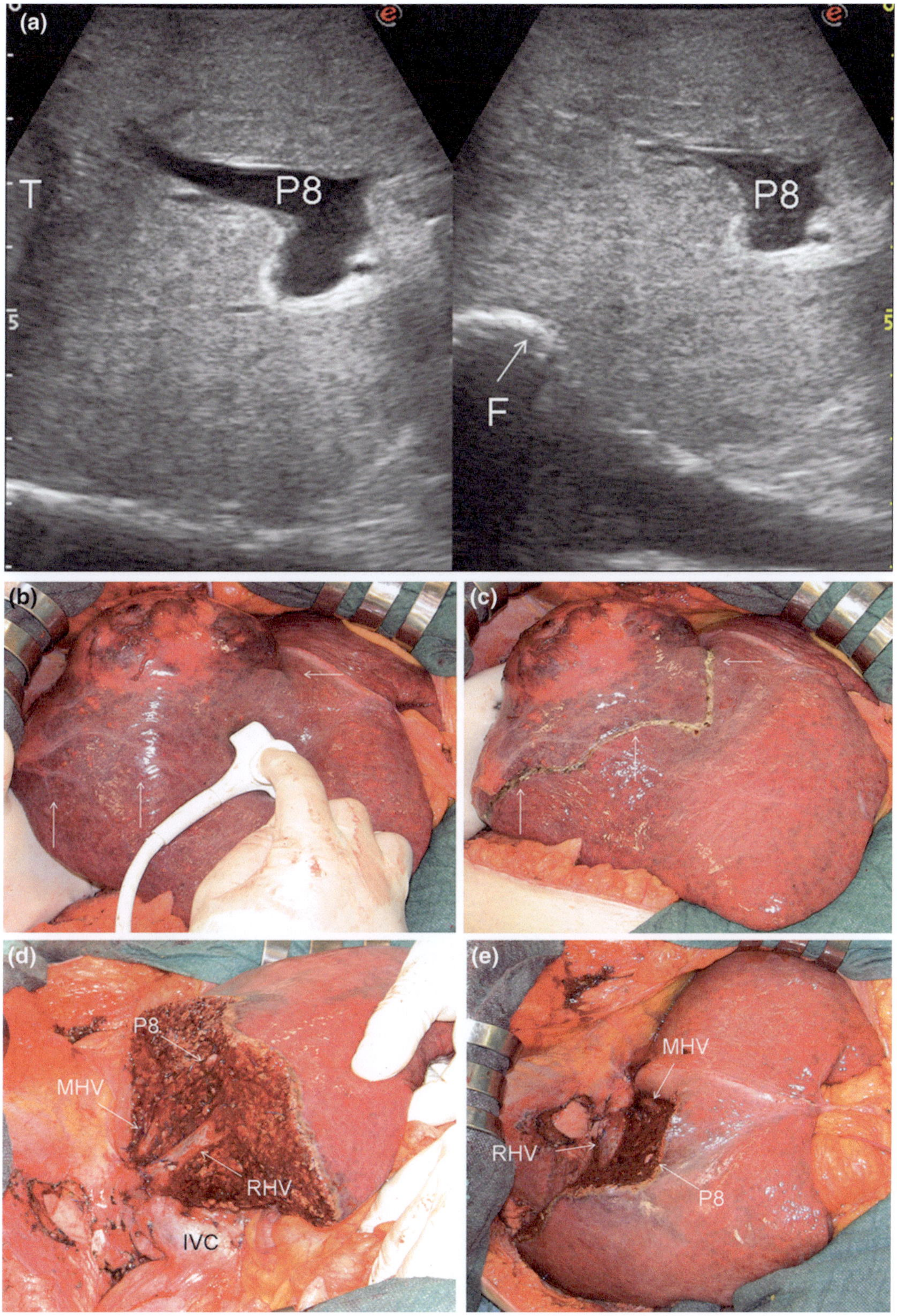
(a)
T
P8
P8
F
(b)
(c)
(d)
P8
MHV
RHV
IVC
(e)
MHV
RHV
P8

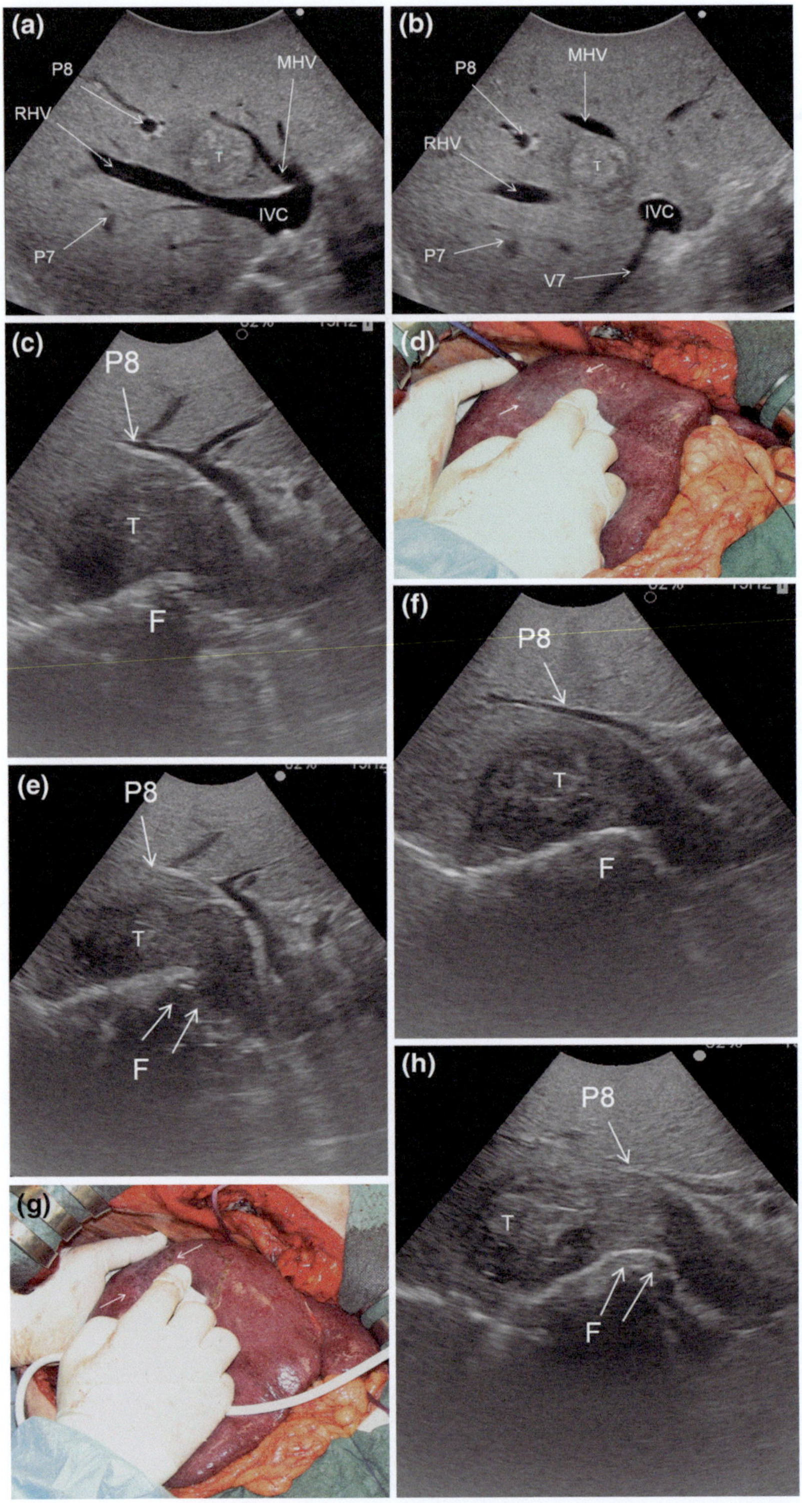
(a)
P8
RHV
MHV
T
IVC
P7
(b)
P8
MHV
RHV
T
IVC
P7
V7
(c)
P8
T
F
(d)
(f)
P8
T
F
(e)
P8
T
F
(h)
P8
T
F
(g)

◀ **Fig. 8.28** **a**, **b** IOUS scans of a tumor (*T*) in segment 8 at the edge with the paracaval portion of segment 1 adjacent to the right hepatic vein (*RHV*) (**a**), being in contact with the middle hepatic vein (*MHV*) (**a**, **b**): the latter is slightly dislodged by the tumor (**a**); **c** IOUS identification of one of the portal branches (*P8*) feeding the tumor (*T*); **d** its compression by means of the probe and the surgeon's finger (*F*) positioned on the opposite side is carried out resulting in a discoloring of the portion compressed (*arrows*); **e** the maneuver is constantly monitored by IOUS in real-time; **f–h** similarly, the maneuver is repeated for the other branch; **i** the area is marked by electrocautery (*arrows*); **j** this picture shows the liver at the end of the segmental resection showing on the cut surface the middle (*MHV*) and the right hepatic veins (*RHV*), and the stump of P8, which are a marking proof of the full anatomicity of the segment removal; inferior vena cava (*IVC*); portal vein to segment 7 (*P7*); hepatic vein draining segment 7 (*V7*) and flowing directly into the IVC

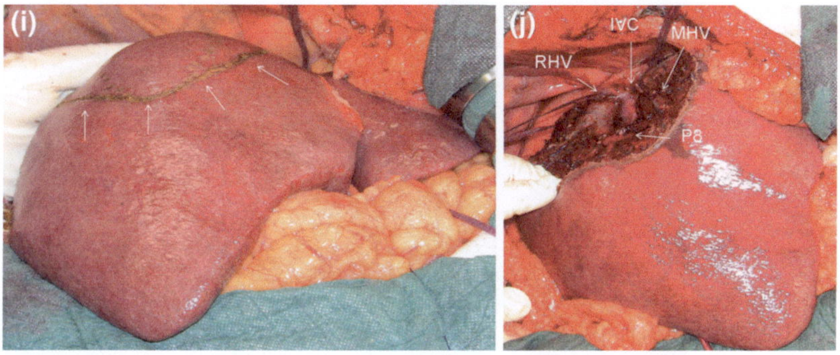

Fig. 8.28 (continued)

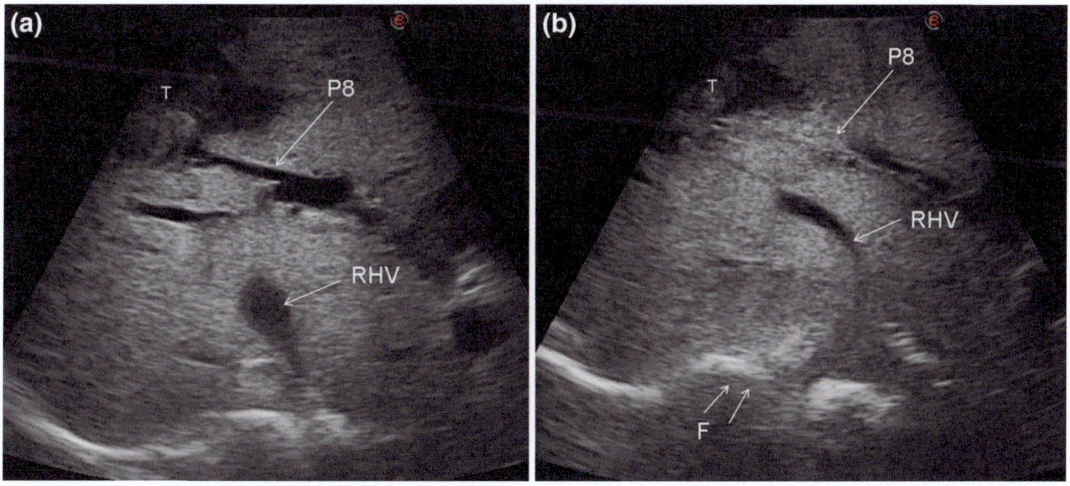

Fig. 8.29 Selection of the scan for compressing the branch to segment 8 (*P8*), which however comprehends the right hepatic vein (*RHV*) (**a**). This results in the compression of both P8 and RHV (**b**), potentially leading to visualize the effect of both transient ischemia and congestion; finger (*F*); tumor (*T*)

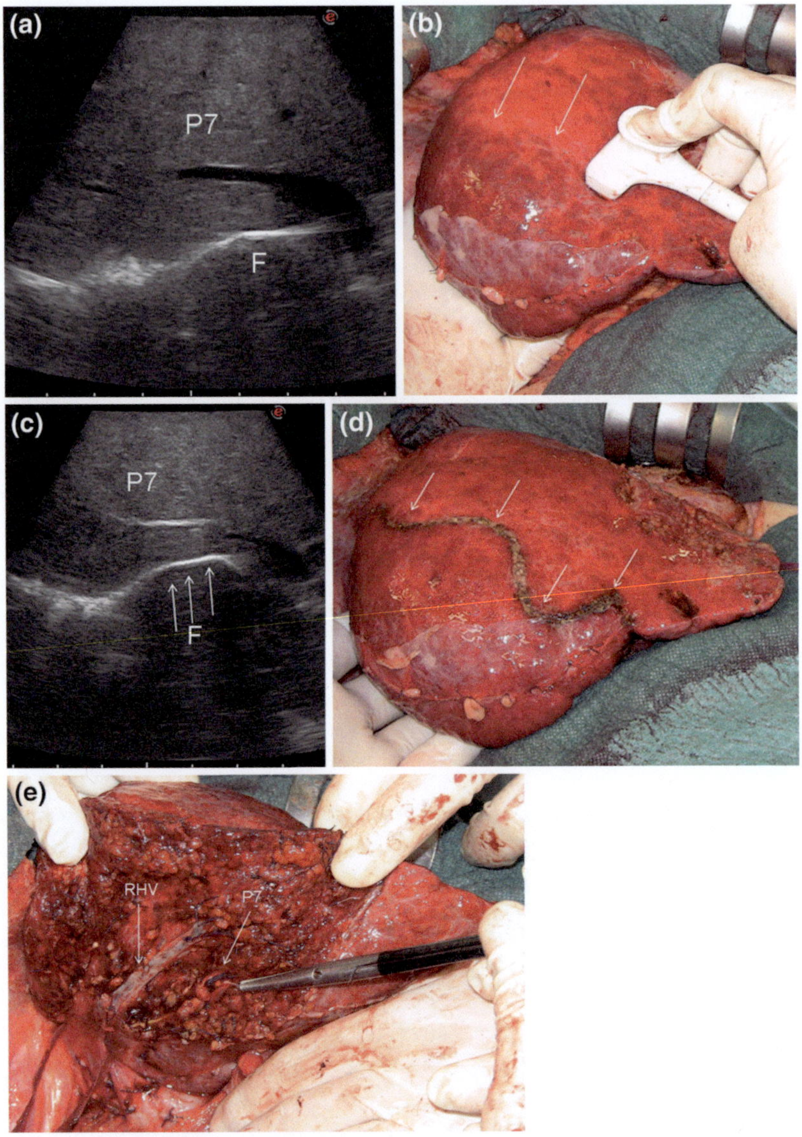

Fig. 8.30 **a** IOUS scan identifying the portal branch (*P7*) feeding the tumor in segment 7; **b** once identified under IOUS guidance, P7 compression is carried out by means of the probe and the surgeon's finger (*F*) positioned on the opposite side, resulting in discoloring of the segmental portion to be removed (*arrows*); **c** the maneuver is monitored under continuous IOUS control; **d** the area is marked by electrocautery (*arrows*); **e** the liver at the end of the segmental resection showing the right hepatic vein (*RHV*) and the stump of P7 as markers of the complete anatomical resection of segment 7

compression site starts to discolor (Figs. 8.26b, f, h, i, 8.27b, 8.28d, g, 8.30b). At this point, the assistant marks the discolored area by electrocautery and the compression is released (Figs. 8.26j, 8.27c, 8.28i, 8.30d).

Hooking of the Portal Branch

Despite, once the compression technique was introduced, the extrahepatic skeletonization and encirclement of the portal branch feeding the inferior portion of segment 4 (P4inf) to perform its selective anatomic resection became less relevant, the following technique deserves a brief description. The segmental portal branches to segment 4 are generally divided into two groups: those for the superior (P4sup) and those for the inferior portion, although the commonest branching pattern can be recognized in merely half of cases [18] (Fig. 8.31). These branches rather than punctured under IOUS guidance, can be approached by dissecting the umbilical portion. Once exposed, the vessel can be encircled with a suture and pulled under IOUS control to verify whether it is P4inf. Then, the proper

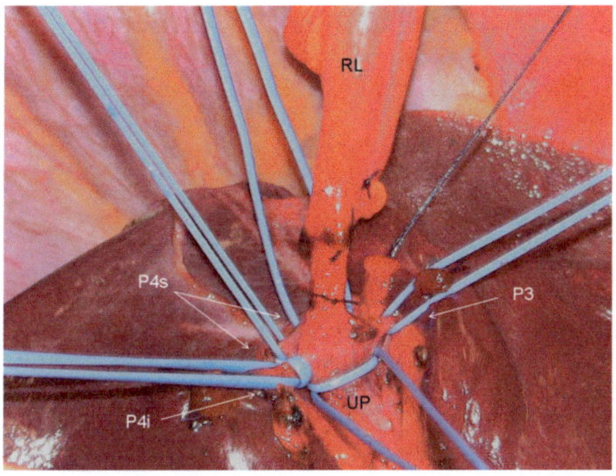

Fig. 8.31 The skeletonization of the branches originating from the umbilical portion (*UP*). It is well evident how in most patients segment 4 recognizes various branches originating from the UP and singularly feeding the inferior portion of segment 4 (*P4i*) and the superior portions of the same segment (*P4s*); portal vein to segment 3 (*P3*); round ligament (*RL*)

portal branch can be ligated and divided and the discolored area which appears on the liver surface should correspond to the S4 inferior, which can be marked by electrocautery to proceed with the liver dissection. This is a peculiar application of the so-called *hooking technique* [19]. Furthermore, the subsegment 4 superior can be resected by simply clamping P4inf, identified by means of the mentioned hooking technique; the discolored subsegment 4 inferior caudally, the plan obtained by IOUS which includes the MHV laterally, and that marked by the falciform ligament medially, delimit the area to be resected. Certainly, the recent introduction of compression also for this portion of the liver has drastically limited the use of this approach, though the hooking technique has retained its role for parenchyma dissection.

Other Techniques

Other methods proposed are balloon catheter inserted transhepatically to occlude the feeding portal branch [20] or, more recently, through the mesenteric vein [21]. Mazziotti et al. proposed segment 8 resection by dividing the liver along the main portal fissure, and subsequently approaching the segment 8 glissonian pedicle intraparenchymally [22]. Other authors have recently suggested ablation of the feeding portal and arterial branches [23–25]. All these alternative techniques are impaired by their invasivity and in some circumstances [23–25] for their irreversible damage to the target, which could imply compulsory extension of the resection area should the first targeted vessel not be the proper one. This extension of the resection area, even if accidental, is exactly what any kind of anatomical segmental resection seeks to avoid.

8.2.1.2 Sectionectomies

Right Posterior Sectionectomy

As for segmentectomies, demarcation of the sectional area to be removed is advocated. Among the methods proposed for obtaining this demarcation, the extrahepatic isolation of the right-sided sectional pedicles consists in careful and meticulous skeletonization of each sectional arterial and portal branch [26]. Alternatively, the three glissonian pedicles in their surrounding fibrous sheath can be encircled as a whole, in association with hepatotomy or not [27]. A further alternative to these established techniques is the compression technique [28]. The hepatic pedicle is encircled with a tourniquet but is not dissected. The portal pedicle for the right posterior section (segments 6–7) is identified by IOUS (Fig. 8.32a) as well as the subsegmental branches of segments 6 and 7; the level targeted for compression is then identified. The surgeon's left hand is placed behind the right hemiliver, once mobilized, while with the right hand the probe is positioned to show P6-7 at the level of interest, which corresponds to the most distal portion of the vessel in relation to its origin, but proximal to the tumor to be removed. Using the left fingertips and the probe itself, the surgeon compresses bilaterally the liver at the targeted position identified in IOUS (Fig. 8.32b). Compression can be repeated to better define the edges of the long demarcation line corresponding to the posterior sectionectomy (Fig. 8.32c, d). In some cases, compression can be carried out using one hand only, which may facilitate the visibility of the edge of the discolored area (Fig. 8.33a–c). When there is no common

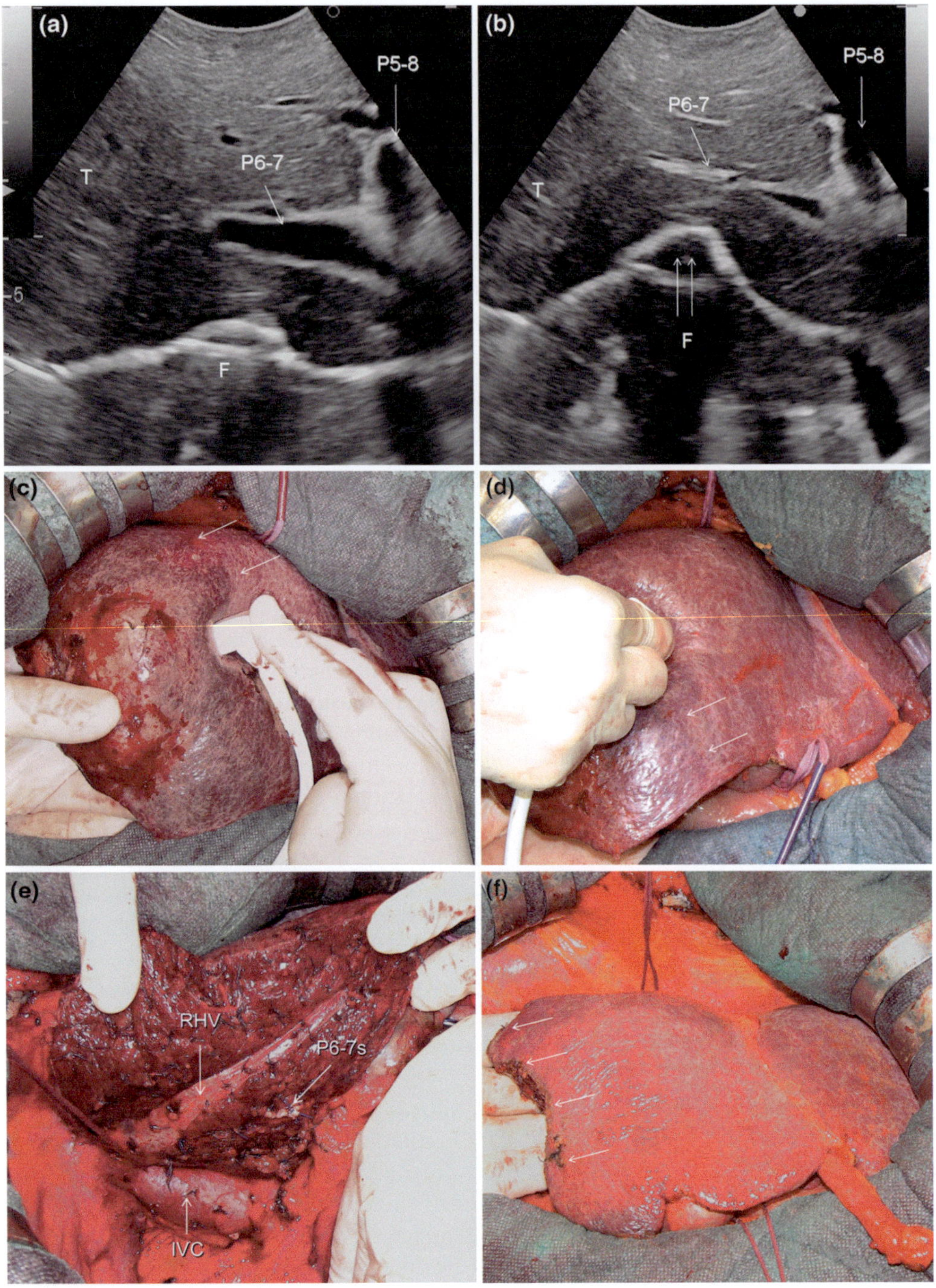

Fig. 8.32 **a** IOUS of the portal branch to the right posterior section (*P6-7*) which is occupied by an HCC (*T*); **b** P6-7 is compressed with the finger (*F*) and the probe paying attention to keeping patent the branch to the right anterior section (*P5-8*); **c**, **d** these pictures show the compression maneuver with the discolored area appearing on the liver surface (*arrows*) progressively in the upper part (**c**) and in the lower one (**d**) disclosing the edge of the right posterior section; **e** then a full anatomical right posterior sectionectomy for an HCC on liver cirrhosis is carried out without any kind of hilar dissection. The full exposure of the right hepatic vein (*RHV*) and the stump of P6-7 (*P6-7s*) are definitive landmarks of the adequacy of the procedure; **f** this image shows the anterior aspect of the liver after resection without any discolored area at the margin (*arrows*)

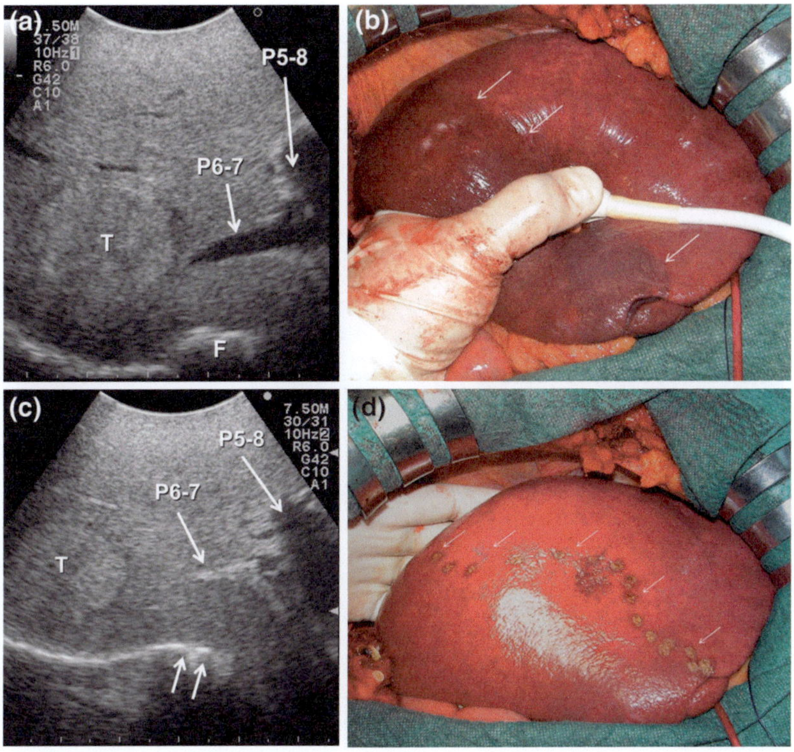

Fig. 8.33 **a** IOUS of the portal branch to the right posterior section (*P6-7*) which is occupied by a colorectal liver metastasis (*T*); **b** the compression maneuver is performed using only the left hand to facilitate the visibility of the discolored margin (*arrows*); **c** P6-7 is compressed with the finger (*F*) and the probe paying attention to keeping patent the branch to the right anterior section (*P5-8*): **d** the marked resection area on the liver surface (*arrows*)

sectional pedicle, the ones to segment 6 and segment 7 are selected and compressed separately as has been reported for segmental resections. Using the probe utilized for compression, the maneuver is constantly monitored in real-time (Figs. 8.32b, 8.33c). Compression is maintained until the surface of the right posterior section lateral to the compression site starts to discolor. At this time the assistant marks the discolored area by electrocautery and the compression is released (Fig. 8.33d). In this way a three-dimensional plane is drawn on the liver surface passing through P6-7 at the level of compression. Liver resection is then carried out following that plane (Fig. 8.32e, f).

Right Anterior Sectionectomy

Similar as for the right posterior section, the hilar dissection and the encirclement of the sectional glissonian pedicles are the most commonly adopted techniques for defining the resection area in a fully anatomical manner. More recently, the *countercompression technique* has been applied for this purpose [15]. P6-7 is identified by IOUS and the level targeted for compression is then detected just after its origin from the right portal branch (RPV) (Figs. 8.34a, 8.35a). Demarcation of the right posterior section is carried out as described in the previous paragraph (Figs. 8.34b, c; 8.35b, c). Similarly, the left portal vein (LPV) is identified by IOUS and the level targeted for compression is then identified just after its origin from the main portal vein (Figs. 8.34d–f, 8.35d–f). The LPV compression is carried out to be released once the Cantlie's line becomes evident by left hemiliver discoloration and it is demarcated by electrocautery (Fig. 8.34g). Once the right anterior section is defined, resection can be carried out without any preventive dissection of the hepatic hilum or encirclement of the sectional pedicles (Figs. 8.34h, 8.35g).

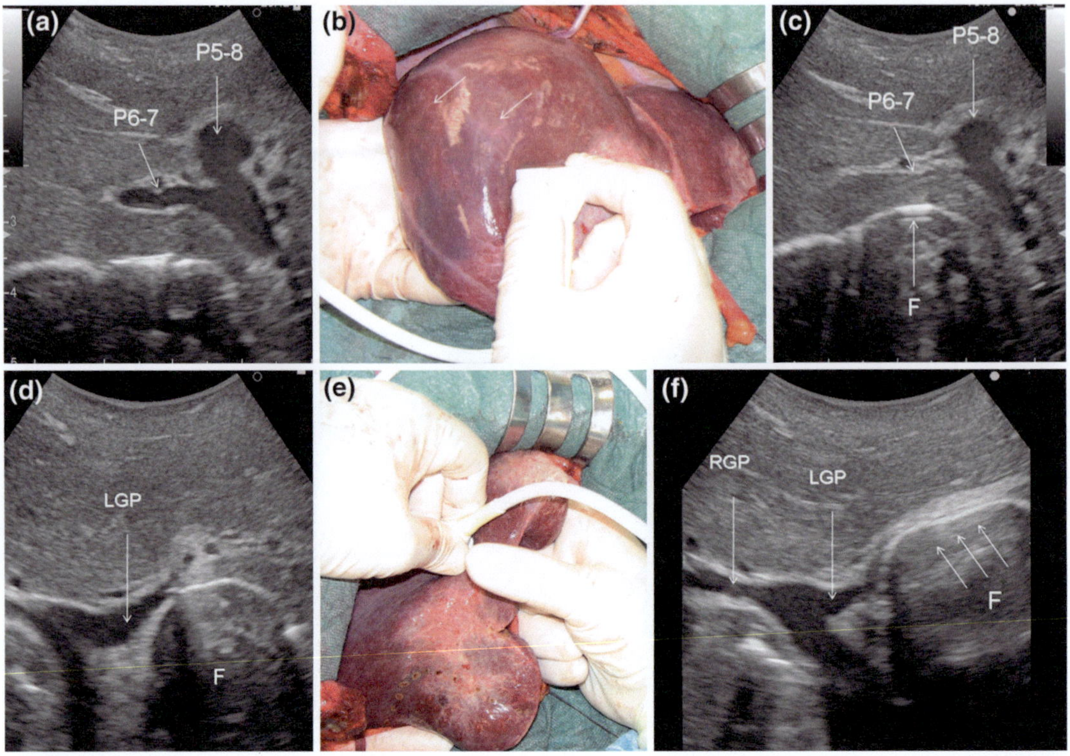

Fig. 8.34 **a** IOUS of the portal branch to the right posterior section (*P6-7*), and to the right anterior section (*P5-8*); **b** the compression maneuver is carried out for P6-7 combining the finger compression and the probe compression and the discolored area starts appearing on the liver surface (*arrows*); **c** the maneuver is monitored under continuous IOUS control; **d** the left glissonian pedicle (*LGP*) is disclosed by IOUS; **e** the compression maneuver is carried out as previously shown; **f** compression of LGP is constantly monitored by IOUS; **g** the margins of the right anterior section obtained with a countercompression modality are obtained and marked on the liver surface (*arrows*); **h** then a full anatomical right anterior sectionectomy is carried out without any kind of hilar dissection. The full exposure of the right hepatic vein (*RHV*), the middle hepatic vein (*MHV*), and the stump of P5-8 (*P5-8s*) are definite landmarks of the adequacy of the procedure; hepatic pedicle (*HP*); right glissonian pedicle (*RGP*)

8.2.2 Limited Resections

As described, selection of anatomical and non-anatomical resection for HCC, although a controversial issue [3–8], is pending in favor of the anatomical approach [5, 9, 10]. Conversely, for CLM limited resection it is commonly accepted as an oncologically adequate approach [2]. Also for limited resections, IOUS guidance plays a fundamental role. Indeed, although there is no need to identify the area of the liver fed by the portal branch to be ligated, once the tumor is identified, the surgeon under IOUS control can relate the electrocautery, positioned on the liver surface, with the tumor edge and any eventual vascular structure close to the tumor itself. Then, the optimal resection area can be drawn on the liver surface being confident of removing what has been planned. To carry out this maneuver the flat and thin tip of the electrocautery is positioned between the probe and the liver surface; this maneuver results in a shadow at the IOUS image which runs deeply just below the electrocautery (Fig. 8.36a–f). Once marked on the liver surface the adequacy of the edge can be further checked with IOUS even without the aid of electrocautery as the air trapped between the probe and the irregular surface of the drawn demarcation line

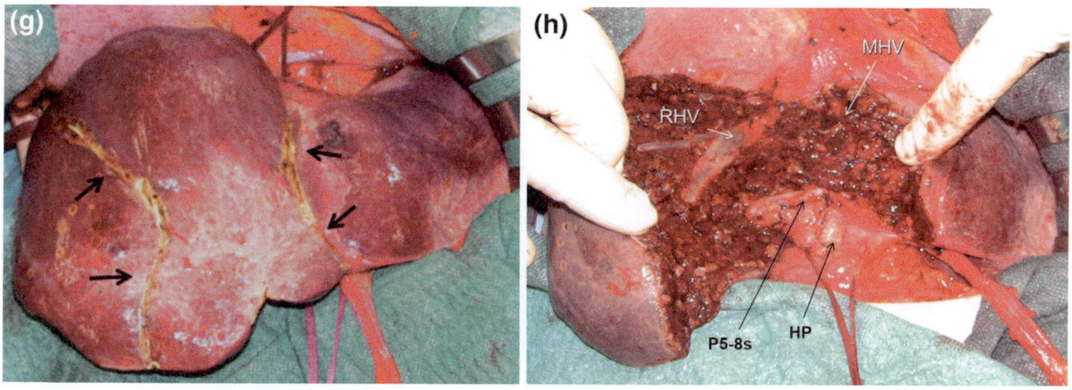

Fig. 8.34 (continued)

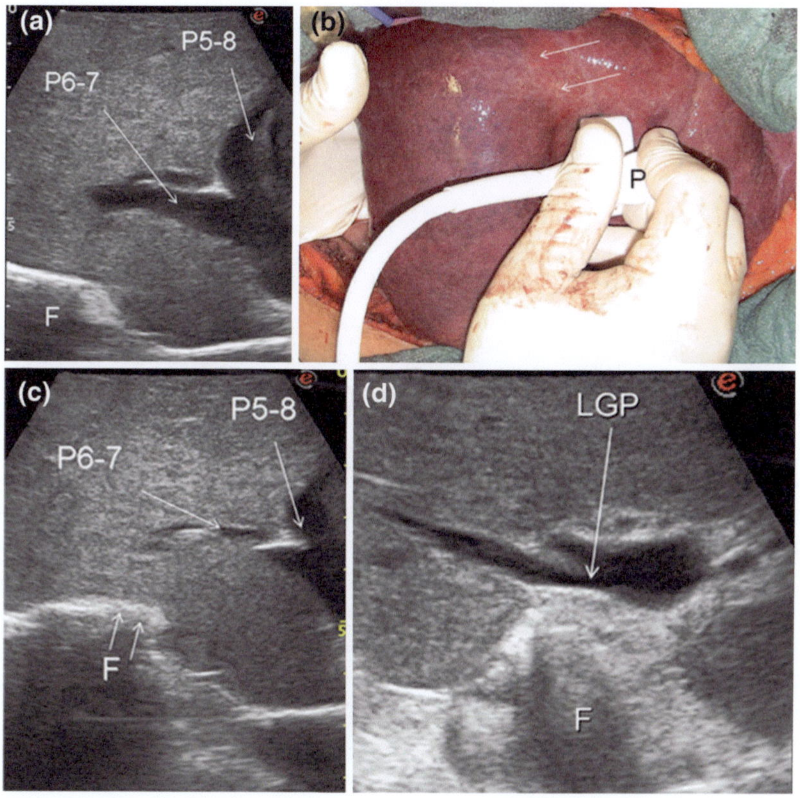

Fig. 8.35 **a** IOUS showing the portal branch to the right posterior section (*P6-7*), and to the right anterior section (*P5-8*); **b** the compression maneuver is carried out for P6-7 combining the finger compression and the probe (*P*) compression and the discolored area starts appearing on the liver surface (*arrows*); **c** the maneuver is monitored under continuous IOUS control; **d** the left glissonian pedicle (*LGP*) is disclosed by IOUS; **e** the compression maneuver is carried out on the left as previously shown; **f** compression of LGP is constantly monitored by IOUS; **g** then a full anatomical right anterior sectionectomy is carried out without any kind of hilar dissection: the full exposure of the right hepatic vein (*RHV*), the middle hepatic vein (*MHV*), and the stumps of P5-8 (*P5-8s*) are definite landmarks of the adequacy of the procedure; hepatic pedicle (*HP*); umbilical portion (*UP*)

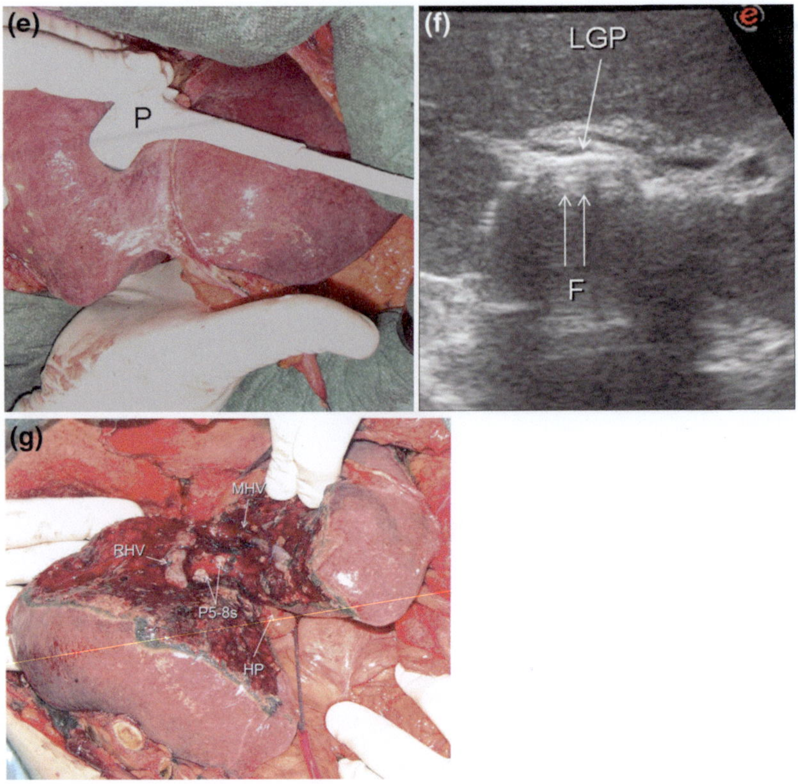

Fig. 8.35 (continued)

can be anyway visualized having at IOUS a similar aspect compared to the images obtained with the electrocautery itself (Fig. 8.37).

At this point, in the event the selected area is on a flat portion of the liver surface, stitches are applied to pull up the dissected margin (*parachute technique*), and the resection of the marked area is started (Fig. 8.38a–e). Inversely, when the expected resection area is at the edge between two opposite sides of the liver, the probe positioned on one side of the liver and the surgeon's fingertip located on the opposite but within the IOUS scanning window allows to define the resection area. Indeed, relations among the electrocautery, the fingertip, and the tumor edge can be precisely estimated, and the dissection plan can be assembled in the surgeon's mind (Fig. 8.39a, b).

The main target to be obtained once the resection area is drawn on the liver surface is that of achieving at the end of dissection the flattest and most regular cut-surface (Figs. 8.36e, 8.38c).

The features of the IOUS probes referred to in Chap. 1, as highlighted in this paragraph, assumes particular relevance. The small size and stability, allowing their easy positioning and handling (Fig. 8.40), lead to disclosing the resection area under complex anatomical conditions as the paracaval portion of the liver (Figs. 8.41a–g, 8.42a–e).

8.3 Liver Parenchyma Dissection

Traditionally, liver tissue has been dissected on straight planes following simple trajectories: for this purpose, conventional subcostal incision which requires the surgeon to assume a visual perspective of the liver surface oblique from caudal to cranial, has been recommended, and

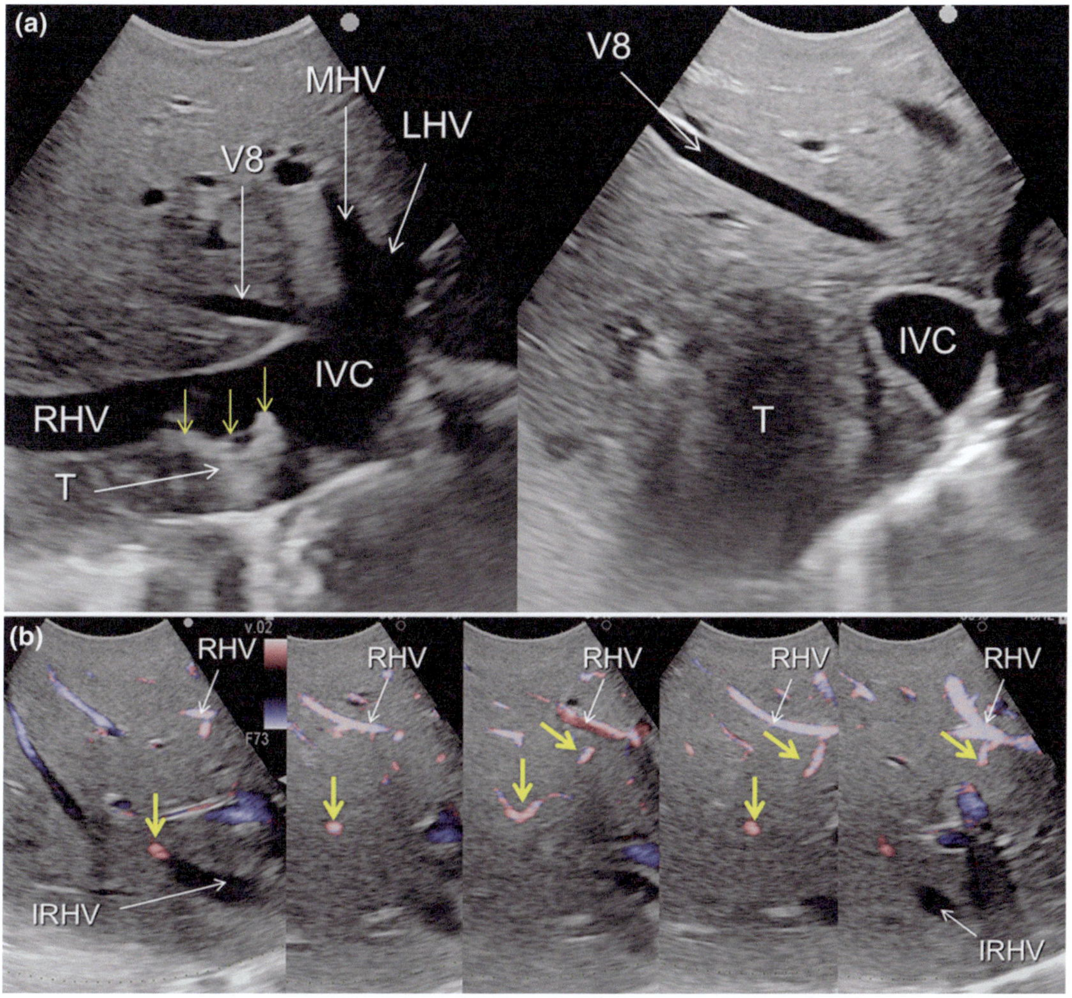

Fig. 8.36 **a** A mass-forming cholangiocellular carcinoma (*MFCCC* here disclosed as *T*) invades the right hepatic vein (*RHV*) at the caval confluence (*yellow arrows*), and below this plane lies in contact with the inferior vena cava (*IVC*); **b** communicating veins (*yellow arrows*) are evident from CFIOUS between the RHV and a thick inferior right hepatic vein (*IRHV*); **c** once having divided the RHV at the caval confluence (*RHVs1*), the resection margins are drawn using the probe (*P*) and the electrocautery (*EC*). The clue is to find a dissection plane allowing preservation of the IRHV; **d** in IOUS the shadow generated by the EC is in between the tumor and the IRHV and approaches the branch to the right posterior section (*P6-7*), which is seen posteriorly compared to the usual scan utilized for looking at this pedicle; **e** resection is carried out sparing the IRHV; on the cut surface the branch to the inferior portion of segment 7 (*P7inf*) has been preserved, and the hepatic stump of the RHV (*RHVs2*) is divided preserving a vascular arch (*dashed yellow arrow*), which should reduce the risk of congested areas keeping open the outflow through the communicating vein and the IRHV; **f** by looking at the anterior portion of the liver there are no congested areas; left hepatic vein (*LHV*); middle hepatic vein (*MHV*); portal branch to the right anterior section (*P5-8*); hepatic vein draining segment 8 (*V8*) and flowing into the common trunk of LHV and MHV

IOUS guidance using the feedback of positioning the surgeon's left hand behind the liver has not been felt essential. Inversely, IOUS guidance allowing to follow the dissection plane in real-time, by placing it constantly in reference to the tumor edge, and with the fingertips of the surgeon's left hand positioned on the opposite side of the dissection plane ''waiting'' for its full

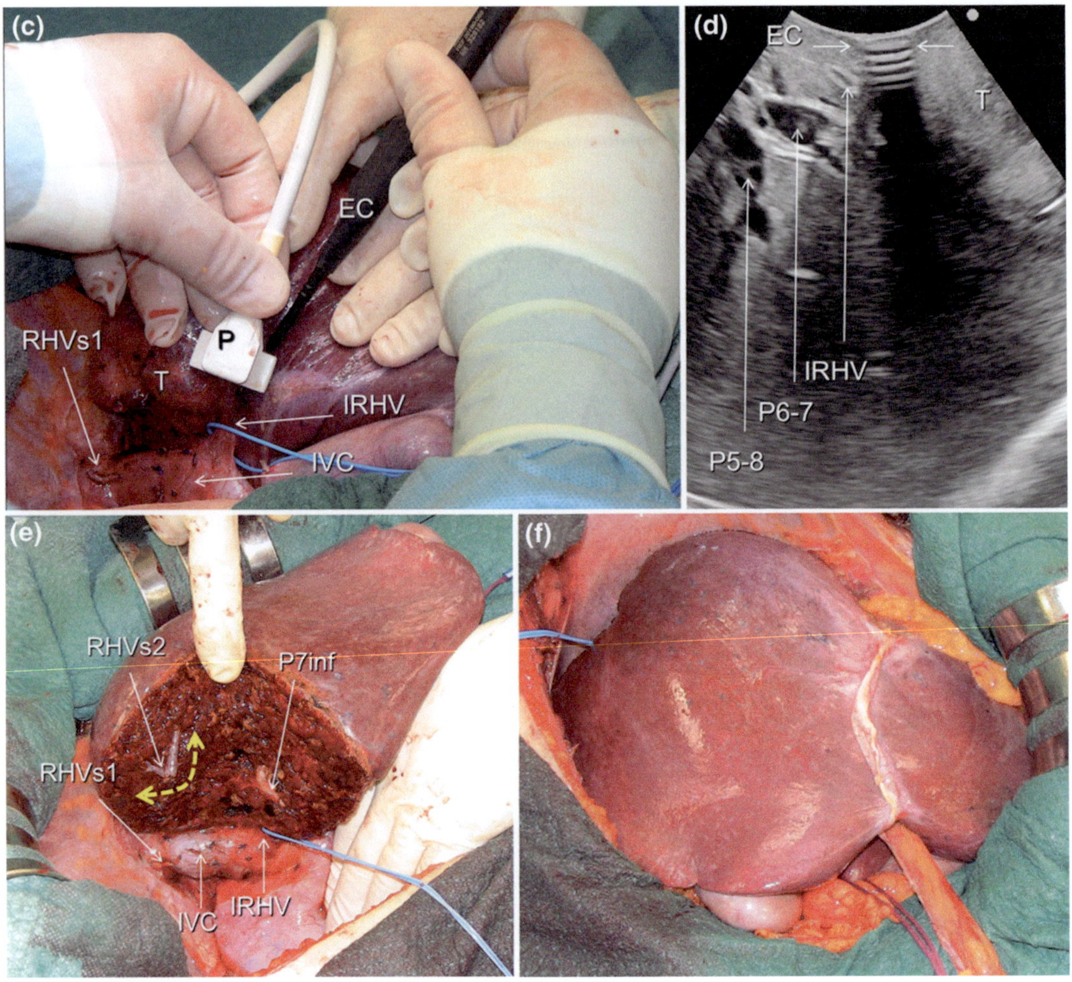

Fig. 8.36 (continued)

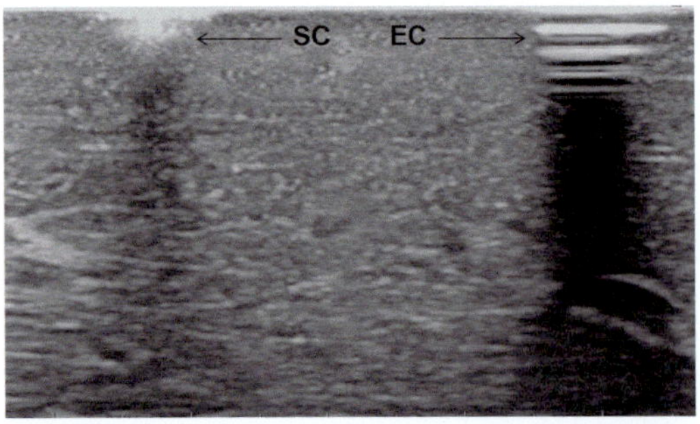

Fig. 8.37 Scar (*SC*) generated by the electrocautery mimicking the shadow produced by the electrocautery (*EC*) itself

accomplishment, has opened the field to new and geometrically more complex trajectories of dissections. Indeed, this constant visual and manual monitoring allows then to modify the trajectory when needed. The dissection plane is constantly visible by IOUS appearing as a more or less intense echogenic line formed by the entrapped air bubbles and clots between the faced cut surfaces (Fig. 8.43a). If the dissection plane is not clearly visible, specifically devised silicon gauze between the facing cut surfaces can be inserted or simply a common gauze can be used (Fig. 8.43b). The latter has the advantage of better visualization but the disadvantage of masking the structures lying posteriorly.

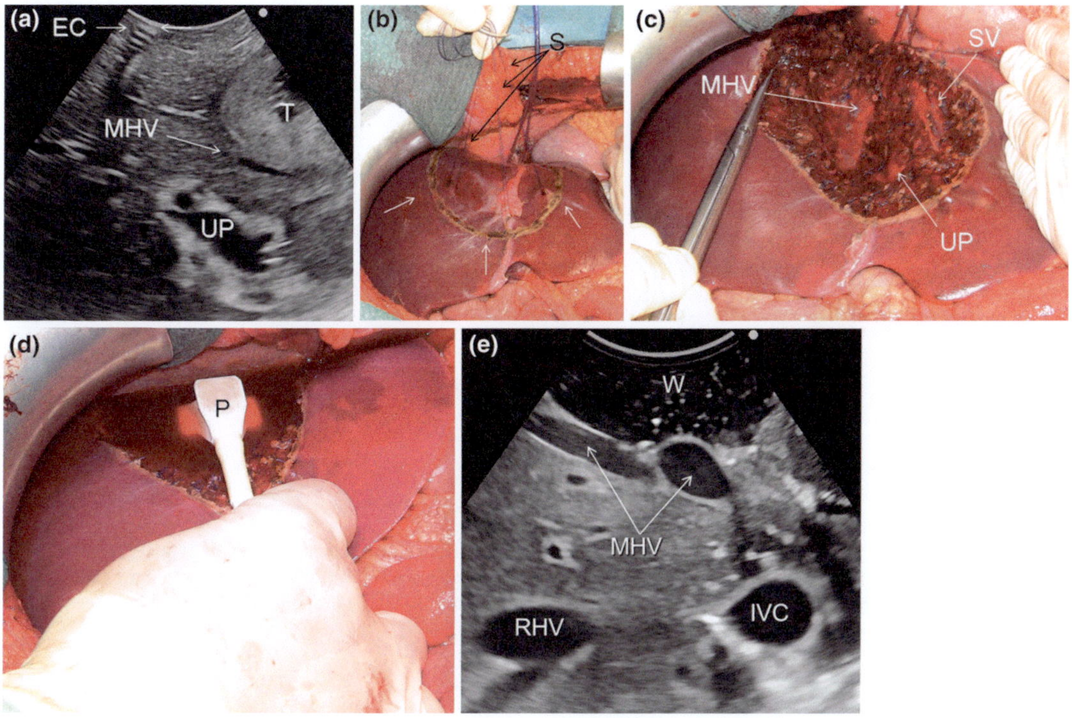

Fig. 8.38 **a** For this lesion in contact with the middle hepatic vein (*MHV*) the resection area is drawn using the electrocautery (*EC*) as usual; **b** the flat surface of the resection area (*arrows*) suggests to put stitches at three of its four cardinal points (*S*) for pulling up the margins while dissection is started (parachute technique); **c** resection is then accomplished using as repeatedly suggested the surgeon's left hand for helping guidance, and resulting in the exposure of the MHV, the scissural vein (*SV*), and the umbilical portion (*UP*); **d** the cut surface is checked with the water-bath technique; **e** from the IOUS the MHV is well visible, as the right hepatic vein (*RHV*) and the inferior vena cava (*IVC*); probe (*P*); water (*W*)

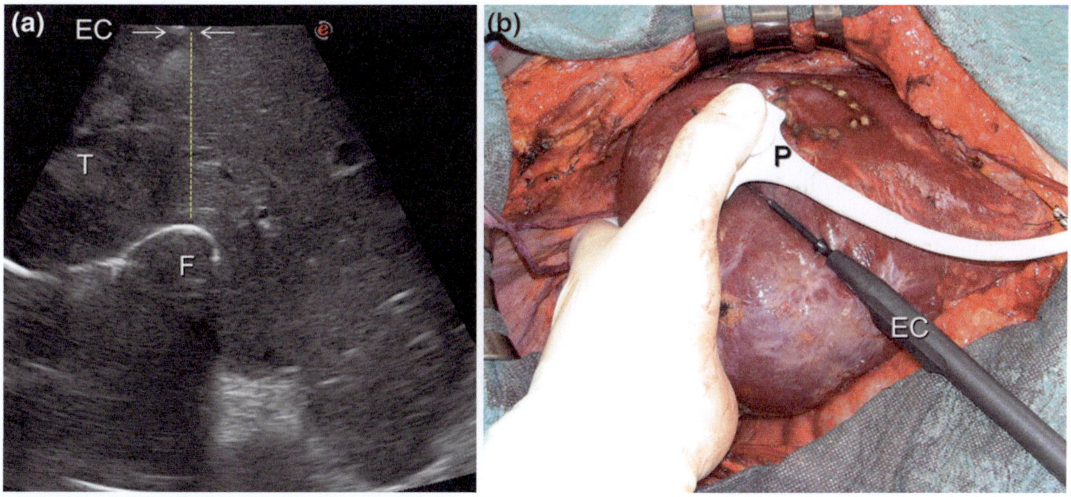

Fig. 8.39 **a** For this lesion the virtual dissection plane delimitated by the finger (*F*) and the electrocautery (*EC*) is quite simple (*dashed yellow arrows*), being at the edge between the anterior and the posterior surfaces of the liver; **b** for this reason there is no need for the parachute technique. Resection is drawn and the surgeon's left hand will provide the traction to open the space between the faced cut surfaces, then allowing to proceed safely with the resection; probe (*P*); tumor (*T*)

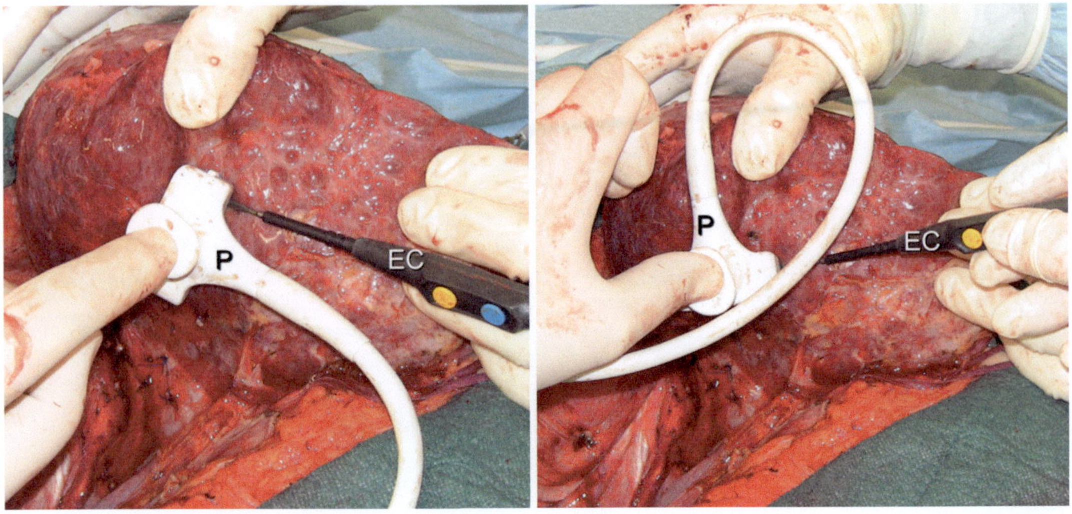

Fig. 8.40 Small size and stability are indispensable features for easily accomplishing those maneuvers which often need to be performed using just one hand; here, it is possible to see how this probe can be maintained adhered to the liver surface despite its irregularity, just fixing it with a fingertip and allowing easy demarcation of the resection area; electrocautery (*EC*); probe (*P*)

In some cases, to better visualize the trajectory of the dissection, the finger can be inserted between the facing cut surfaces. The latter also has the advantage of allowing the palpation of the lesion with the fingertip once the dissection gets closer to it (Fig. 8.44). All these maneuvers allow the surgeon to keep to the proper dissection plane. Recognizing a wrong dissection plane early, permits prompt modification and avoidance of possibly incomplete tumor removal (Fig. 8.45) or damaging structures which need to be preserved (Fig. 8.46a–e), or in case of multinodular patterns to miss resection of some lesions (Fig. 8.47). In this way it is possible to carry out a rounded trajectory of the dissection plane around the tumor allowing its complete removal even with tumor exposure, and enabling to spare important vascular structures. This results in conservative but radical treatments, and in a lower rate of major hepatectomies.

It is worth to repeat how the role of the surgeon's left hand is important in giving direction to the dissection of the liver as guided by IOUS, and in fact hanging the liver, anticipating what has then been proposed for driving the right hepatectomy by an anterior approach [29].

Artifacts in IOUS showing the dissection plane can sometimes mask structures such as portal branches which should be ligated or conversely retained. The so-called *hooking technique* has been devised to better visualize the targeted point where the portal branch should be divided [30]. When the glissonian sheath is exposed and skeletonized, it is encircled with a stitch (Fig. 8.48a). Then under IOUS control, the stitch hooking the exposed vessel is gently pulled up (Fig. 8.48b), which stretches the portal branch slightly and the traction point is demonstrated clearly by IOUS (Figs. 8.48c, 8.49a, b). If the exposed portal branch is not clearly visible in IOUS because it has collapsed, the portal triad is unclamped. If the target site is correct, the portal branch is ligated and divided and resection is completed under IOUS guidance. Conversely, if the exposed vessel was not the targeted one, it is spared and useless sacrifice of further liver parenchyma is avoided.

The hooking technique is particularly useful in ventral or dorsal subsegmentectomy of segment 8 (Fig. 8.50a, b). The portal trunk to this segment may show a bifurcation in its dorsal branch and ventral trunk just close to the origin

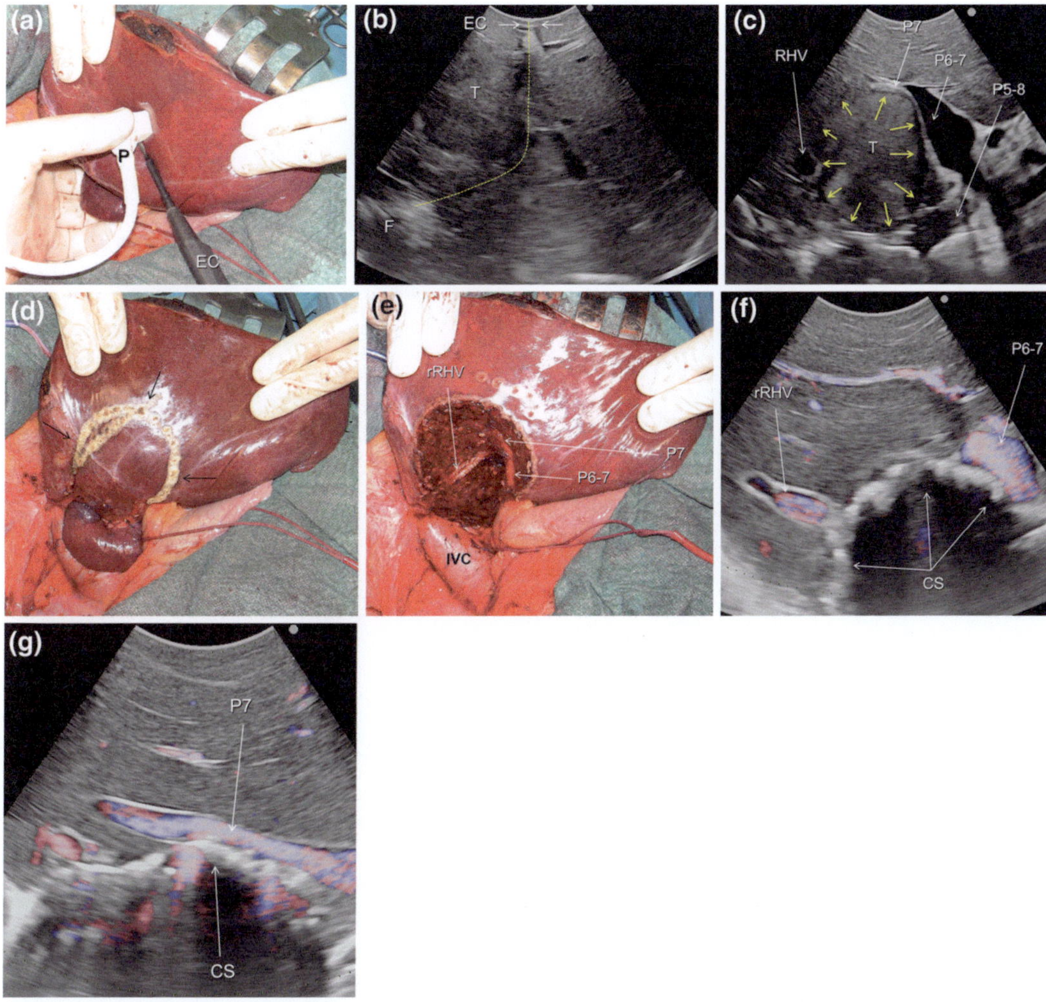

Fig. 8.41 **a** Relevance of probe stability once the surgeon with his left-hand fingertips positioned at the edge between segments 2 and 1 (where the Arantius' ligament runs) somehow hooks the caudate lobe, while with the same hand fixes the probe (*P*) on the liver surface, then drawing the resection area using the electrocautery (*EC*); **b** from IOUS, EC and surgeon's fingertip (*F*) delineated the virtual plane (*dashed yellow line*) to remove the tumor (*T*) located in the paracaval portion; **c, d** in spite the complex position of the lesion in IOUS, which is in contact (*yellow arrows*) with the right hepatic vein (*RHV*) and the portal branch to the right posterior section (*P6-7*), having as a sort of roof the portal branch to the right anterior section (*P5-8*) (**c**), the planned resection is particularly limited (*arrows*) (**d**); **e** on the cut surface P6-7 and the RHV, which has been patched with bovine pericardium for partial tumor invasion (rRHV), are exposed together with the branch to segment 7 (*P7*), which has been preserved too; P5-8 is exposed too but masked in the picture by P6-7; **f, g** from CFIOUS the rRHV (**f**), P6-7 (**f**), and P7 (**g**) are perfectly patent; cut surface (*CS*); inferior vena cava (*IVC*)

of the portal vessel to segment 5. In this case, there is a risk of ligating and dividing the portal branch of segment 5 instead of the planned subsegmental branch of segment 8 which would lead to segment 5 becoming devascularized. The hooking technique under IOUS control enables confirmation of the branch that was encircled, and then the surgeon can decide with certainty whether to ligate it. This technique is also useful in case of tumor thrombus in major

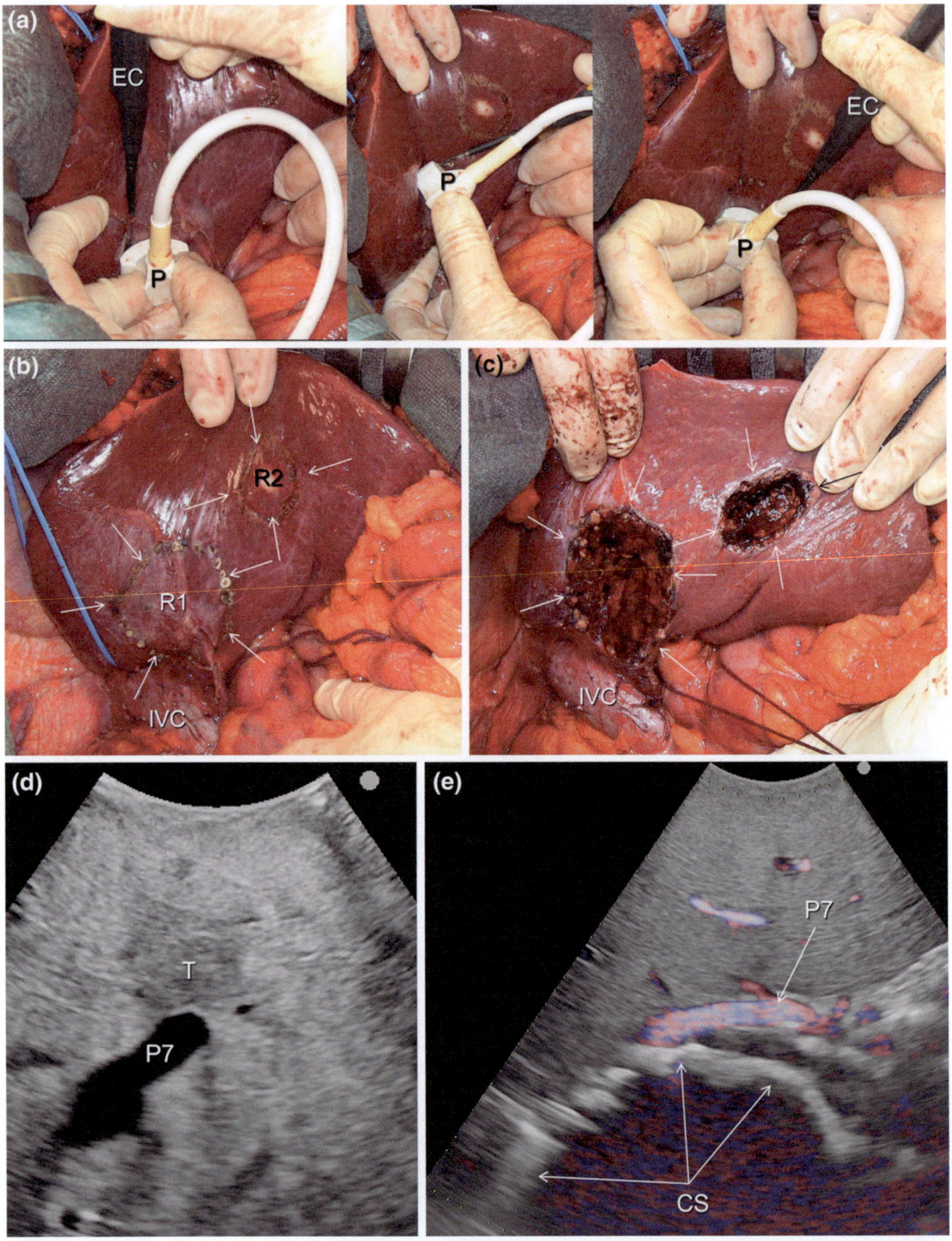

Fig. 8.42 **a** From *left* to *right*: drawing with the probe (*P*) and the electrocautery (*EC*) of a resection area in the paracaval portion of the liver; **b** the resection areas (*R1* and *R2*) are then drawn (*arrows*); **c** limited resections are carried out (*arrows*); **d**, **e** in IOUS the tumor (*T*) before resection (*R1*) is shown in contact with the portal branch to segment 7 (*P7*) (**d**), which was spared and remained patent at the postresectional check with CFIOUS (**e**); cut surface (*CS*); inferior vena cava (*IVC*)

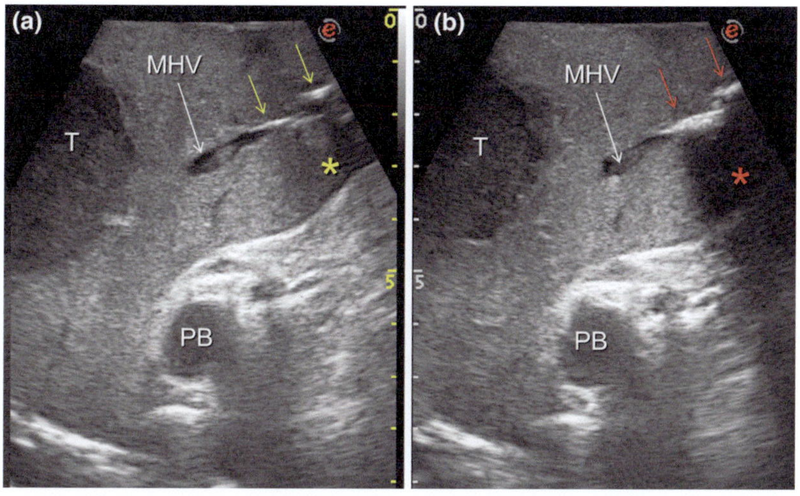

Fig. 8.43 **a** The dissection line (*yellow arrows*), as it appears facing each other the cut surfaces: this generates moderate posterior artifacts (*) but makes less evident the dissection plane; **b** the dissection line (*red arrows*) as it appears putting a gauze between the facing cut surfaces: this modality generates strong posterior artifacts acting as a true barrier to the ultrasound (*) but makes more evident the dissection plane; middle hepatic vein (*MHV*); portal bifurcation (*PB*); tumor (*T*)

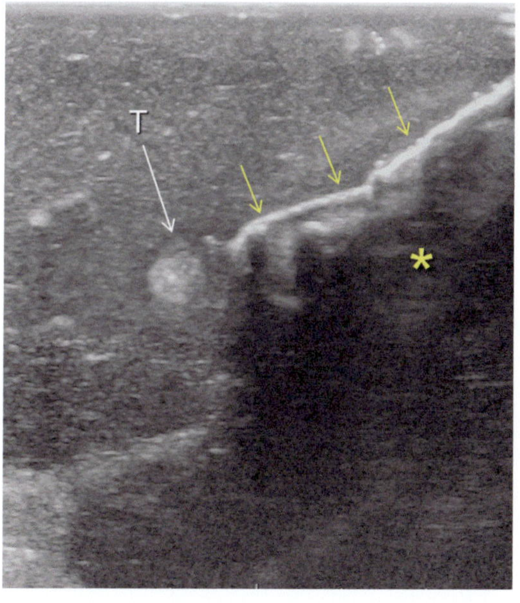

Fig. 8.44 The finger inserted between the facing cut surfaces can more clearly make visible the dissection plane (*yellow arrows*), and, despite the strong artifacts (*), it allows the surgeon to feel and when closer even palpate the lesion to confirm the proper dissection plane: this is particularly useful for tiny lesions (*T*) as the one represented here

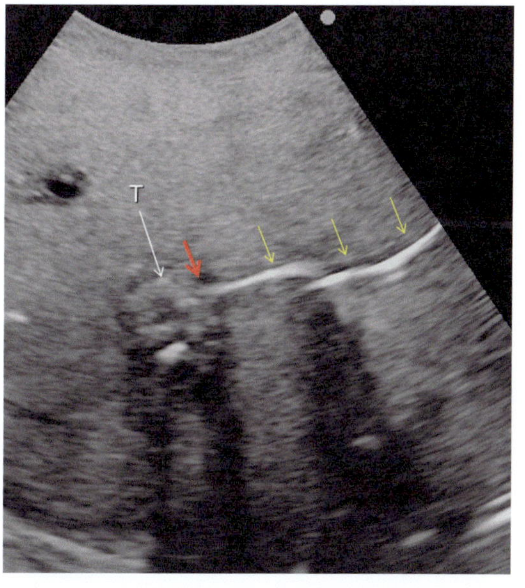

Fig. 8.45 Following the dissection plane is fundamental for avoiding tumor division and thus leaving residual neoplastic tissue: IOUS showing the dissection plane (*yellow arrows*) having encountered the tumor (*T*) (*red arrow*), and needing to be modified

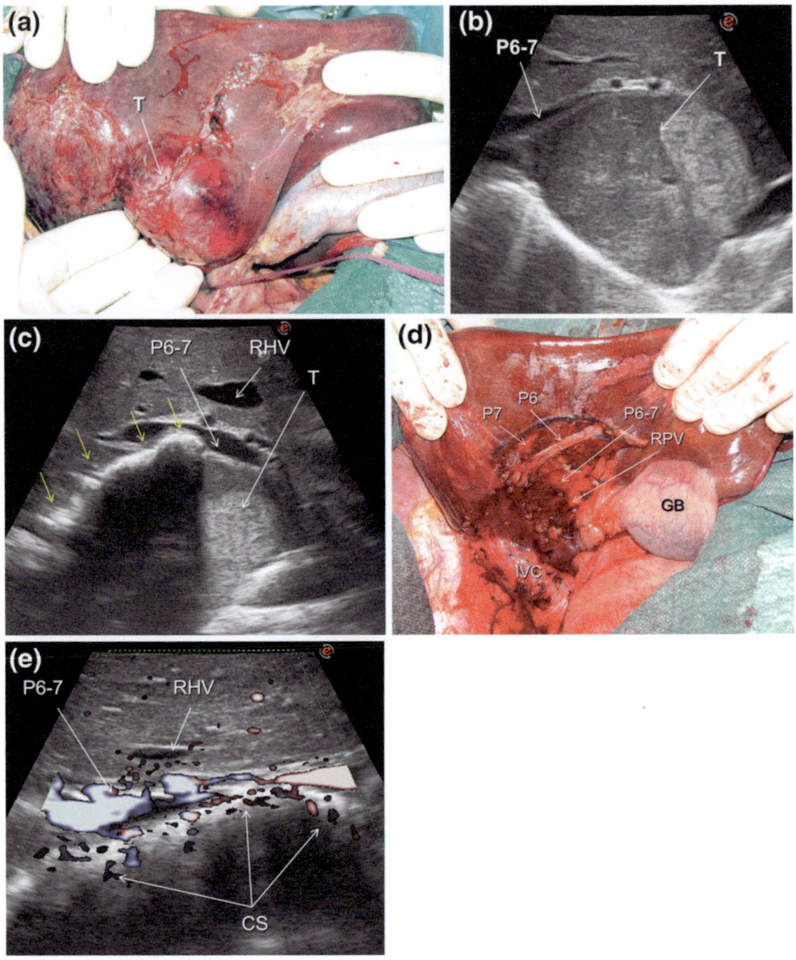

Fig. 8.46 **a** A large HCC (*T*) occupying the right-sided paracaval portion of segment 1 and the caudate process; **b** IOUS shows a tumor with a typical mosaic pattern, dislodging and compressing the portal pedicle to the right posterior section (*P6-7*); **c** the dissection plane (*yellow arrows*) has to be followed carefully to avoid damaging of the major vascular structures: in this sense IOUS allows keeping it under constant control; **d** once the tumor has been removed on the cut surface, P6-7 and the branches feeding segments 6 (*P6*) and 7 (*P7*) are well exposed as the right portal branch (*RPV*); **e** CFIOUS confirms the patency of the exposed vessels; gallbladder (*GB*); right hepatic vein (*RHV*)

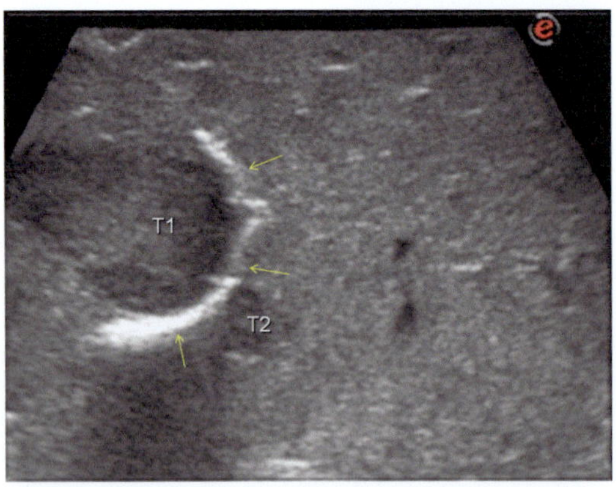

Fig. 8.47 Monitoring the dissection plane is fundamental also for avoiding to inadvertently miss tumor removal: IOUS clearly shows the dissection line (*yellow arrows*) would miss a tiny lesion (*T2*) adjacent to the main one (*T1*) in a patient with multiple bilobar colorectal liver metastases (at the end 25 lesions will be removed)

portal branches [31]. Here, once the portal branch is skeletonized, it is encircled with a stitch and, under IOUS control, the stitch is gently pulled up. This traction stretches the portal branch slightly and the traction point is demonstrated clearly by IOUS (Fig. 8.51a–c). If the traction point is not at the level of the tumor thrombus it is possible to ligate the portal branch and proceed with the liver resection being sure that the thrombus is going to be entirely removed. Of course this method can also be applied similarly for more peripheral portal branches (Fig. 8.52a–i).

During liver dissection the backflow bleeding from the hepatic veins causes significant blood loss. Therefore, limiting its occurrence is a

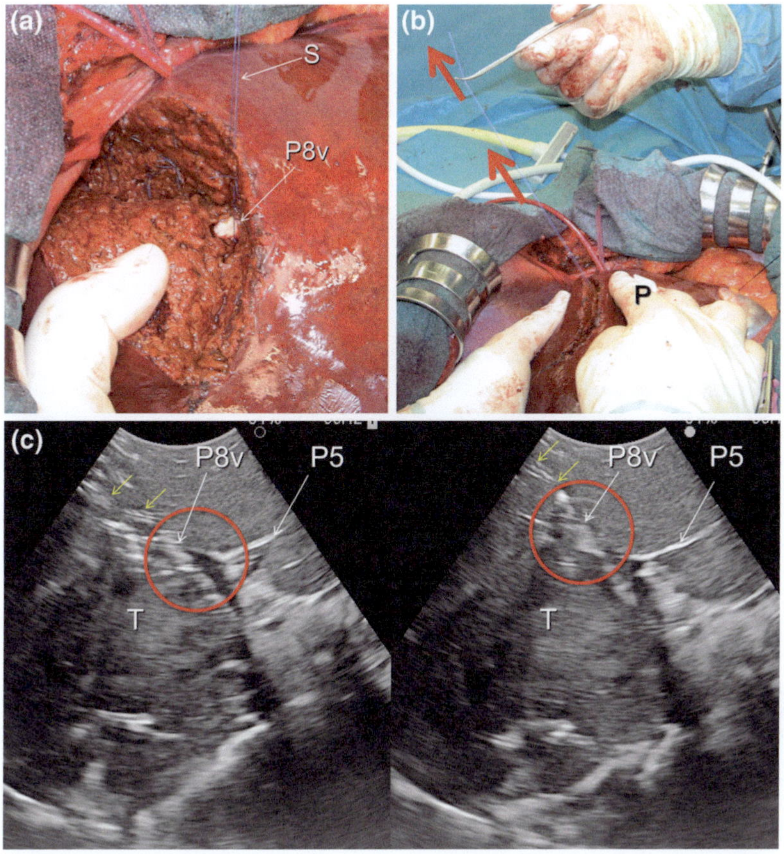

Fig. 8.48 **a** The glissonian pedicle of segment 8 ventral (*P8v*) has appeared on the dissection plane and is encircled with a suture (*S*) for ligation; **b** however, before ligating and dividing the pedicle, IOUS is used and the suture is pulled up (*red arrows*) under its control; **c** on the left in IOUS the *yellow arrows* indicate the dissection plane through which the suture is passing and the *red circle* points out the site that should move in case the pedicle is the one the surgeon is thinking he has encircled (P8v rather than the pedicle to segment 5 superior which is herein indicated as P5); on the right, once the suture is pulled up the site moves up (*red circle*) stretching P8v confirming that the latter is the encircled pedicle: then, its ligation and division can be carried out safely; probe (*P*); tumor (*T*)

priority in liver resections. The surgeon's left hand hanging the liver other than driving the dissection contributes in controlling such backflow bleeding. However, as mentioned here and in Chap. 7, IOUS can play a role in this sense too. Indeed, an ultrasound-guided technique has recently been described for controlling backflow bleeding from the RHV during right-sided liver resection [32]. The technique is simple and is now applied to every hepatic vein. Once the hepatocaval confluence is exposed anteriorly, dissection can proceed until the right surface of the extrahepatic RHV is exposed in case the RHV has to be controlled, the left surface of the extrahepatic LHV for the LHV itself, and the right-anterior surface of the MHV for the MHV itself (Figs. 8.11, 8.53a, b). The surgeon's fingertips compress the vessel at the exposed side, and the effectiveness of finger compression is checked by CFIOUS (Figs. 8.18, 8.54a–d).

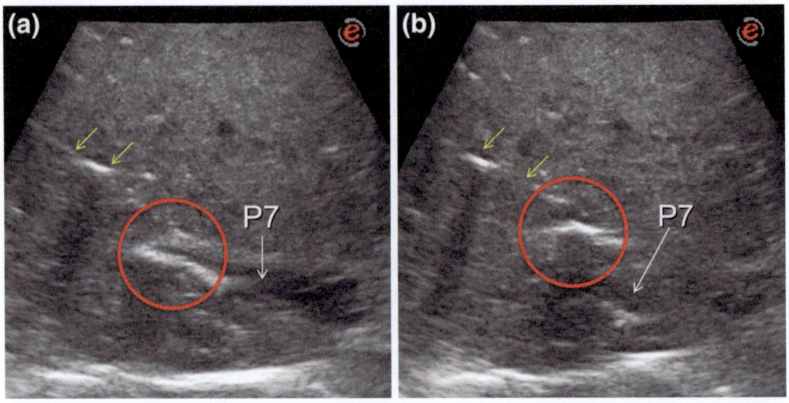

Fig. 8.49 **a** In this IOUS the *yellow arrows* indicate the dissection plane through which the suture should have passed and the *red circle* points out the site that should move in case the pedicle is the one the surgeon is thinking he has encircled (glissonian pedicle to segment 7 herein indicated as P7); **b** once the suture is pulled up, the site moves up (*red circle*) stretching P7 and confirming that this is the encircled pedicle: then, its ligation and division can be carried out safely

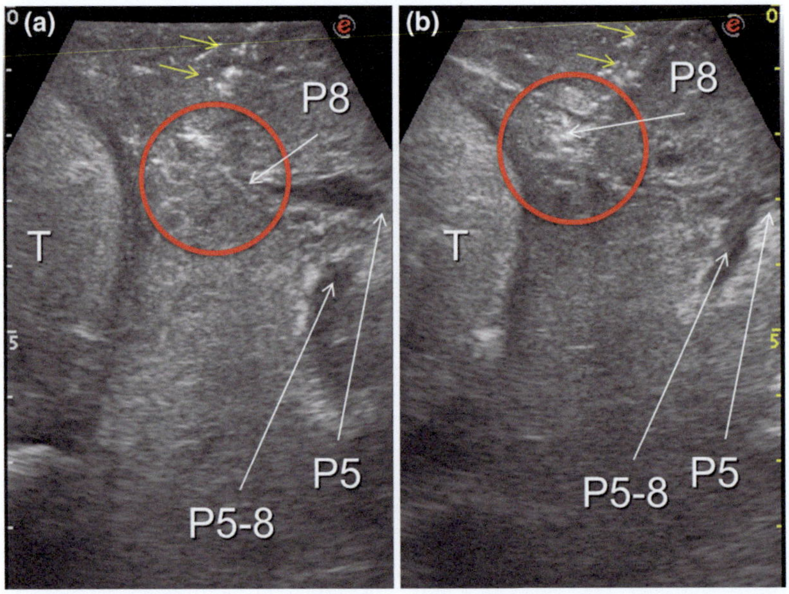

Fig. 8.50 **a** In this IOUS the *yellow arrows* indicate the dissection plane through which the suture should have passed and the *red circle* points out the site that should move in case the pedicle is the one the surgeon is thinking he has encircled (glissonian pedicle to segment 8 herein indicated as P8); **b** once the suture is pulled up, the site moves up (*red circle*) stretching P8, and confirming this is the encircled pedicle: then, its ligation and division can be carried out safely; portal branch to segment 5 (*P5*); portal branch to the right anterior section (*P5-8*); tumor (*T*)

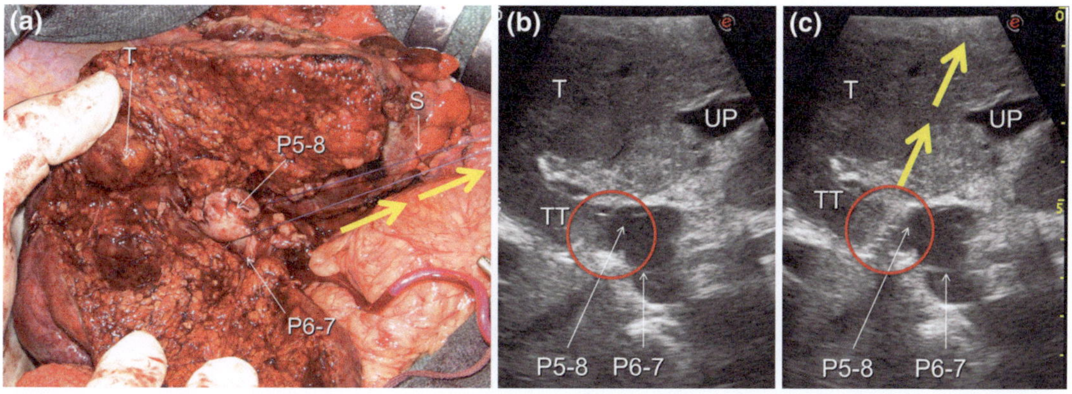

Fig. 8.51 **a** During the dissection for performing a right anterior sectionectomy in a patient with an HCC with portal vein thrombosis in the pedicle to the right anterior section (*P5-8*), the latter is skeletonized and encircled with a suture (*S*) at its origin; the suture will be gently pulled up (*yellow arrows*) under IOUS guidance; **b** in IOUS the margin of the tumor thrombus (*TT*) is well visible within P5-8 (*red circle*); **c** once the suture is slightly pulled up, not to risk dividing the thrombus, the site moves up (*red circle*) stretching P5-8 just before the edge of the thrombus: therefore, the level of the encirclement is suitable for ligation with no risk of thrombus division and incomplete removal; portal branch to the right posterior section (*P6-7*); tumor (*T*); umbilical portion (*UP*)

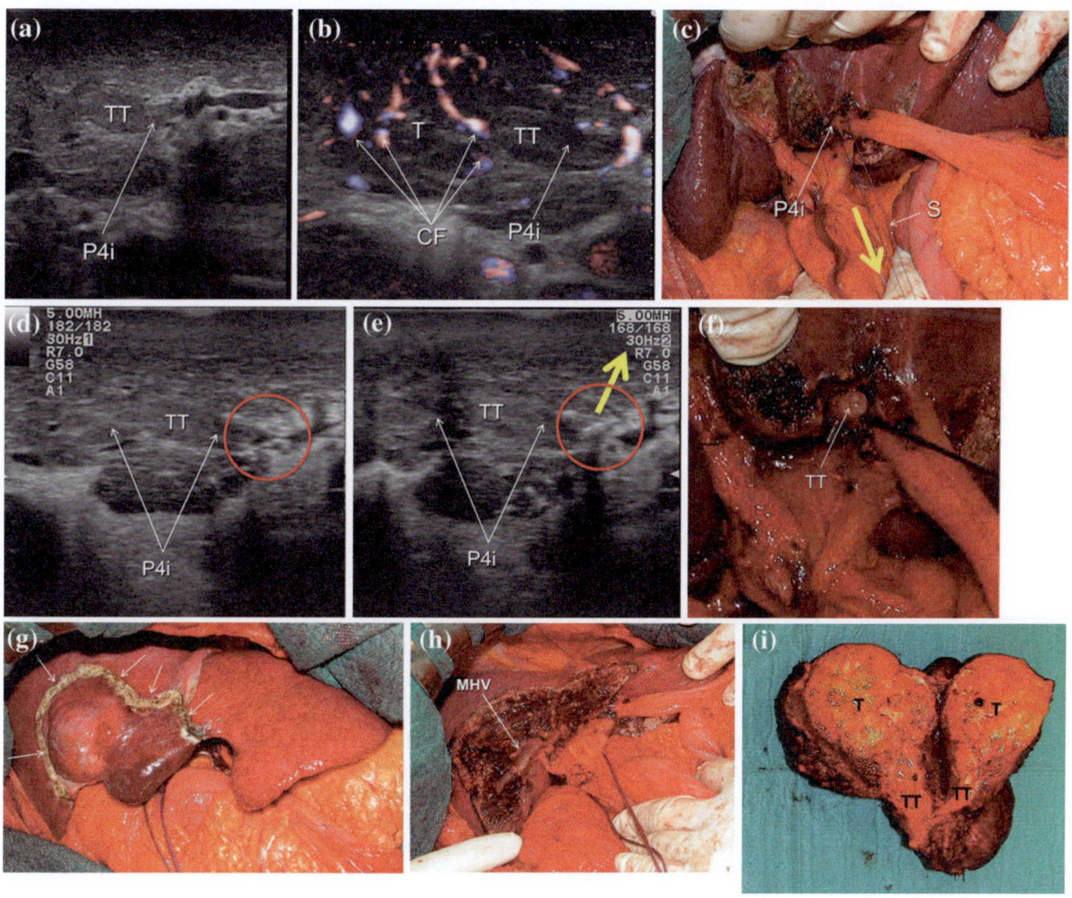

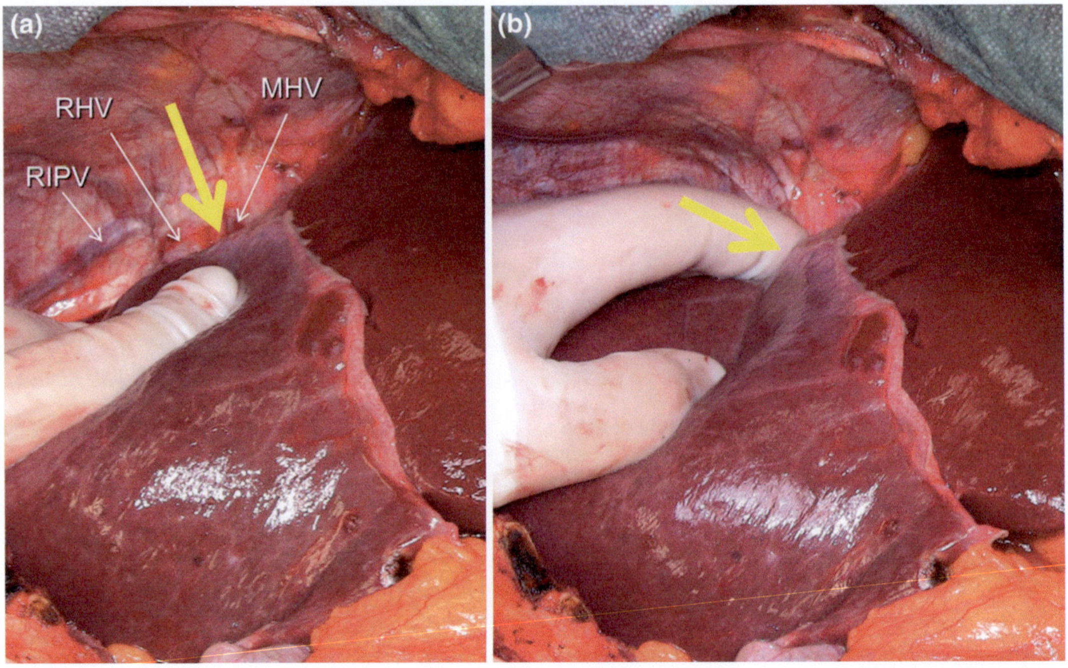

Fig. 8.53 **a** The *yellow arrow* points to the space between the right (*RHV*) and middle hepatic vein (*MHV*); **b** the finger is allocated in that fossa (*yellow arrow*) enabling the surgeon to compress the MHV and reduce backflow bleeding if needed: this maneuver, together with a low central venous pressure maintained by the anesthesiologist, reduces the need for clamping the vein; right inferior phrenic vein (*RIPV*)

8.3.1 Other Methods for Liver Dissection Guidance

Dissection guidance has become possible through tracking systems which combine the position of the dissecting instruments and software reconstructing three-dimensional liver images based on preoperative CT or MRI or three-dimensional ultrasound [33]. These approaches offer real-time and continued guidance of liver dissection, rather than simple IOUS guidance, which can be done repeatedly but does not provide information if dissection is not interrupted for ultrasound check. However, the little data provided so far are not sufficient to disclose a real advantage of the approach, which on the other hand, seems rather complex. A free line between the tracking system and the trackers allocated on the ultrasound probe and the used dissecting instrument has to be maintained, otherwise data registration for navigation is interrupted. In this sense, tracking systems can be optical for which a free line sight has to be maintained between the instruments or electromagnetic system, which on the other hand, is sensitive to disturbances originated by the

◀**Fig. 8.52** **a** IOUS in presence of an HCC occupying segment 4 inferior in the feeding portal branch (*P4i*) discloses a tumor thrombus (*TT*); **b** CFIOUS confirms the hypervascular pattern (*CF*) of the tumor from which the thrombus is originating; **c** P4i is encircled at its origin and gentle traction will be applied to the suture (*S*) under IOUS guidance before eventual ligation and division; **d** IOUS showing the site which is expected to be the level of encirclement (*red circle*); **e** once gentle traction is applied (*yellow arrow*) it is confirmed that the site of encirclement is not at the level of the tumor thrombus (*red circle*); **f** once the vein is divided, the integrity of the tumor thrombus is confirmed; **g** the resection area is marked (*arrows*); **h** an anatomical resection of segment 4 inferior is carried out having properly exposed the distal portion of the middle hepatic vein (*MHV*); **i** the specimen confirms the integrity of the tumor thrombus which has been entirely removed

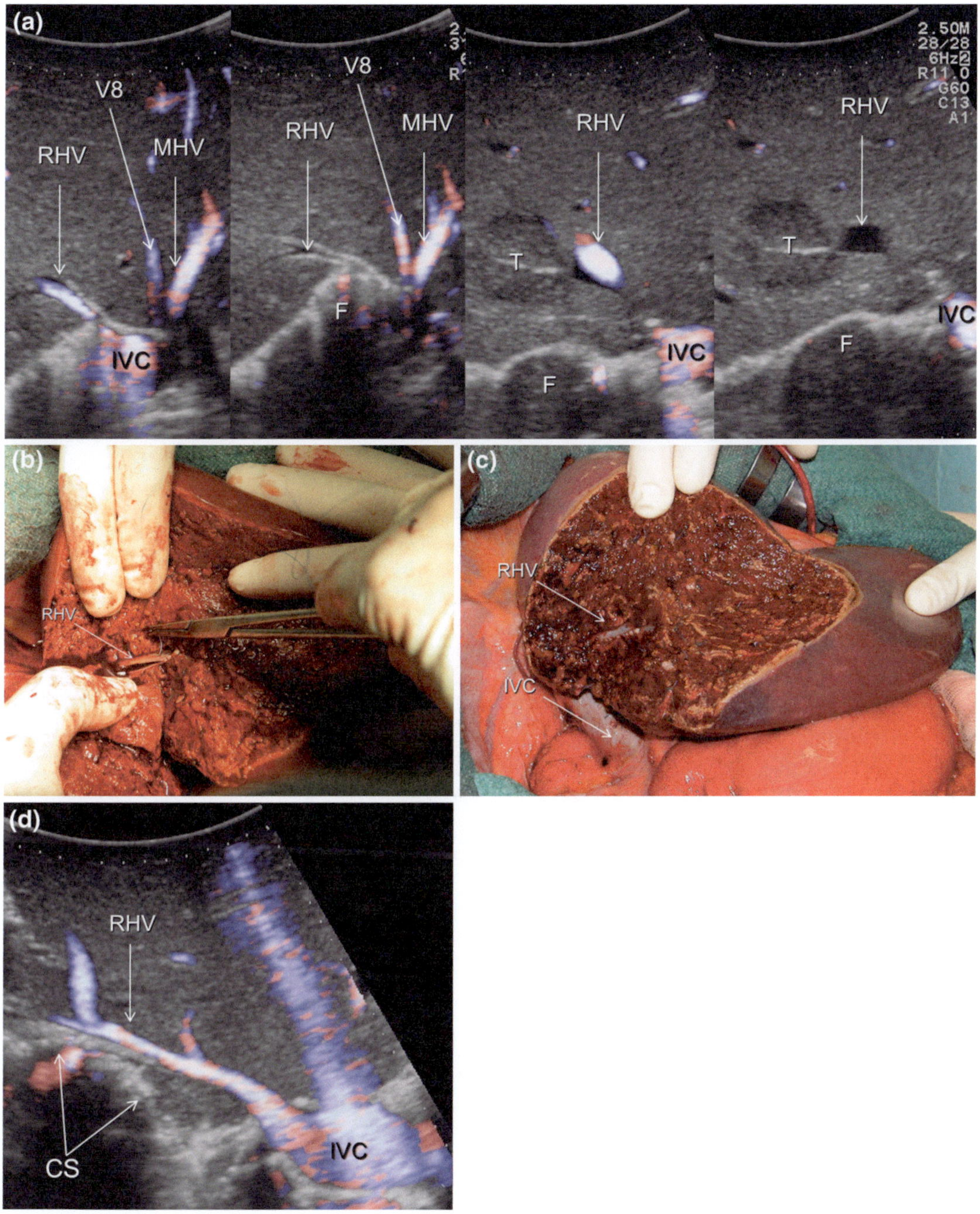

Fig. 8.54 **a** Patient with a colorectal metastasis (*T*) in contact with the right hepatic vein (*RHV*) but relatively distant from the caval confluence; once (on the *left*), at the caval confluence, and above the tumor location, the RHV is compressed with the finger (*F*) the color-flow disappears from the lumen and this is confirmed (on the *right*) at the level of the tumor-vein contact; **b** despite the relatively minimal contact, the detachment has been associated with a minimal wall resection for which a running suture has been needed for reconstruction. This has been done just compressing the RHV at the caval confluence with no need for clamping although the vein was previously encircled; **c** the cut surface at the end of the resection with the RHV reconstructed by direct suture; **d** CFIOUS confirms the regular patency of the reconstructed RHV which is facing the cut surface (*CS*); inferior vena cava (*IVC*); middle hepatic vein (*MHV*); hepatic vein draining segment 8 (*V8*) and flowing into the MHV at caval confluence

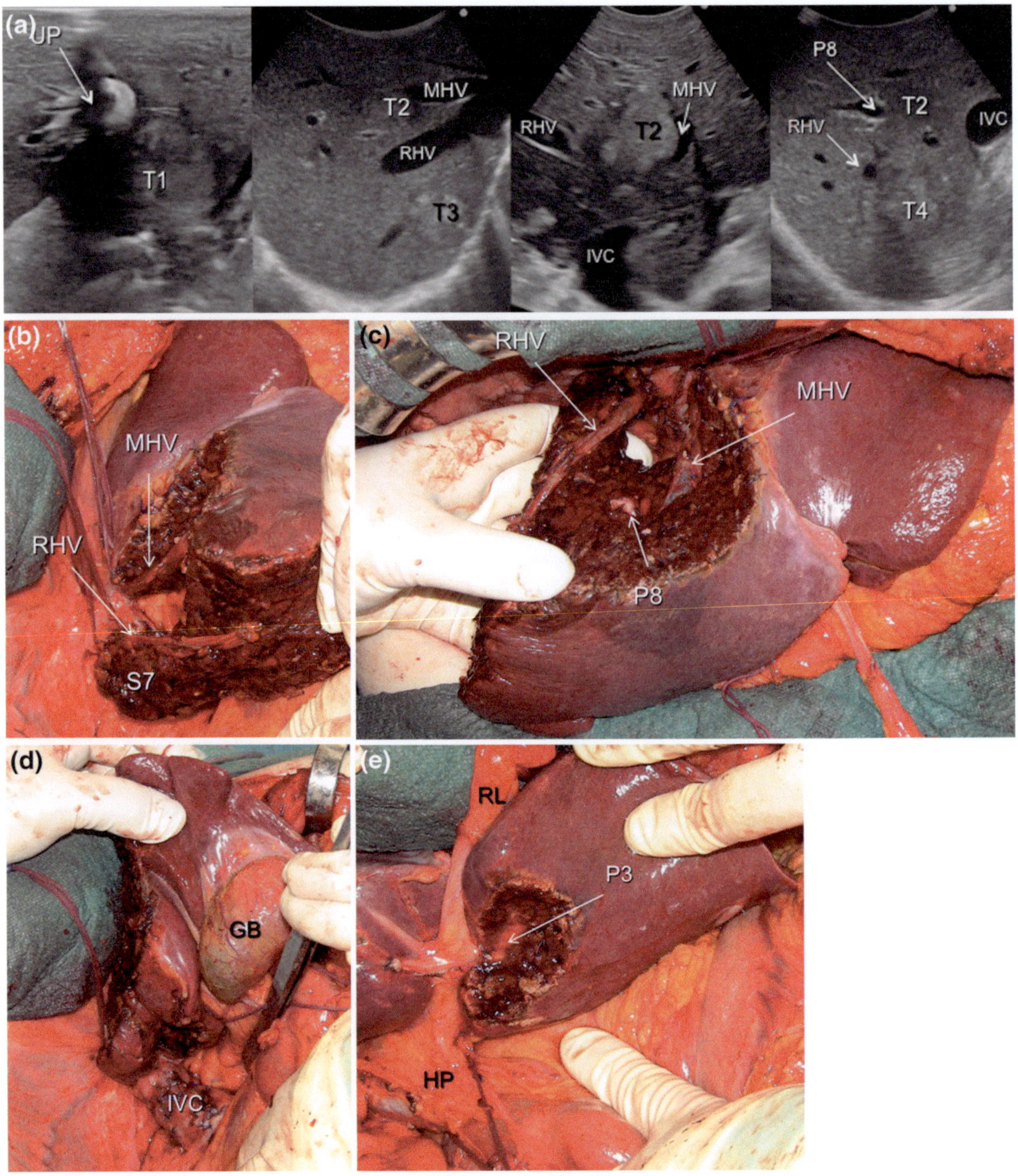

Fig. 8.55 **a** Multiple colorectal liver metastases of which one (*T1*) was below and in contact with the umbilical portion (*UP*) in segment 3, another (*T2*) was in contact with the middle hepatic vein (*MHV*), the right hepatic vein (*RHV*), and the portal branch to segment 8 (*P8*), occupying segment 8, and the paracaval portion of segment 1, a third (*T3*) was in segment 7, and a fourth (*T4*) was just behind and in contact with the RHV along its mid-tract; **b**, **c** the hepatectomy consisted in a partial resection of segments 6 and 7 enlarged to the entire segment 8 and the paracaval portion including the caudate lobe; the RHV at caval confluence remained sustained by a portion of segment 7 (*S7*), which was preserved with its portal pedicle, while the MHV was fully exposed; **d** the paracaval portion was removed; **e** the tumor in segment 3 was removed exposing on the cut surface the segmental portal pedicle (*P3*); gallbladder (*GB*); hepatic pedicle (*HP*); inferior vena cava (*IVC*); round ligament (*RL*)

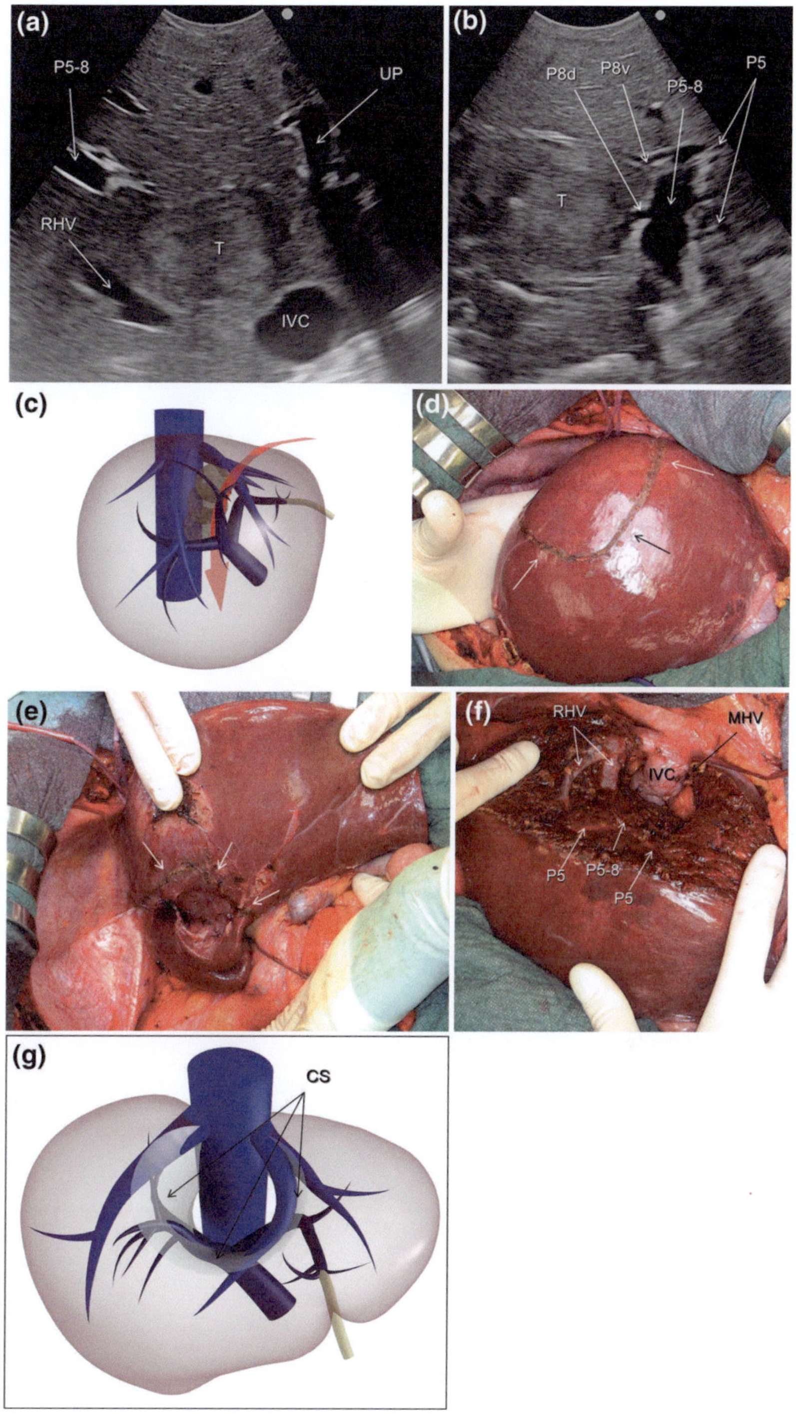

Fig. 8.56 **a**, **b** Single colorectal liver metastasis (*T*) located, as shown by IOUS, behind (**a**) and above (**b**) the pedicle to the right anterior section (*P5-8*), adjacent to the right hepatic vein (*RHV*) and the umbilical portion (*UP*) and just in front the inferior vena cava (*IVC*) (**a**); the tumor was fed by the pedicles originating from P5-8 to segment 8 ventral (*P8v*) and dorsal (*P8d*) (**b**); **c** the presentation can be assimilated to those suitable for the liver tunnel (see Chap. 7) procedure, which was planned with a main dissection plane represented by the *red arrow*; **d**, **e** the drawn resection area (*arrows*) visualized frontally (**d**), and posteriorly (**e**); **f** at the end on the cut surface pedicles to segment 5 (*P5*) the dorsal aspect of P5-8, the RHV and the middle hepatic vein (*MHV*) were exposed together with the IVC; **g** schematically a liver tunnel was accomplished; cut surface (*CS*)

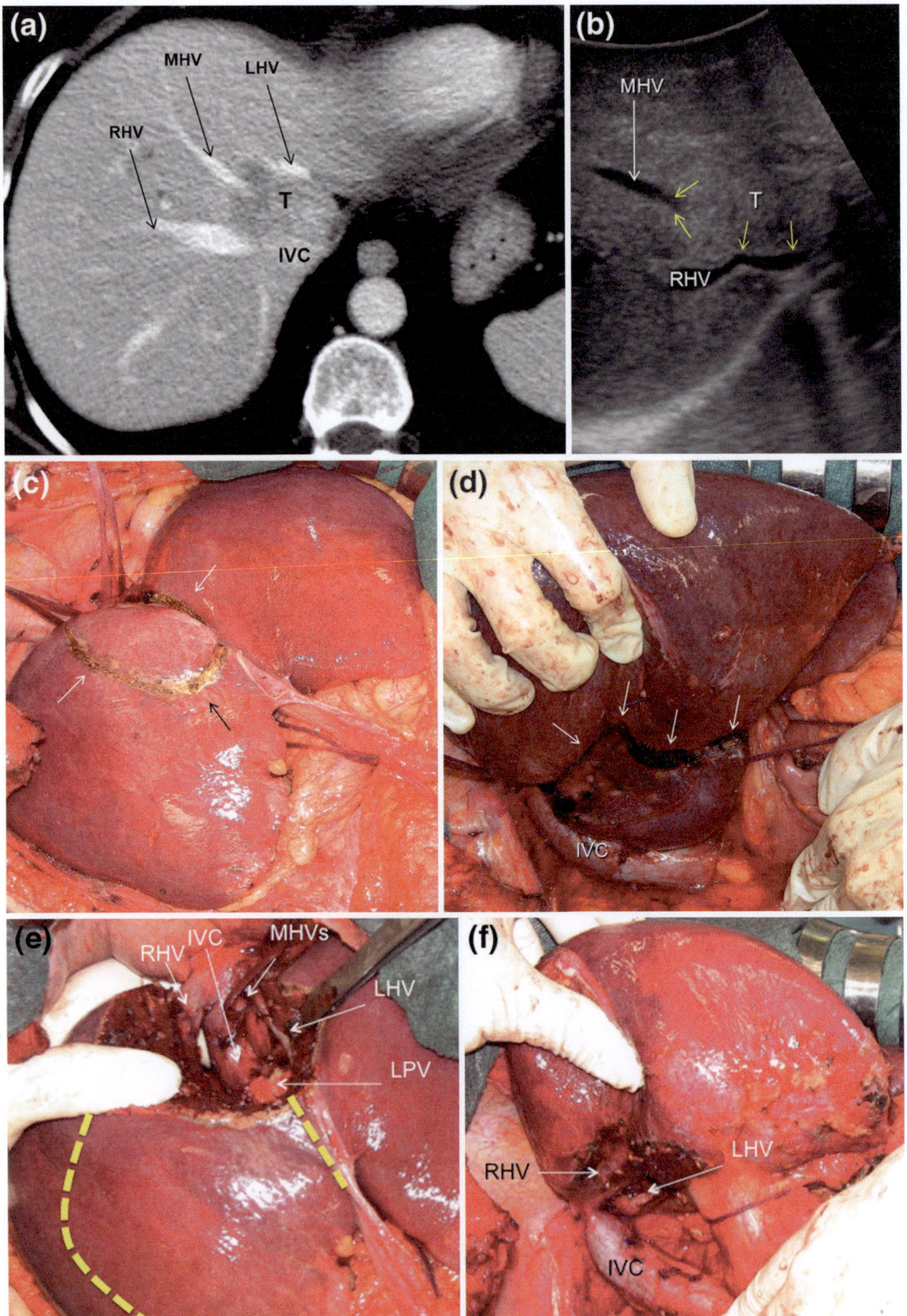
(a)
MHV
LHV
RHV
T
IVC
(b)
MHV
T
RHV
(c)
(d)
IVC
(e)
RHV
IVC
MHVs
LHV
LPV
(f)
RHV
LHV
IVC

Fig. 8.57 **a** This patient had a single mass-forming cholangiocarcinoma (*T*), which, as shown in this computed tomography, was located in the paracaval portion of segment 1, being in contact at the caval confluence with the inferior vena cava (*IVC*), the right hepatic vein (*RHV*), and the left hepatic vein (*LHV*), and invading the middle hepatic vein (*MHV*); **b** in IOUS the lesion appears slightly hyperechoic and appeared invading the MHV (*yellow arrows*), and in close contact with the RHV (*yellow arrows*); **c**, **d** the presentation having communicating veins (*CV*) at IOUS between RHV and MHV, can be assimilated to those suitable for the liver tunnel procedure associated with a mini-mesohepatectomy (see Chap. 7), as it was planned drawing the resection areas accordingly both anteriorly (**c**) and posteriorly (**d**) (*arrows*); **e** at the end, on the cut surface the left portal vein (*LPV*), the LHV, the RHV, and the IVC are fully exposed: the stump of the MHV (*MHVs*) was also visible. The *dashed yellow lines* point out the area actually drained by the CV connecting the MHV hepatic stump with the adjacent hepatic veins; **f** posteriorly the RHV and the LHV can be visualized; **g** specimen with the resected tract of the MHV; **h**, **i** outline of the performed operation which consisted in a mini-mesohepatectomy with liver tunnel, and was feasible because of the presence of CV (see Chap. 7); cut surface (*CS*)

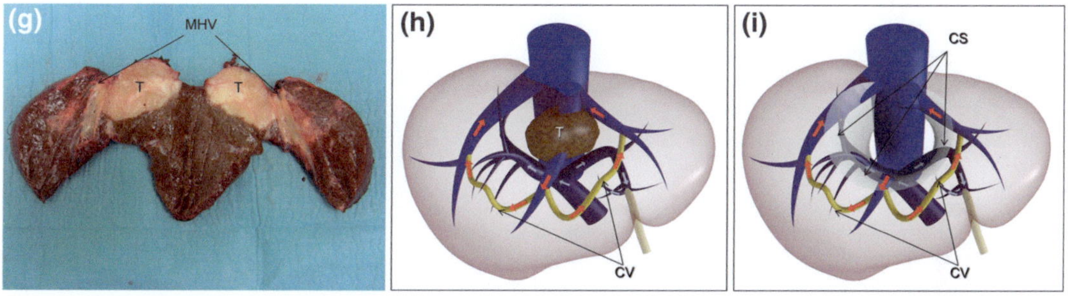

Fig. 8.57 (continued)

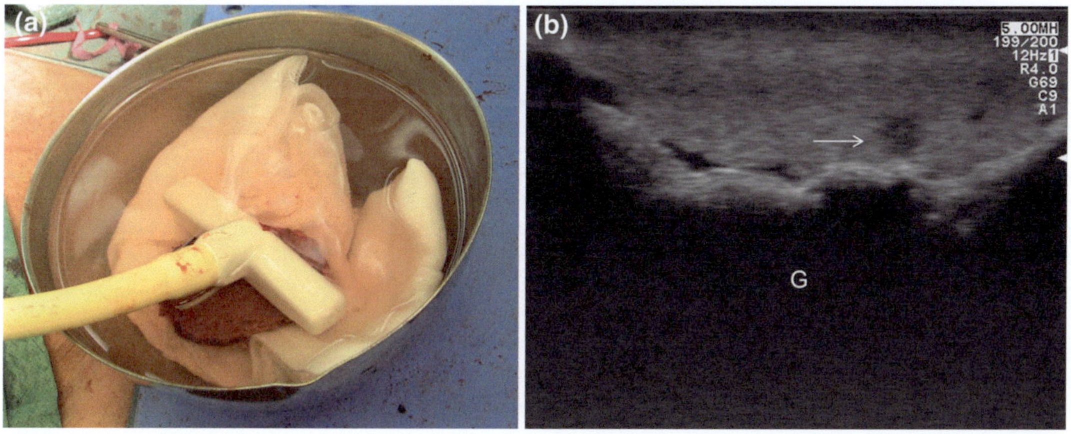

Fig. 8.58 The water-bath technique for checking the surgical specimen just removed (**a**) the whole inclusion of the targeted nodule, as confirmed by IOUS (*arrow*) (**b**); gauzes (*G*)

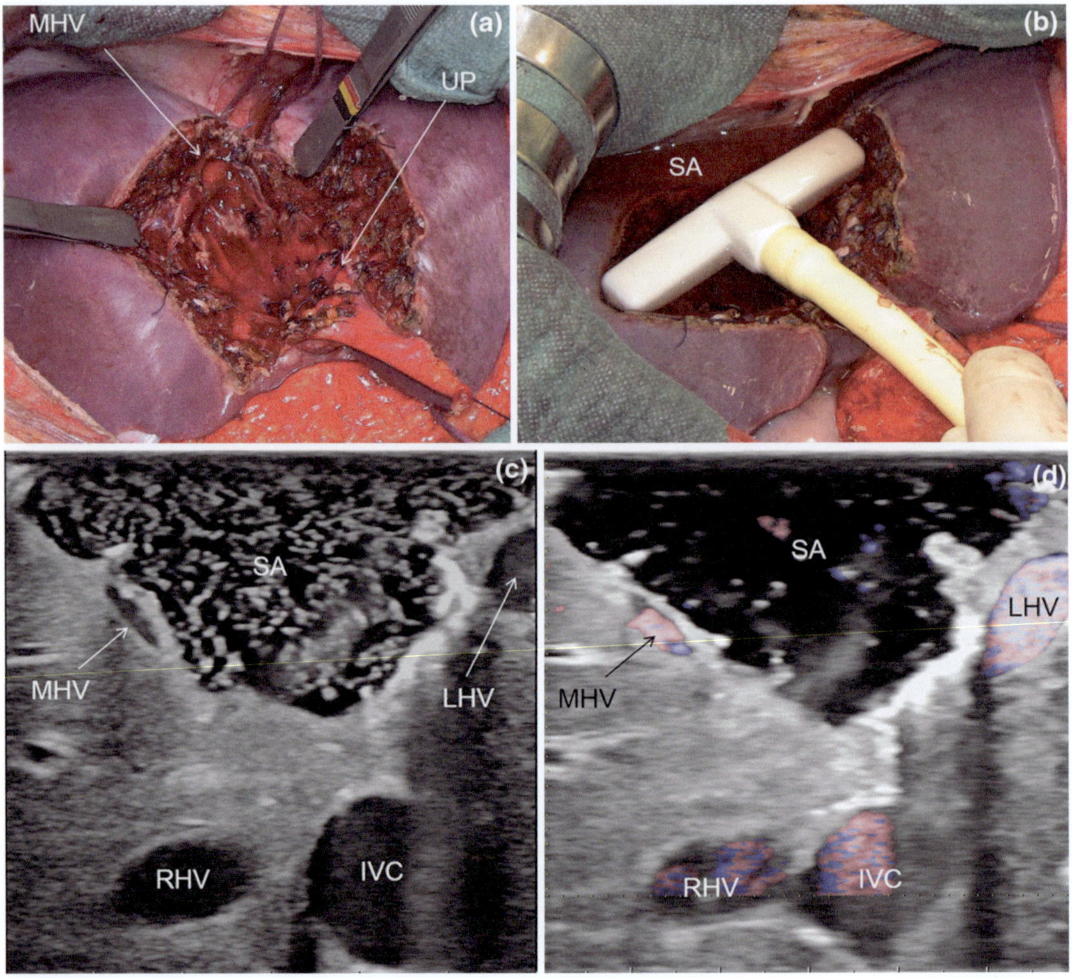

Fig. 8.59 In case of doubt as to whether there is some residual tumor in the remnant liver or the patency of the exposed vessel has to be checked (**a**), then the cut surface filled with saline (*SA*) is re-explored by IOUS (**b**); exploration is carried out in B-mode (**c**) and in CFIOUS mode (**d**) confirming the absence of residual disease, and of the patency of the middle hepatic vein (*MHV*), and the left hepatic vein (*LHV*); inferior vena cava (*IVC*); right hepatic vein (*RHV*); umbilical portion (*UP*)

surgical instruments themselves. In one of the few reports, the lack of communication between the elements connected via an infrared-based optical line was responsible for the failure of navigation in 4 % of treated patients [34]. Another problem concerning the use of these navigation systems is in the reduction of precision once dissection gets deeper into the liver due to organ shifting and deformation, which makes the data less reliable. This is the major limitation of this approach since it fails to provide information at the point where it is most needed. In neurological or head-and-neck surgery the targets are fixed and the results seem more consistent with the objectives [35, 36], but in abdominal surgery there is no similar facilitating situation. More recently, a further modification has been introduced in the original setting of inserting under ultrasound guidance an electromagnetic sensor into the liver close to the tumor to be removed [37], with the aim of overcoming the problem of decreasing the

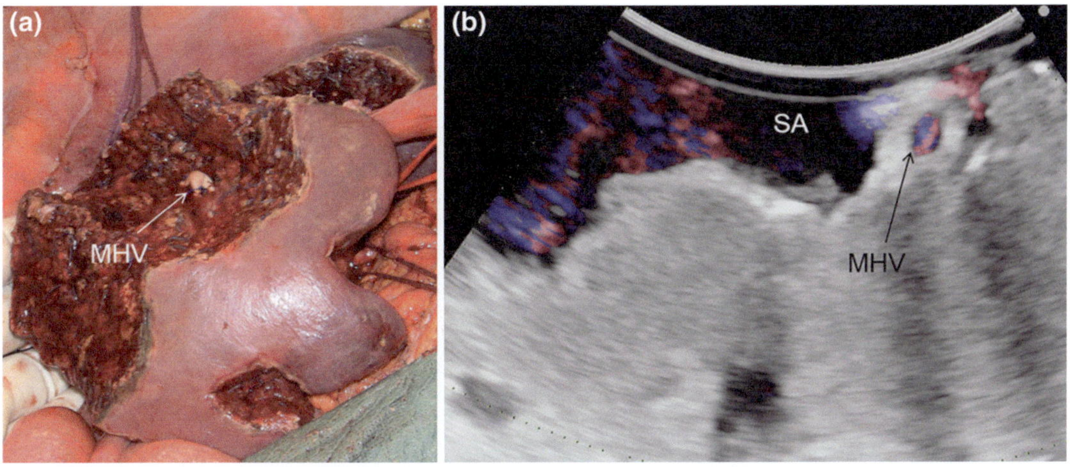

Fig. 8.60 In vascular reconstruction accomplished with a patch of bovine pericardium (**a**), the patency of the vessel has to be checked by CFIOUS (**b**); therefore, the cut surface is filled with saline (*SA*), and re-explored confirming the patency of the reconstructed middle hepatic vein (*MHV*)

precision of the navigation in proceeding deeper into the liver.

Some concerns have been raised concerning the possible addition of complexity to the proposed method. On the other hand, some authors try to overcome the problem of the readability of the organ shifting and deformation during surgical maneuvers by adding a framework which makes feasible the updating of the three-dimensional preoperative models with the intraoperative new data [38]. This may provide improvements to overcome organ deformation and shifting. However, the need for adjunctive instruments in the surgical theater, the use of a three-dimensional ultrasound modality, certainly more complex than bi-dimensional ultrasound, and the related costs, even in the event that the actual technical drawbacks will be solved, make uncertain the advantages of this implementation compared to the use of the herein described ultrasound guidance. The latter, in expert hands, clearly provides enhanced conservativity in hepatectomies (Figs. 8.55a–e, 8.56a–g, 8.57a–i), maintaining and improving the oncological radicality, which should be considered the gold standard in terms of ''navigated'' liver surgery—all this with relatively inexpensive technology which is a valid parameter in times of cost constraints. Rather than searching for more complex technologies, the challenge is to implement those existing and moreover to provide an educational program for the next generations of surgeons, applying ultrasound for surgical maneuvers.

8.4 Postresectional Control

There are two possibilities given by IOUS after nodule removal: (a) the ''*water bath*'' technique which consists in real-time control of proper resection of the targeted nodule verifying its complete inclusion in the specimen once removed from the liver [39] (Fig. 8.58a, b), and (b) checking the cut surface refilled with saline to avoid artifacts generated by residual air bubbles and clots (Figs. 8.38a–e, 8.59a–d). The latter can be useful also for checking vessel patency in case of reconstruction (Fig. 8.60a, b). In those patients in which major resections are needed, color-Doppler IOUS allows proper positioning of the remnant liver till the in- and outflow are normal in terms of velocity and waveform at color-Doppler [40] (Fig. 8.61a, b).

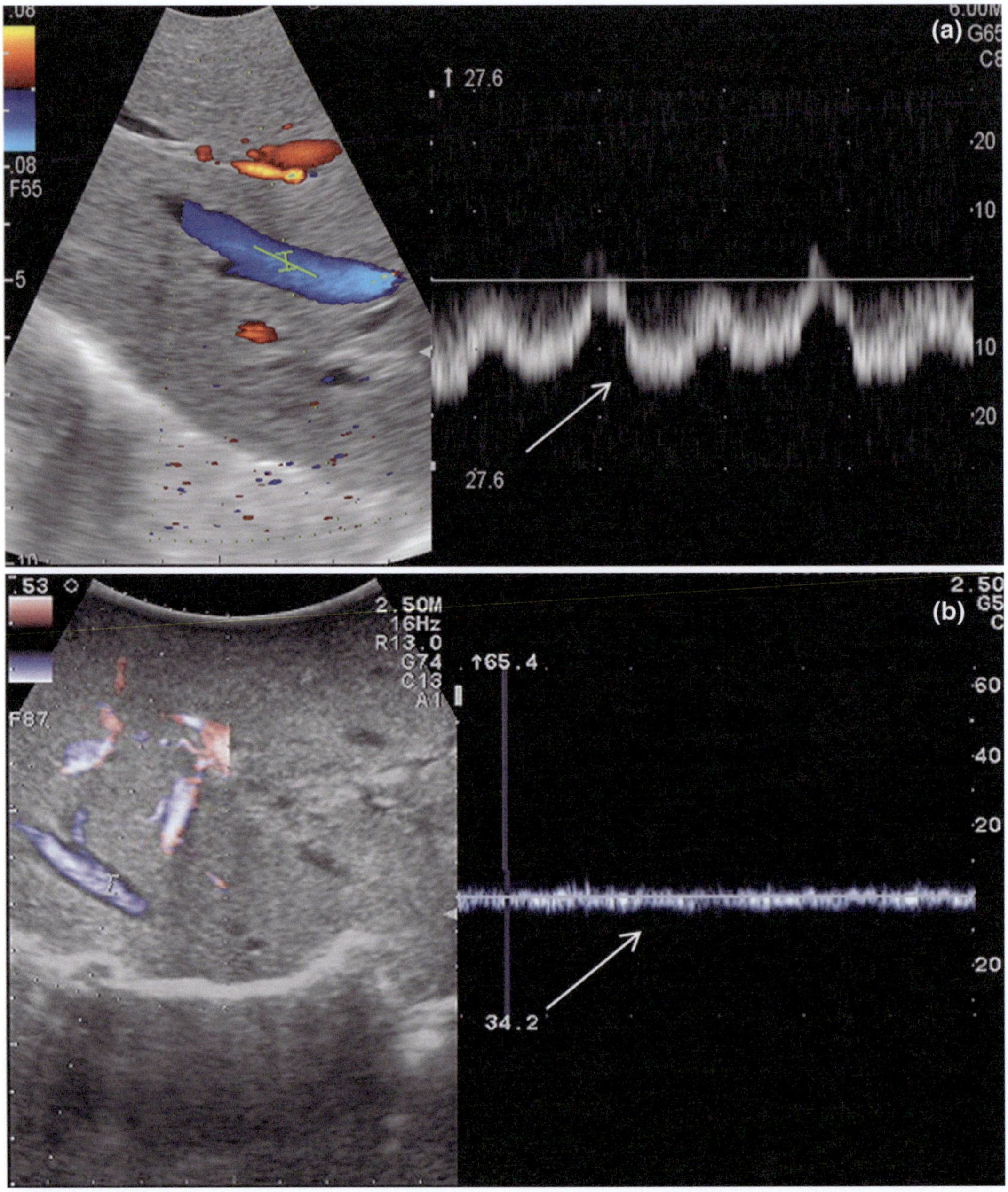

Fig. 8.61 In right hepatectomy, the proper repositioning of the remaining liver is performed by checking with color-Doppler whether the outflow is featured by a triphasic waveform (*arrow*) at velocimetry (**a**), or inversely is demodulated (*arrow*) (**b**); in the latter case, the remaining liver should be repositioned to search for a position featured by the pattern in (**a**)

References

1. Torzilli G, Montorsi M, Palmisano A et al (2006) Right inferior phrenic vein indicating the right hepatic vein confluence into the inferior vena cava. Am J Surg 192:690–694
2. Sarpel U, Bonavia AS, Grucela A et al (2009) Does anatomic versus nonanatomic resection affect recurrence and survival in patients undergoing surgery for colorectal liver metastasis? Ann Surg Oncol 16:379–384
3. Wakai T, Shirai Y, Sakata J et al (2007) Anatomic resection independently improves long-term survival in patients with T1–T2 hepatocellular carcinoma. Ann Surg Oncol 14:1356–1365
4. Regimbeau JM, Kianmanesh R, Farges O et al (2002) Extent of liver resection influences the outcome in patients with cirrhosis and small hepatocellular carcinoma. Surgery 131:311–317
5. Eguchi S, Kanematsu T, Arii S et al (2008) Comparison of the outcomes between an anatomical subsegmentectomy and a nonanatomical minor hepatectomy for single hepatocellular carcinomas based on a Japanese nationwide survey. Surgery 143:469–475
6. Cho YB, Lee KU, Lee HW et al (2007) Anatomic versus non-anatomic resection for small single hepatocellular carcinomas. Hepatogastroenterology 54:1766–1769
7. Kaibori M, Matsui Y, Hijikawa T et al (2006) Comparison of limited and anatomic hepatic resection for hepatocellular carcinoma with hepatitis C. Surgery 139:385–394
8. Tanaka K, Shimada H, Matsumoto C et al (2008) Anatomic versus limited nonanatomic resection for solitary hepatocellular carcinoma. Surgery 143:607–615
9. Hasegawa K, Kokudo N, Imamura H et al (2005) Prognostic impact of anatomic resection for hepatocellular carcinoma. Ann Surg 242:252–259
10. Ueno S, Kubo F, Sakoda M et al (2008) Efficacy of anatomic resection vs non-anatomic resection for small nodular hepatocellular carcinoma based on gross classification. J HBP Surg 15:493–500
11. Makuuchi M, Yamazaki S, Hasegawa H et al (1980) Ultrasonically guided liver surgery. Jpn J Ultrason Med 7:45–49
12. Takayama T, Makuuchi M, Watanabe K et al (1991) A new method for mapping hepatic subsegment: counterstaining identification technique. Surgery 109:226–229
13. Torzilli G, Makuuchi M (2004) Ultrasound-guided finger compression in liver subsegmentectomy for hepatocellular carcinoma. Surg Endosc 18:136–139
14. Torzilli G, Procopio F, Cimino M et al (2010) Anatomical segmental and subsegmental resection of the liver for hepatocellular carcinoma: a new approach by means of ultrasound-guided vessel compression. Ann Surg 251:229–235
15. Torzilli G, Procopio F, Palmisano A et al (2009) New technique for defining the right anterior section intraoperatively using ultrasound-guided finger counter-compression. J Am Coll Surg 209:e8–e11
16. Torzilli G, Procopio F, Palmisano A et al (2011) Total or partial anatomical resection of segment 8 using the ultrasound-guided finger compression technique. HPB (Oxford) 13:586–591
17. Torzilli G, Cimino M, Del Fabbro D et al (2013) Anatomical resection of segment 8 by means of ultrasound-guided vessel compression. Ann Surg Oncol 20(2):474
18. Onishi H, Kawarada Y, Das BC et al (2000) Surgical anatomy of the medial segment (S4) of the liver with special reference to bile ducts and vessels. Hepatogastroenterology 47:143–150
19. Torzilli G, Makuuchi M (2001) Ultrasound-guided liver subsegmentectomy: the peculiarity of segment 4. J Am Coll Surg 193:706–708
20. Shimamura Y, Gunvén P, Takenaka Y et al (1986) Selective portal branch occlusion by balloon catheter during liver resection. Surgery 100:938–941
21. Ou JR, Chen W, Lau WY (2007) A new technique of hepatic segmentectomy by selective portal venous occlusion using a balloon catheter through a branch of the superior mesenteric vein. World J Surg 31:1240–1242
22. Mazziotti A, Maeda A, Ercolani G et al (2000) Isolated resection of segment 8 for liver tumors: a new approach for anatomical segmentectomy. Arch Surg 135:1224–1229
23. Lupo L, Gallerani A, Aquilino F et al (2003) Anatomical hepatic resection using radiofrequency thermoablation in the treatment of primary or secondary liver tumors. Tumori 89:105–108
24. Santambrogio R, Costa M, Barabino M et al (2008) Laparoscopic radiofrequency of hepatocellular carcinoma using ultrasound-guided selective intrahepatic vascular occlusion. Surg Endosc 22:2051–2055
25. Curro G, Bartolotta M, Barbera A et al (2009) Ultrasound-guided radiofrequency-assisted segmental liver resection: a new technique. Ann Surg 250:229–233
26. Makuuchi M, Hashikura Y, Kawasaki S et al (1993) Personal experience of right anterior segmentectomy (segments V and VIII) for hepatic malignancies. Surgery 114:52–58
27. Takasaki K, Kobayashi S, Tanaka S et al (1990) Highly anatomically systematized hepatic resection with Glissonean sheath code transection at the hepatic hilus. Int Surg 75:73–77
28. Torzilli G, Procopio F, Donadon M et al (2011) Anatomical right posterior sectionectomy: a further expansion of the ultrasound-guided compression technique. Updates Surg 63:91–95
29. Belghiti J, Guevara OA, Noun R et al (2001) Liver hanging maneuver: a safe approach to right hepatectomy without liver mobilization. J Am Coll Surg 193(1):109–111

30. Torzilli G, Takayama T, Hui AM et al (1999) A new technical aspect of ultrasound-guided liver surgery. Am J Surg 178:341–343
31. Torzilli G, Montorsi M, Gambetti A et al (2005) Utility of the hooking technique for cases of major hepatectomy. Surg Endosc 19:1156–1157
32. Torzilli G, Donadon M, Palmisano A et al (2007) Back-flow bleeding control during resection of right-sided liver tumors by means of ultrasound-guided finger compression of the right hepatic vein at its caval confluence. Hepatogastroenterology 54:1364–1367
33. Chopra SS, Hunerbein M, Eulenstein S et al (2008) Development and validation of a three dimensional ultrasound based navigation system for tumor resection. Eur J Surg Oncol 34:456–461
34. Beller S, Hunerbein M, Eulenstein S et al (2007) Feasibility of navigated resection of liver tumors using multiplanar visualization of intraoperative 3-dimensional ultrasound data. Ann Surg 246:288–294
35. Hohlweg-Majert B, Schon R, Schmelzeisen R et al (2005) Navigational maxillofacial surgery using virtual models. World J Surg 29:1530–1538
36. Hamada H, Hayashi N, Asahi T et al (2005) Efficacy of a navigation system in neuro-endoscopic surgery. Minim Invasive Neurosurg 48:197–201
37. Beller S, Eulenstein S, Lange T et al (2009) Upgrade of an optical navigation system with a permanent electromagnetic position control: a first step towards ''navigated control'' for liver surgery. J Hepatobiliary Pancreat Surg 16:165–170
38. Dagon B, Baur C, Bettschart V (2008) A framework for intraoperative update of 3D deformable models in liver surgery. Conf Proc IEEE Eng Med Biol Soc 2008:3235–3238
39. Makuuchi M (1987) Abdominal intraoperative ultrasonography. Igaku-Shoin, Tokyo
40. Ogata S, Kianmanesh R, Belghiti J (2005) Doppler assessment after right hepatectomy confirms the need to fix the remnant left liver in the anatomical position. Br J Surg 92:592–595

Intraoperative Cholangio Ultrasound in the Study of the Biliary Tree

9

Guido Torzilli, Fabio Procopio, and Angela Palmisano

9.1 Introduction

It has been shown how IOUS is able to provide precise details about the anatomy of intrahepatic bile ducts, even when not dilated (see Chap. 3), and their variants with their centripetal bifurcation pattern as compared to the portal branches (Fig. 9.1). This aspect is crucial in liver surgery as major hepatectomies are at major risk for biliary complications and among them those at major risk of damage are the left-sided hepatectomies, due to the possibility of having a right posterior section draining into the left bile duct [1] (Fig. 9.2). Other than IOUS, also CEIOUS may play a role in this sense since it provides a negative image of the biliary tree as compared to the enhanced surrounding liver parenchyma (Fig. 9.3). On the other hand, bile duct injury during major hepatectomy occurs in 8 % of patients and in 22 % of left-sided major resection [2]. These complications are often life-threatening and, in the experience of Lo et al. [2], 39 % of patients with biliary complications died. Help in reducing this risk is achieved by performing intraoperative cholangiography (IOC) and intraparenchymatous division of the bile ducts peripherally to the confluence of the main bile ducts and the confluence of those draining the caudate lobe. IOC, in particular, still represents the gold standard for studying the anatomy of the biliary tract as well as for guiding reconstruction in case of bile duct resection. Moreover, with the advent of living donation, IOC is the standard reference for evaluating preoperative imaging [3]. IOUS in this sense does not play a central role within the current surgical practice, if not for guiding intraoperatively dilated bile duct drainage [4]. However, we believe that IOUS could play an important role for the following indications:

1. resection guidance for biliary tumors;
2. providing details about the integrity of the intrahepatic biliary tree after a resection; and
3. proper drainage of the bile duct stump.

9.2 Resection Guidance for Biliary Tumors

Concerning resection guidance, with the exclusion of the mass-forming type of cholangiocarcinoma for which the role of IOUS guidance is similarly relevant as for CLM, the above-mentioned limitations are actually real and linked to the features of the target. Indeed, perihilar cholangiocarcinomas are generally isoechoic (see Chap. 4), and thus less visible even by IOUS (Fig. 9.4a). However, more important, these tumors tend to expand within the bile duct wall frustrating any attempt to

G. Torzilli (✉) · F. Procopio · A. Palmisano
Department of Hepatobiliary Surgery,
Humanitas Research Hospital-IRCCS,
University of Milan-School of Medicine,
Via A. Manzoni 56, 20089, Rozzano, MI, Italy
e-mail: guido.torzilli@humanitas.it;
guido.torzilli@unimi.it

G. Torzilli (ed.), *Ultrasound-Guided Liver Surgery*,
DOI: 10.1007/978-88-470-5510-0_9, © Springer-Verlag Italia 2014

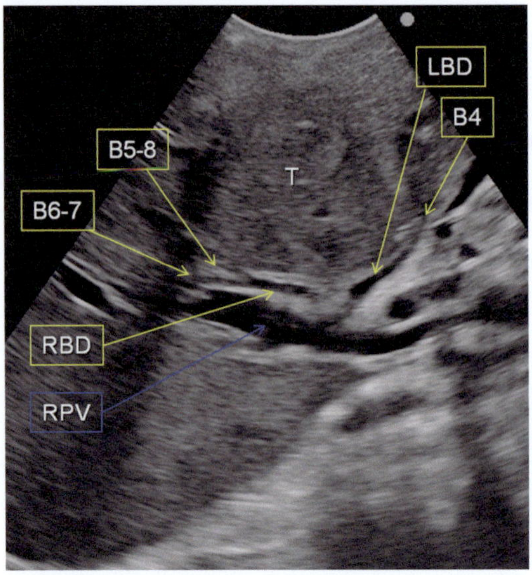

Fig. 9.1 IOUS can provide anatomical details of the intrahepatic biliary tree even if not dilated, with details of its centripetal bifurcation pattern: in a single scan one can recognize the right bile duct (*RBD*), the one draining the right anterior (*B5-8*), the one draining the right posterior (*B6-7*), the left bile duct (*LBD*), and the duct draining segment 4 (*B4*), while only the right portal vein (*RPV*) is to be seen

disclose the real tumor margin in a reliable way (Fig. 9.4b), and thus accounting for the still considerable rate of palliative resections [5]. This limitation together with the low visibility of the main lesion impacts also the capability of IOUS to disclose an eventual vascular encasement by the tumor (Figs. 9.4c–e, 9.5a, b), which accounts for the need of extemporary vascular reconstruction, in spite of the encouraging results of such a policy [5]. However, as IOUS can recognize the intrahepatic biliary tree anatomy, it can also play a role in avoiding its damage by providing fundamental information for planning the surgical strategy (see Chap. 7) or guiding the liver dissection (see Chap. 8) (Fig. 9.6a–g). Another aspect which is relevant both for planning the surgical strategy and guiding the resection is its ability of reveal even minimal bile duct dilation: this is particularly the case for tumor-vessel relationships for establishing the risk of tumor invasion of the glissonian sheath, and, as a consequence, the need for its resection and for the extension of the

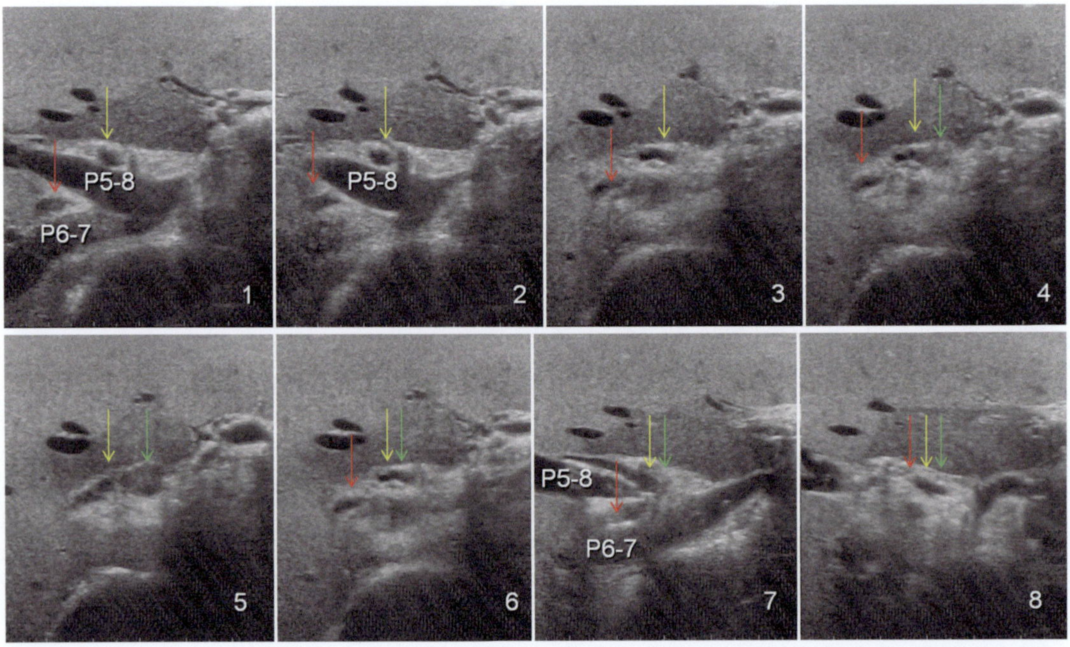

Fig. 9.2 IOUS images from 1 to 8 show how in this patient the right anterior bile duct (*B5-8* indicated by *yellow arrow*) is flowing into the left bile duct (*green arrow*) which together meet the right posterior bile duct (*B6-7* indicated by *red arrow*) in frame number 8; portal branch to the right anterior section (*P5-8*); portal branch to the right posterior section (*P6-7*)

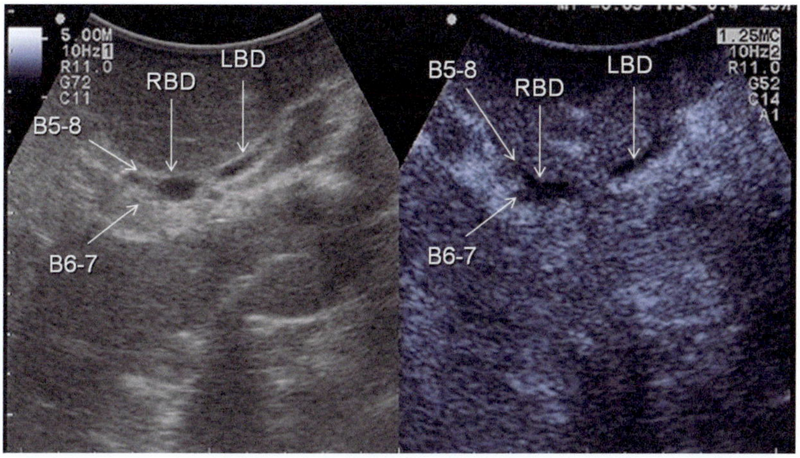

Fig. 9.3 On the left, IOUS of the intrahepatic biliary confluence showing the right anterior bile duct (*B5-8*), the right posterior bile duct (*B6-7*), the right (*RBD*) and the left bile ducts (*LBD*), and, on the right, the same scan by CEIOUS

resection area according to the criteria mentioned earlier [6] (see Chap. 7). IOUS allows the precise definition of this occurrence in patients with tumors in contact with an intrahepatic glissonian sheath (Fig. 9.7) but also its exclusion (Figs. 9.8, 9.9).

9.3 Intrahepatic Biliary Tree Integrity

Confirming biliary tree integrity is important in case of suspected damage after surgical dissection and is crucial to avoid postoperative morbidity and the consequent need for invasive procedures and even repeated surgery. A simple and self-made contrast agent can be employed for this purpose and which can be visualized by IOUS—becoming a true *intraoperative cholangio ultrasound* (IOCUS). The contrast agent consists of a compound of air and saline. Their ratio varies from that of pure air (Fig. 9.10) in having the same amounts of saline and air (Fig. 9.11a–c). The higher the concentration of injected air, the higher is the pressure with which the contrast is injected, the more evident will be a parenchymatous effect (Fig. 9.12), and the less clear will be the anatomical detail, and vice versa (Fig. 9.13). Indeed, the lower the air concentration, the lower is also the presence of those artefacts that can interfere with anatomical evaluation (Fig. 9.14a–c). The other important aspect to be taken into account, as just mentioned, is the pressure with which the compound is injected. Even pure air, if injected slowly thus enabling its slow flowing into the bile ducts and the progressive mixture with the bile juice, may provide anatomical details with sufficient panoramicity for disclosing the entire biliary tree (Fig. 9.15) or for checking the integrity of the biliary tract draining a certain part of the liver (Figs. 9.16a–c, 9.17a–d, 9.18a–e).

9.4 Proper Drainage of the Bile Duct Stump

Guiding the biliary reconstruction is fundamental for ensuring a proper patient's outcome once a bile duct has been resected and the proper biliary drainage has to be restored. This is particularly true in patients operated for perihilar cholangiocarcinoma, in whom the proper function of each residual segment is crucial, both to rule out morbidity linked to an undrained portion of the liver as well as to maintain the critical

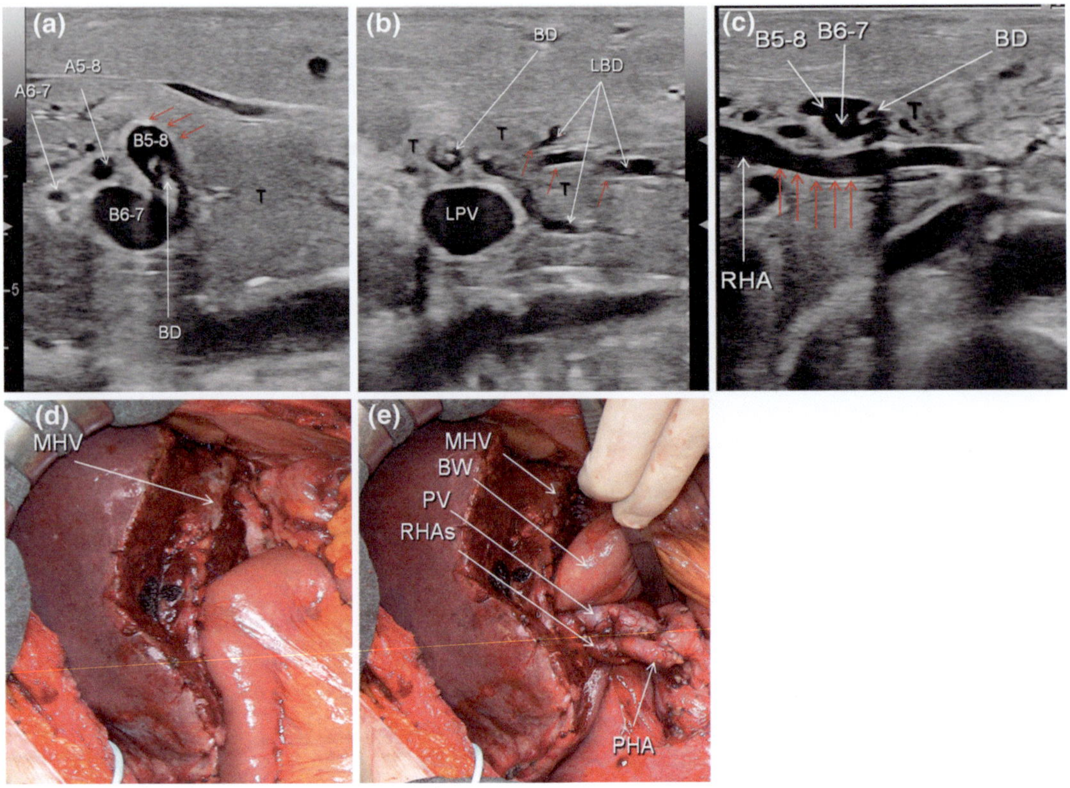

Fig. 9.4 **a** IOUS image of the main lesion (*T*) which is slightly hypoechoic compared to the surrounding liver, with undefined margins especially with regard to their intramural extension (*red arrows*) at the level of the right anterior (*B5-8*) and right posterior (*B6-7*) bile ducts, in which the biliary drainage is visible (*BD*); **b** the tumor extends to the left bile duct (*LBD*), but there are no reliable criteria to establish precisely the extent of the intramural extension (*red arrows*); **c** the right hepatic artery, passing in contact with the tumor except a slightly reduced caliper and an unusual straightness (*red arrows*), does not show in IOUS other aspects which could help to define whether it is invaded by the tumor or not; **d** with the bile duct stump frozen section free of tumor, a right hepatectomy together with segment 1 was carried out; **e** the right hepatic artery was resected, and, in absence of a left hepatic artery suitable for being tilted and anastomosed with its stump (*RHAs*), the latter was anastomosed to the proper hepatic artery (*PHA*), which remained long; hepatic artery to the right anterior section (*A5-8*); hepatic artery to the right posterior section (*A6-7*); bowel (*BW*); left portal vein (*LPV*); middle hepatic vein (*MHV*); portal vein (*PV*)

volume for a functioning liver parenchyma, and preventing liver failure. In this sense, IOCUS can be adopted both for providing an anatomical detail for disclosing each bile duct draining the remaining segments (Fig. 9.19a–f), and for disclosing a parenchymatous phase which should be considered sufficient for ruling out the risk of undrained liver portions (Figs. 9.20, 9.21).

9.5 Summary and Conclusion

IOCUS comes at no extra costs, not only because ultrasound is used anyway for staging and guidance, but also because the contrast agents used are air or a compound of air and saline. The advantages of ultrasound versus IOC

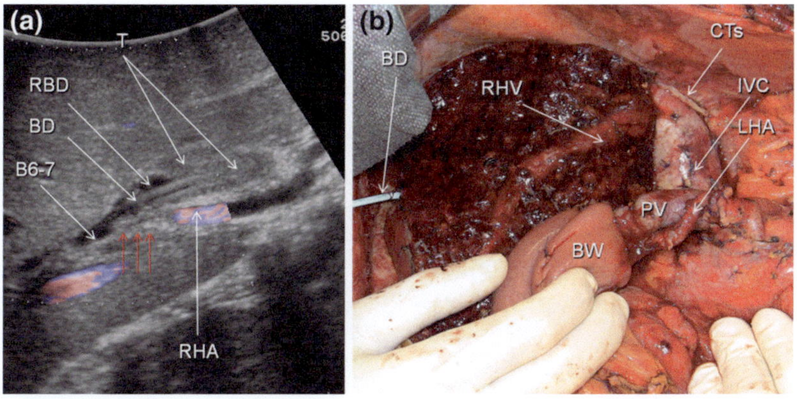

Fig. 9.5 **a** IOUS image showing the main lesion (*T*) which is isoechoic in relation to the surrounding liver, with undefined margins especially with regard to its intramural extension at the level of the right bile duct (*RBD*) just at the level of the confluence of the right posterior bile duct (*B6-7*); furthermore, the right hepatic artery (*RHA*) has stopped (*red arrows*); **b** a left trisectionectomy together with the left hepatic artery (*LHA*) tilting to revascularize the stump of the right posterior hepatic artery was carried out; biliary drainage (*BD*); bowel (*BW*); stump of the common trunk of the middle and left hepatic veins (*CTs*); inferior vena cava (*IVC*); portal vein (*PV*)

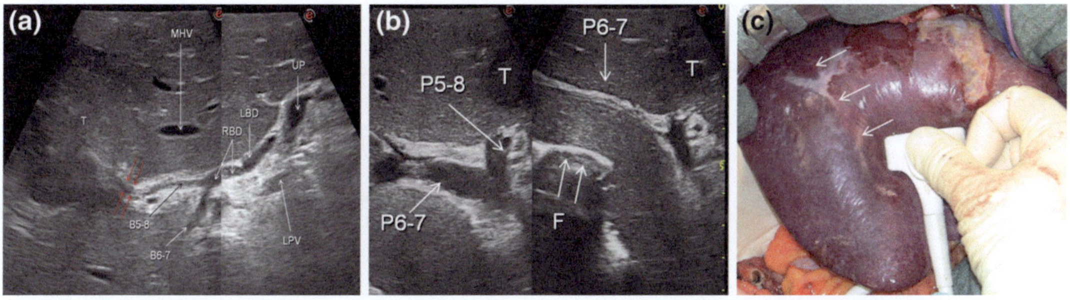

Fig. 9.6 **a** IOUS image showing the main lesion (*T*) infiltrating the right anterior pedicle including its bile duct (*B5-8*) (*red arrows*); despite this, IOUS was able to also perfectly disclose the anatomy of the biliary tree showing the right-sided confluence of B5-8 and the bile duct from the right posterior section (*B6-7*) into the right bile duct (*RBD*), and the confluence of the latter with the left bile duct (*LBD*) into the common bile duct; **b–d** then, a right anterior compression sectionectomy was planned as described in Chap. 8, by compressing the right posterior portal branch (*P6-7*) (**b**), which made evident the right-sided demarcation line on the liver surface (*arrows*) (**c**), compressing the left portal vein (*LPV*) (**d**), and marking also the related demarcation line; **e** dissection was carried out (*yellow arrows*) approaching the middle hepatic vein (*MHV*) first, and then the B5-8 distant from its confluence with B6-7; **f** once the right anterior pedicle was reached and encircled, before its division, the hooking technique was performed as previously described (see Chap. 8), to confirm the preservation of B6-7 (*red circles* focus the point of encirclement and traction, *yellow arrows* the dissection line); **g** then a right anterior sectionectomy was carried out; finger (*F*); hepatic pedicle (*HP*); portal branch to the right anterior section (*P5-8*); stump of the portal branch to the right anterior section (*P5-8 s*); right hepatic vein (*RHV*); round ligament (*RL*); umbilical portion (*UP*)

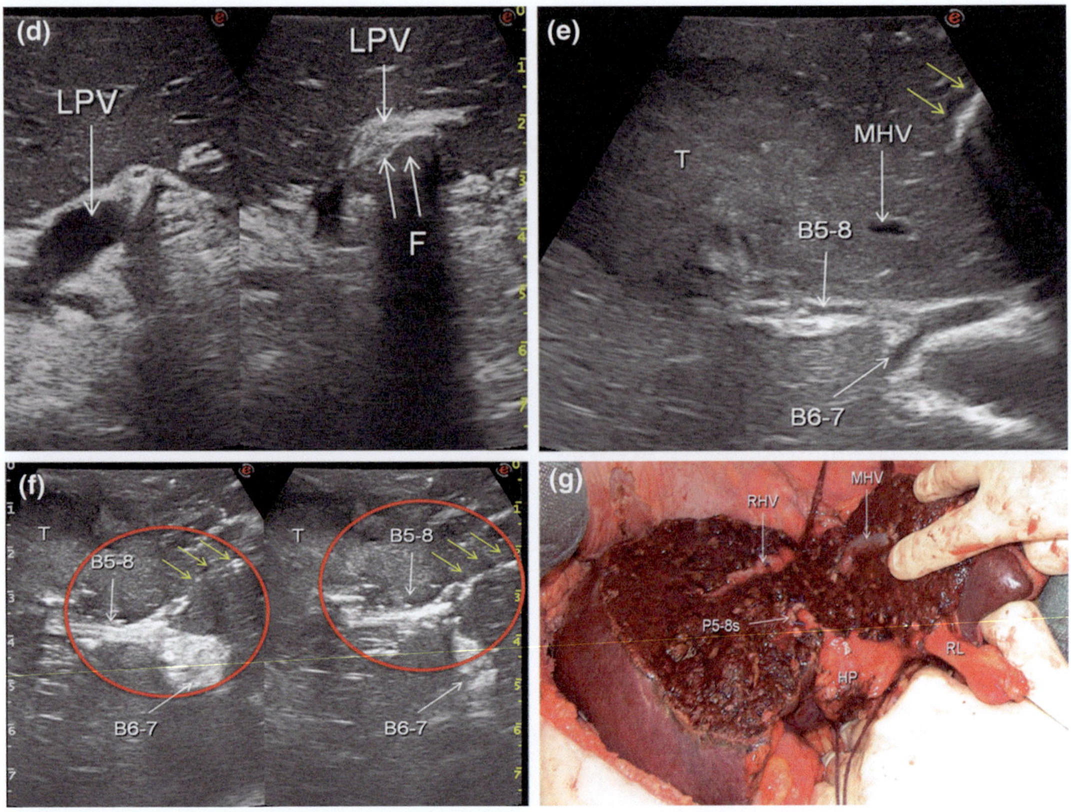

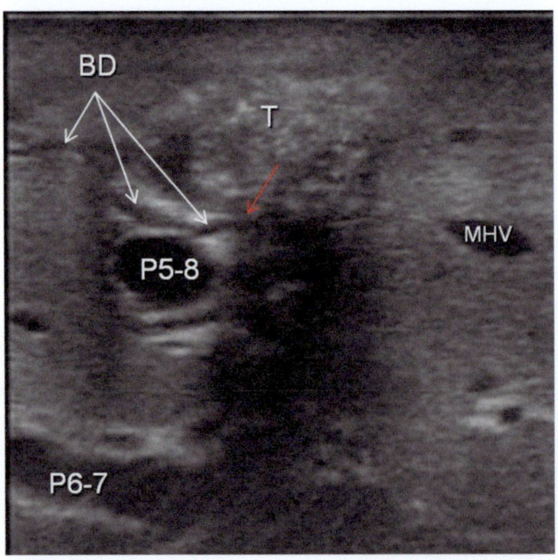

Fig. 9.7 A bile duct (*BD*) infiltrated (*red arrow*) by a tumor (*T*) and thus visible with its peculiar serpiginous path; middle hepatic vein (*MHV*); portal branch to the right anterior section (*P5-8*); portal branch to the right posterior section (*P6-7*)

in terms of cost saving have already been pointed out in regard to laparoscopic cholecystectomy [7].

Compared to IOC, which bears the disadvantage of radiation risk, IOCUS does not disclose just the biliary tree, but also the context in which a problem has eventually occurred. In that sense, IOCUS plays a role in resection guidance even in such patients. Other procedures have been recently promoted as alternatives to IOC, such as intraoperative exploration of biliary anatomy using indocyanine green (ICG) fluorescence imaging . This technique seems promising and has been validated experimentally and clinically [8, 9]. However, the reported experience was limited to the recognition of biliary anatomy without any additional information concerning relations with surrounding structures. Furthermore, although fluorescence imaging

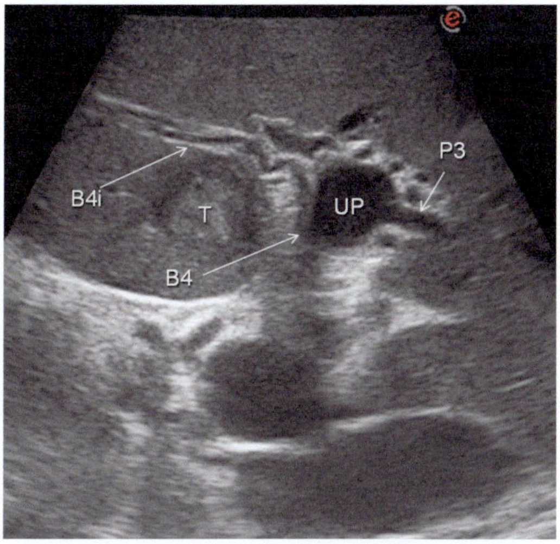

Fig. 9.8 IOUS is able to disclose that despite the adjacency to the tumor (*T*), and somehow a serpiginous path, the bile duct draining segment 4 inferior (*B4i*), and that draining the entire segment 4 (*B4*) are not invaded; portal branch to segment 3 (*P3*); umbilical portion (*UP*)

allows to avoid x-ray, as well as canulation of the cystic duct, it requires an infrared camera.

The main drawback of IOCUS consists in the need for an experienced operator in advanced ultrasound and thus may be of limited value. However, ultrasound has helped surgeons in reducing major morbidity in laparoscopic cholecystectomy [10], and it is now considered in several reports the gold standard for this operation rather than IOC [11]. This has happened in spite of the more difficult learning curve with ultrasound compared to IOC [12]. The same applies for IOCUS in liver surgery and the herein reported experience should act as proof of its reliability and promote its more extensive use.

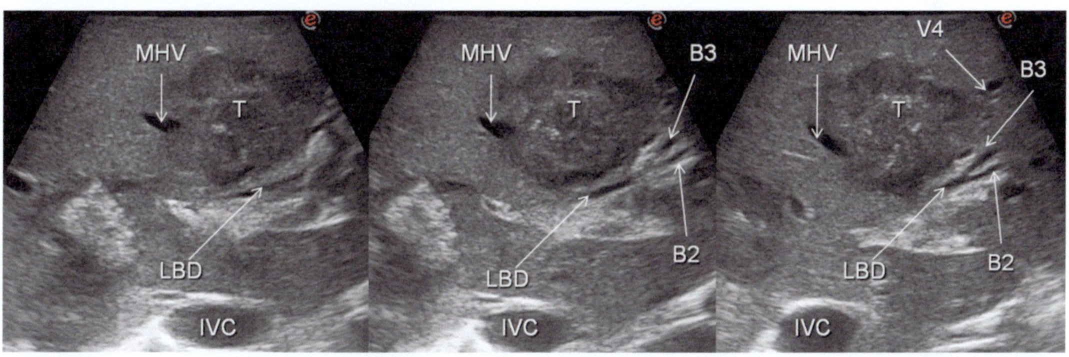

Fig. 9.9 Lack of contact between the tumor (*T*), the left bile duct (*LBD*), and the bile ducts draining segment 3 (*B3*) and 2 (*B2*) is well demonstrated in IOUS; inferior vena cava (*IVC*); middle hepatic vein (*MHV*); vein draining segment 4 (*V4*)

Fig. 9.10 Air is directly injected into the bile duct stump under IOUS guidance

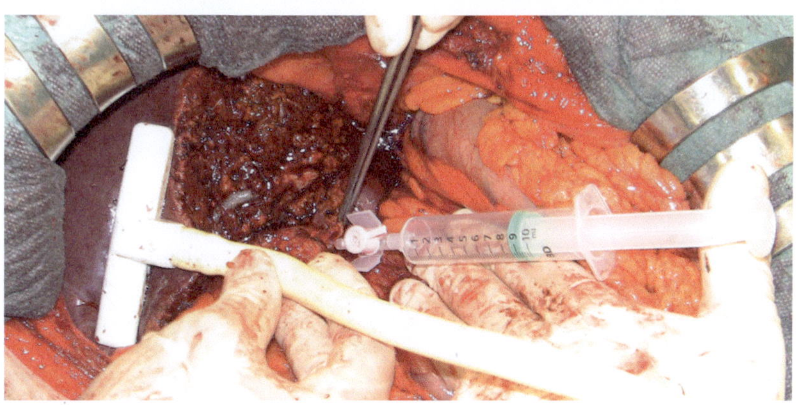

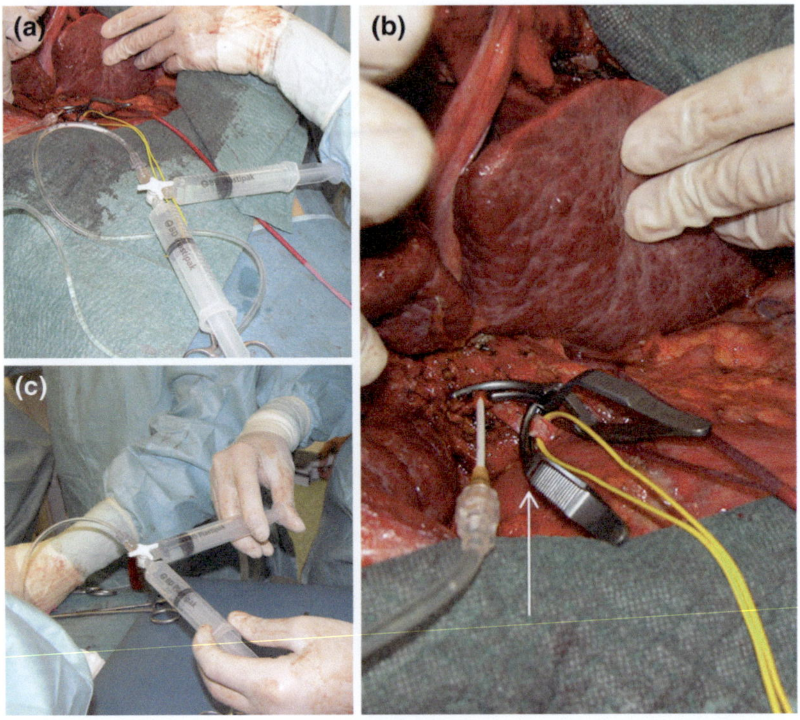

Fig. 9.11 Two syringes filled, respectively, with air and saline are prepared and connected to each other and with a deaerated tube (**a**), cannulating the cystic duct with the coledochus, which is clamped (*arrow*) (**b**), then the air and the saline are mixed in order to be injected (**c**)

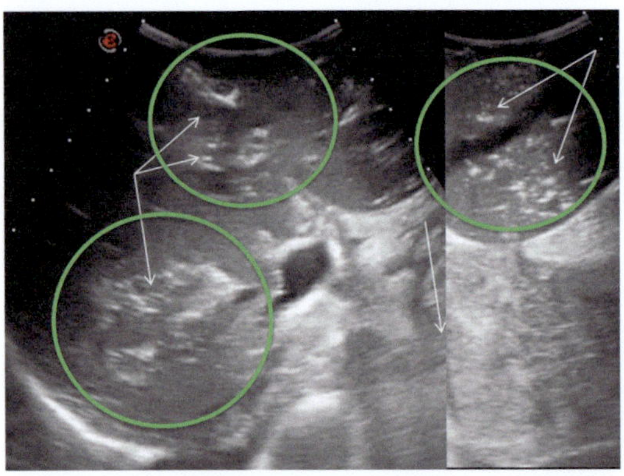

Fig. 9.12 Once enough pure air is injected strongly into the biliary tree, the effect obtained gives a parenchymatous contrast (*arrows* and *green circles*)

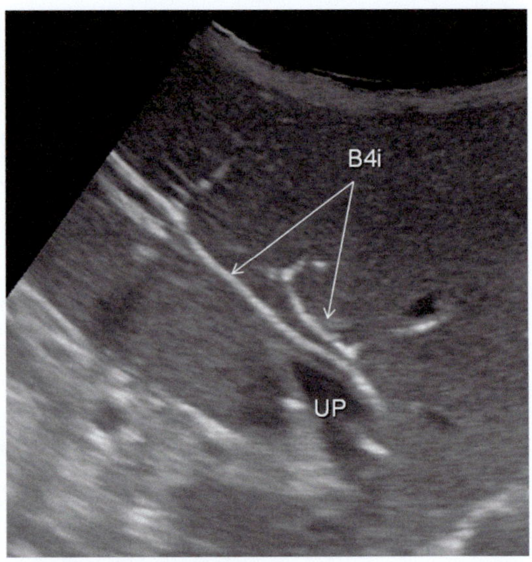

Fig. 9.13 Once air and saline are mixed and injected gently into the biliary tree, the effect obtained gives anatomical details as in this case showing the bile ducts draining the segment 4 inferior (*B4i*); umbilical portion (*UP*)

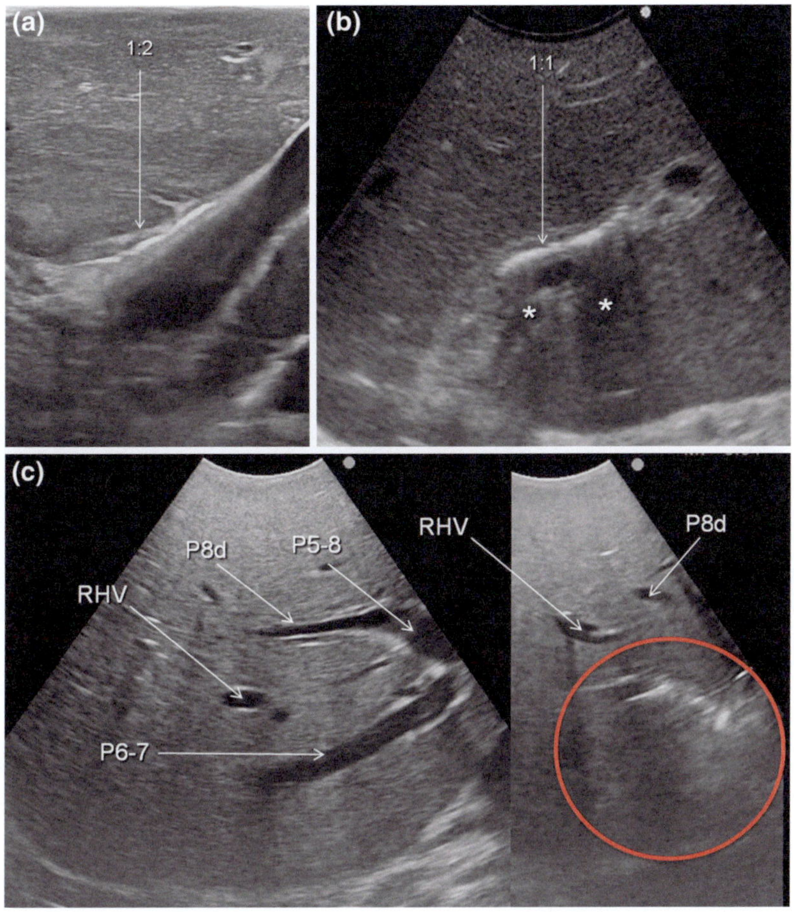

Fig. 9.14 Once air and saline are mixed and injected gently, the anatomical details vary depending on the concentration of the two components having more anatomical detail once the ratio air/saline is 1:2 (**a**), with some artifacts (*) at a ratio of 1:1 (**b**), or strong artifacts (*red circle*) if pure air is injected (**c**); portal branch to subsegment 8 dorsal (*P8d*); portal branch to the right anterior section (*P5-8*); portal branch to the right posterior section (*P6-7*); right hepatic vein (*RHV*)

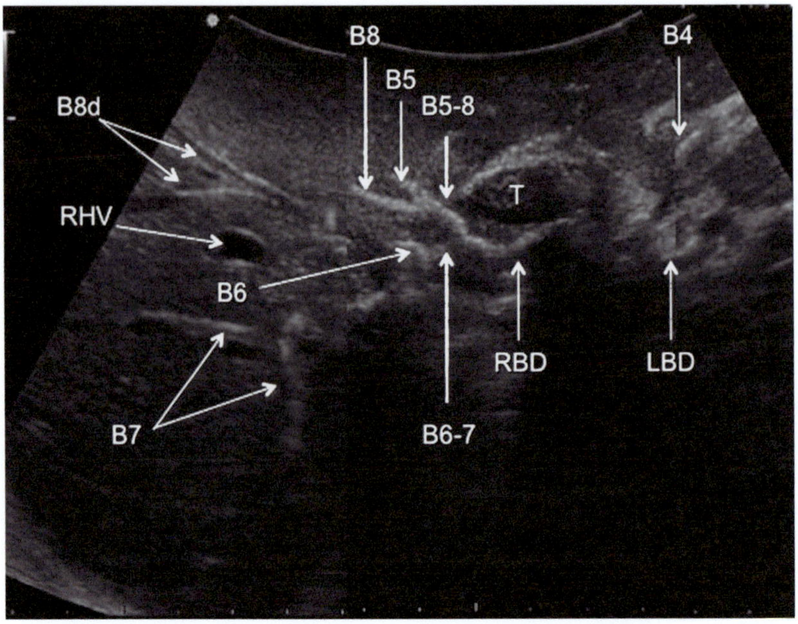

Fig. 9.15 Once pure air is injected slowly and gently allowing its mixture with the bile juice, the anatomical details can be obtained together with a panoramicity which allows visualizing most of the intrahepatic biliary tree; bile duct draining segment 4 (*B4*); bile duct draining segment 5 (*B5*); bile duct draining segment 6 (*B6*); bile ducts draining segment 7 (*B7*); bile duct draining segment 8 (*B8*); bile duct draining subsegment 8 dorsal (*B8d*); bile duct draining the right anterior section (*B5-8*); bile duct draining the right posterior section (*B6-7*); left bile duct (*LBD*); right bile duct (*RBD*); right hepatic vein (*RHV*)

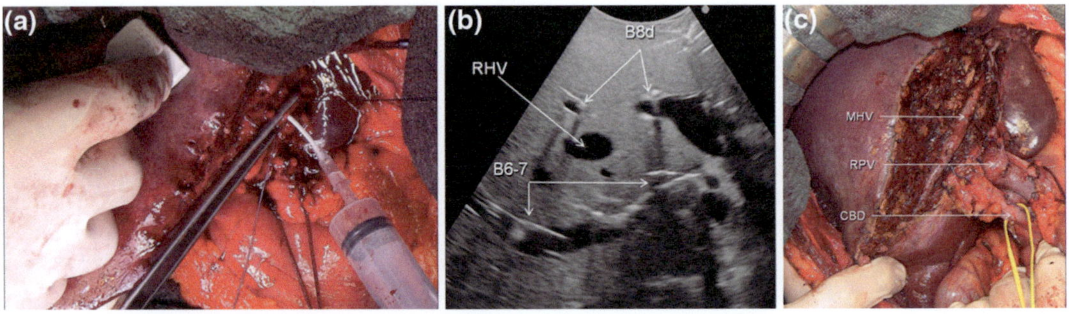

Fig. 9.16 After a left hepatectomy in which the dissection has given the impression of having approached too close to the biliary confluence, the injection of air into the biliary stump (**a**), the visualization by IOCUS of the contrast effect disclosing the bile duct draining the right posterior section (*B6-7*), and that draining the segment 8 dorsal (*B8d*) (**b**), demonstrate the preservation of the proper biliary drainage of the right hemiliver (**c**); common bile duct (*CBD*); middle hepatic vein (*MHV*); *right portal* vein (*RPV*)

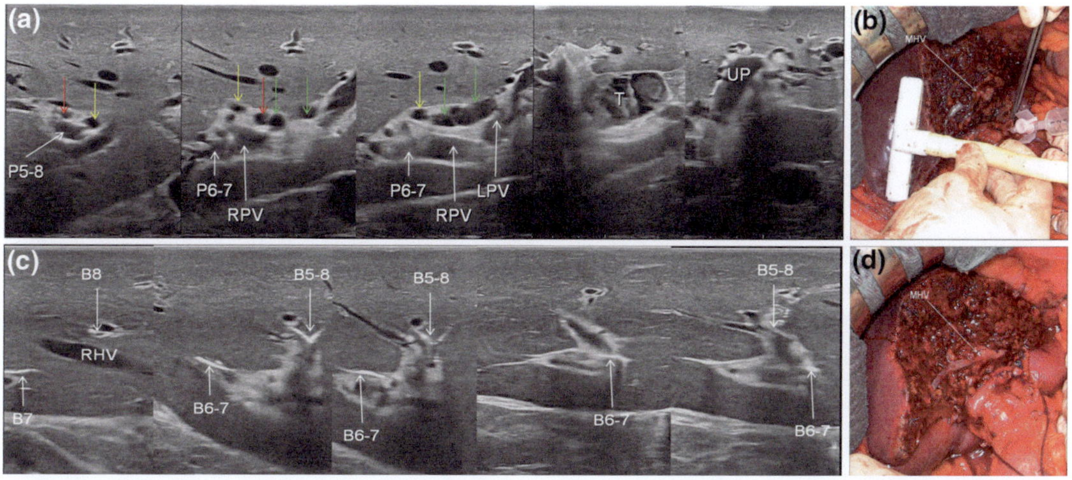

Fig. 9.17 **a** In this patient, operated for an intraductal cholangiocarcinoma (*T*), IOUS disclosed from the left to the right, the bile duct draining the right posterior section (B6-7 here indicated by *red arrow*) flowing into the left bile duct (*green arrow*), and then flowing together with the bile duct draining the right anterior section (B5-8 here indicated by *yellow arrow*) into the common bile duct; **b** once a left hepatectomy is carried out, confirmation of the proper division of the LBD is obtained by injecting slowly air into the bile duct stump; **c** B6-7 and B5-8 ducts are well followed up to those draining segments 7 (*B7*) and 8 (*B8*); **d** the left hepatectomy is then safely concluded; left portal vein (*LPV*); middle hepatic vein (*MHV*); portal branch to the right anterior section (*P5-8*); portal branch to the right posterior section (*P6-7*); right hepatic vein (*RHV*); right portal vein (*RPV*); umbilical portion (*UP*)

Fig. 9.18 **a** In this patient, IOUS shows an HCC (*T*) located between the umbilical portion (*UP*) and the middle hepatic vein (*MHV*) which it is in contact with, while the vein approaches its confluence into the inferior vena cava (*IVC*); **b** a transverse scan further details the relation between tumor, MHV, and UP; **c** finger (*F*) compression of the segment 4 pedicle (*P4*) is carried out and the segment edges are visible on the liver surface; **d** before removal of the specimen, a bile duct stump just above the left glissonian pedicle (*LGP*) is injected with air and the bile duct draining the right posterior section (*B6-7*), the right anterior section (*B5-8*), segment 3 (*B3*), and segment 2 (*B2*) are visualized confirming the preserved integrity of the remnant biliary tree; **e** a fully anatomical segmentectomy of segment 4 is then carried out; hilar pedicle (*HP*); right glissonian pedicle (*RGP*); round ligament (*RL*) ▶

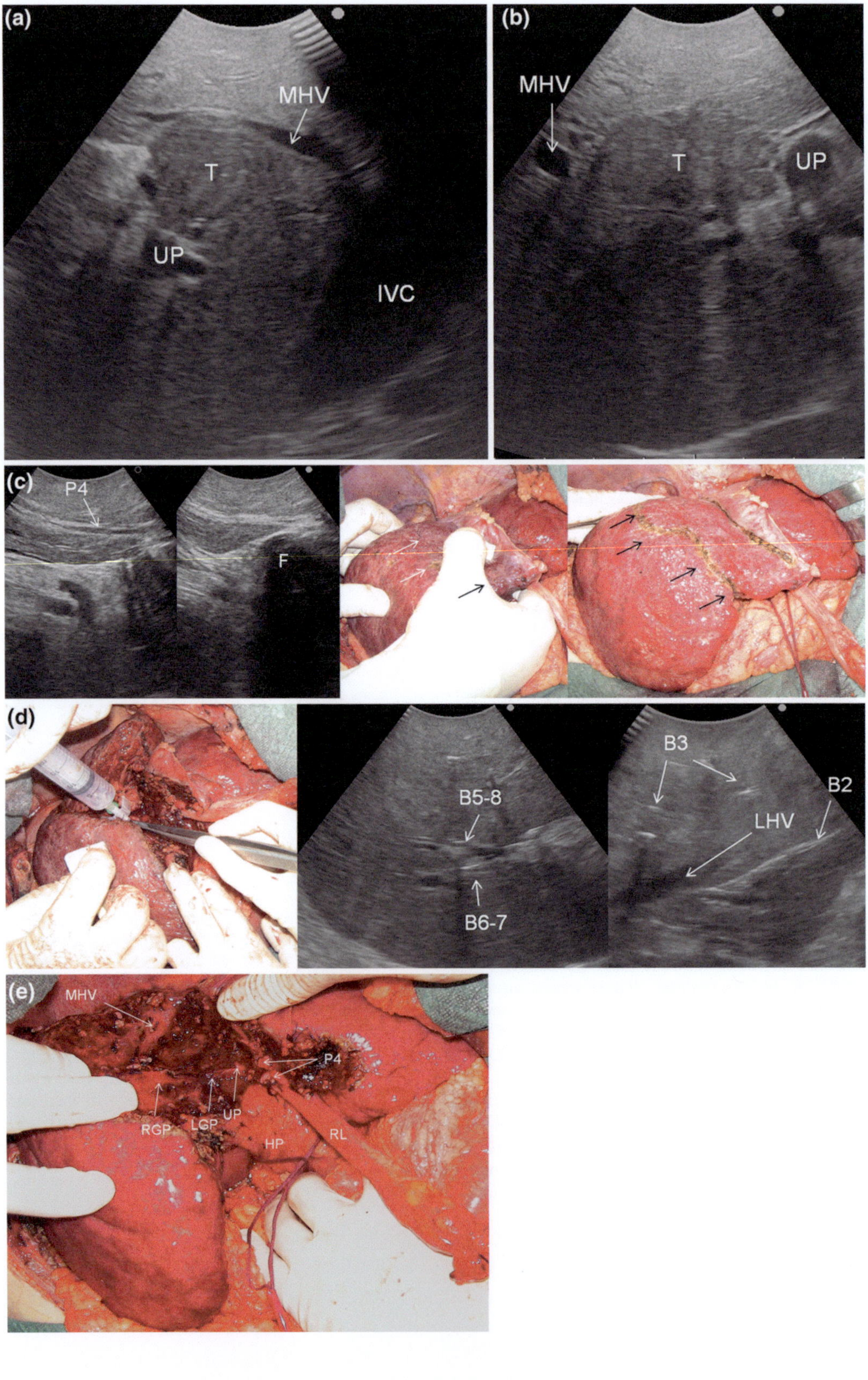
(a)
MHV
T
UP
IVC
(b)
MHV
T
UP
(c)
P4
F
(d)
B5-8
B6-7
B3
B2
LHV
(e)
MHV
P4
RGP
LGP
UP
HP
RL

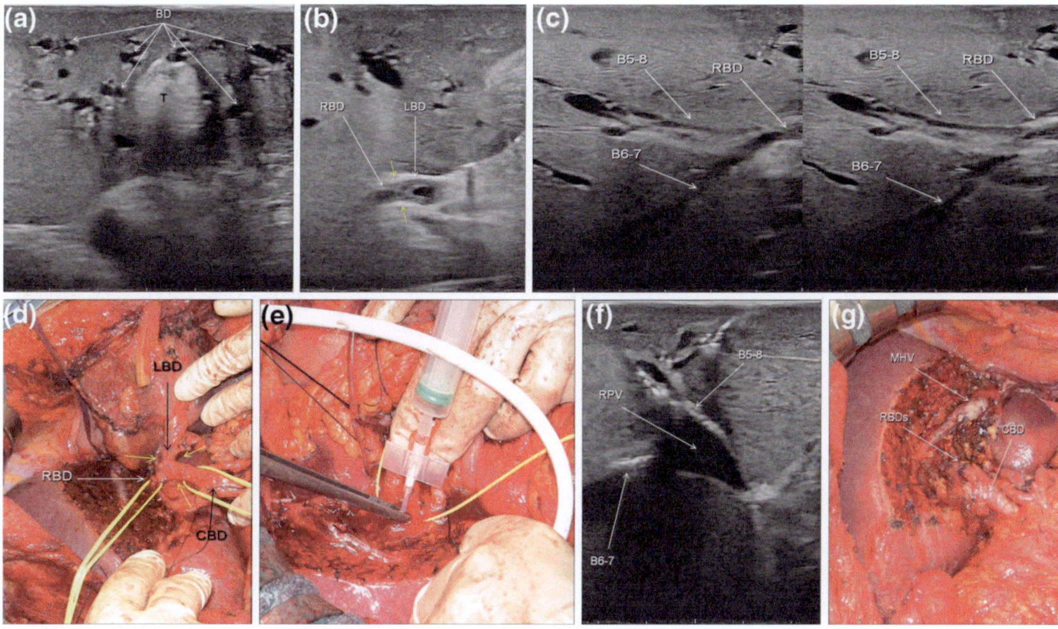

Fig. 9.19 **a–c** In this patient, IOUS shows a cholangiocarcinoma (*T*) determining bile duct (*BD*) dilation in the left liver (**a**), having associated with the wall thickening of the left bile duct (*LBD*) up to its confluence (*yellow arrows*) together with the right bile duct (*RBD*) into the common bile duct (*CBD*) (**b**); **c** on the right, apart from a wall thickening of the RBD, there are no signs of dilation of the ducts draining the right anterior (*B5-8*) and posterior (*B6-7*) sections; **d** left hepatectomy is almost concluded, remaining to be removed the biliary confluence (*yellow arrows*); **e** IOCUS with air is carried out by gentle injection from the hepatic stump after resection; **f** in IOCUS, B5-8 and B6-7 are well disclosed; **g** the operation is completed by end-to-end biliary reconstruction enabled by the negative frozen section on both sides, the wideness of the stumps, and the redundant length of the CBD; right bile duct stump (*RBDs*); right portal vein (*RPV*)

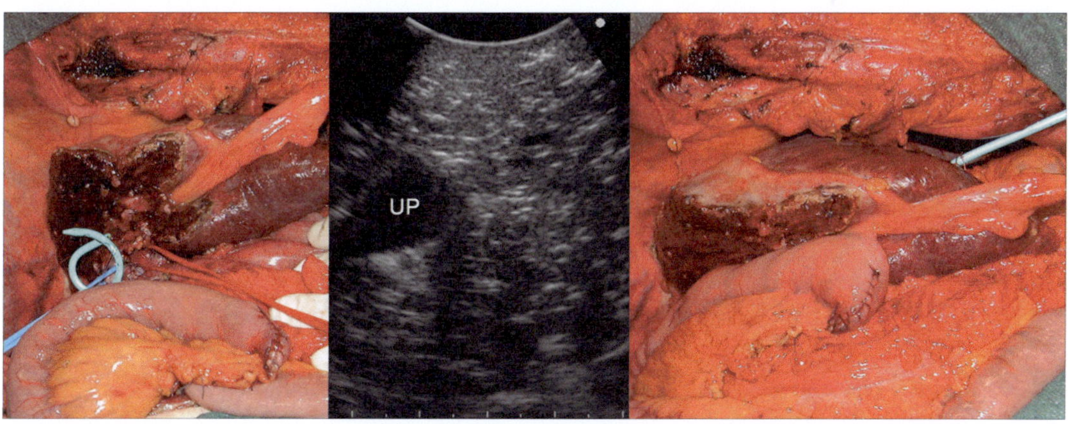

Fig. 9.20 Before hepatico-jejunostomy after right hepatectomy extended to segment 4 inferior and segment 1 for a perihilar cholangiocarcinoma (*left*), IOCUS confirms proper drainage by means of a parenchymatous phase (*center*), and then the anastomosis is carried out (*right*); umbilical portion (*UP*)

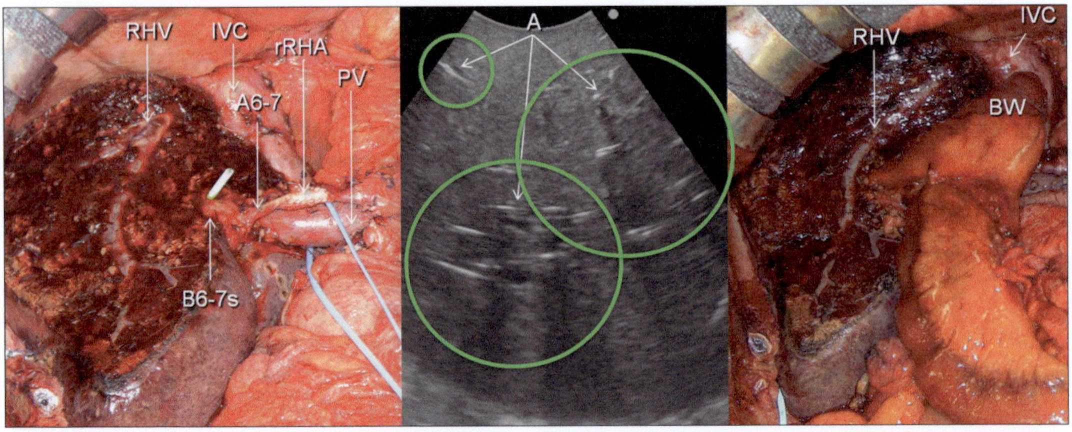

Fig. 9.21 Before hepatico-jejunostomy after left trisectionectomy extended to segment 1 for a perihilar cholangiocarcinoma (on the *left*), IOCUS confirms proper drainage by means of a parenchymatous phase (*green circles*), and then the anastomosis was carried out (on the *right*); air (**a**); hepatic artery to the right posterior section (*A6-7*); stump of the bile duct draining the right posterior section (*B6-7 s*); bowel (*BW*); inferior vena cava (*IVC*); portal vein (*PV*); reconstructed (with patch of bovine pericardium) right hepatic artery (*rRHA*); right hepatic vein (*RHV*)

References

1. Mizumoto R, Suzuki H (1988) Surgical anatomy of the hepatic hilum with special reference to the caudate lobe. World J Surg 12:2–10
2. Lo CM, Fan ST, Liu CL et al (1998) Biliary complications after hepatic resection: risk factors, management, and outcome. Arch Surg 133:156–161
3. Lee VS, Krinsky GA, Nazzaro CA et al (2004) Defining intrahepatic biliary anatomy in living liver transplant donor candidates at mangafodipir trisodium-enhanced MR cholangiography versus conventional T2-weighted MR cholangiography. Radiology 233:659–666
4. Torzilli G, Makuuchi M, Komatsu Y et al (1999) US guided biliary drainage during hepatico-jejunostomy for diffuse bile duct carcinoma. Hepatogastroenterology 46:863–866
5. Nagino M, Nimura Y, Nishio H et al (2010) Hepatectomy with simultaneous resection of the portal vein and hepatic artery for advanced perihilar cholangiocarcinoma: an audit of 50 consecutive cases. Ann Surg 252:115–123
6. Torzilli G, Del Fabbro D, Palmisano A et al (2005) "Radical but conservative" is the main goal for ultrasonography-guided liver resection: prospective validation of this approach. J Am Coll Surg 201:517–528
7. Torzilli G, Procopio F, Botea F et al (2009) One-stage ultrasonographically guided hepatectomy for multiple bilobar colorectal metastases: a feasible and effective alternative to the 2-stage approach. Surgery 146:60–71
8. Tagaya N, Shimoda M, Kato M et al (2010) Intraoperative exploration of biliary anatomy using fluorescence imaging of indocyanine green in experimental and clinical cholecystectomies. J Hepatobiliary Pancreat Surg 17:595–600
9. Mitsuhashi N, Kimura F, Shimizu H et al (2008) Usefulness of intraoperative fluorescence imaging to evaluate local anatomy in hepatobiliary surgery. J Hepatobiliary Pancreat Surg 15:508–514
10. Machi J, Oishi AJ, Tajiri T et al (2007) Routine laparoscopic ultrasound can significantly reduce the need for selective intraoperative cholangiography during cholecystectomy. Surg Endosc 21:270–274
11. Machi J, Johnson OJ, Deziel DJ et al (2009) The routine use of laparoscopic ultrasound decreases bile duct injury: a multicenter study. Surg Endosc 23:384–388
12. Perry KA, Myers JA, Deziel DJ (2008) Laparoscopic ultrasound as the primary method for bile duct imaging during cholecystectomy. Surg Endosc 22:208–213

Part IV
Liver Transplantation

Liver Transplantation from Deceased Donors

10

Matteo Cescon, Fabio Piscaglia, Alessandro Cucchetti, and Antonio Daniele Pinna

Doppler ultrasonography (US) provides an accurate assessment of the hepatic vasculature in liver transplantation (LT). It can be performed perioperatively or at the bedside. The evaluation of the hepatic vessels includes color and spectral Doppler analysis. ColorDoppler provides information regarding the presence and direction of flow, as well as the location of turbulent flow in a post-stenotic segment. Spectral analysis describes the direction, velocity, and phasicity of flow.

10.1 Hepatic Artery Complications

There are several possible sites of hepatic artery (HA) anastomosis. In orthotopic whole LT, the most frequent anastomosis is between the donor celiac or common HA, and the recipient HA at either the bifurcation into left and right hepatic arteries or the origin of the gastroduodenal artery. When the recipient HA cannot be used, the anastomosis can be performed on the recipient aorta with a donor artery interposition graft, on the recipient splenic artery or on an accessory HA. The presence of a donor accessory artery requires a second anastomosis. In split LT, the anastomosis is variably performed between the donor right, left, proper or common HA, and the recipient right, left, proper or common HA, with or without interposition vascular grafts. Knowledge of the type of anastomosis is important because stenosis frequently occurs at this site. HA complications include thrombosis, stenosis, and pseudoaneurysm. Biliary ischemia is often the consequence of HA thrombosis or stenosis [1, 2], with development of non-anastomotic biliary strictures or leaks.

On Doppler US, the normal HA has a low resistance waveform with continuous diastolic flow and a resistance index (RI, defined as peak systolic velocity minus end-diastolic velocity, all divided by peak systolic velocity) ranging between 0.60 and 0.80. The systolic peak has a rapid, almost vertical shape, with an early peak and a highest peak (Fig. 10.1). For the measurement of systolic acceleration time, the early peak is to be used. For the measurement of RI, the highest peak is to be used (Figs. 10.2 and 10.3). An RI lower than 0.50 in any hepatic arterial vessel indicates HA thrombosis or stenosis, with a sensitivity of 60 % and a specificity of 77 % [3, 4]. A prolonged systolic

M. Cescon (✉) · F. Piscaglia · A. Cucchetti · A. D. Pinna
General Surgery and Transplantation Unit, Department of Medical and Surgical Sciences, University of Bologna, Via Massarenti 9, 40138 Bologna, Italy
e-mail: matteo.cescon@unibo.it

F. Piscaglia
e-mail: fabio.piscaglia@unibo.it

A. Cucchetti
e-mail: aleqko@libero.it

A. D. Pinna
e-mail: antoniodaniele.pinna@aosp.bo.it

G. Torzilli (ed.), *Ultrasound-Guided Liver Surgery*,
DOI: 10.1007/978-88-470-5510-0_10, © Springer-Verlag Italia 2014

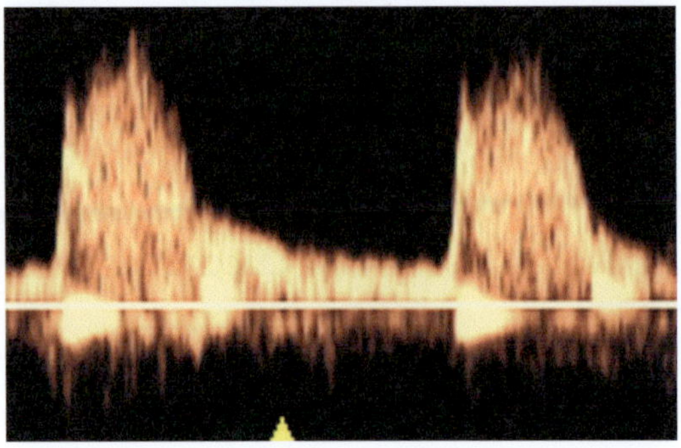

Fig. 10.1 Arterial Doppler ultrasound waveform showing both early and highest systolic peaks (early and highest systolic peaks may be coincident or not coincident, as represented in this instance)

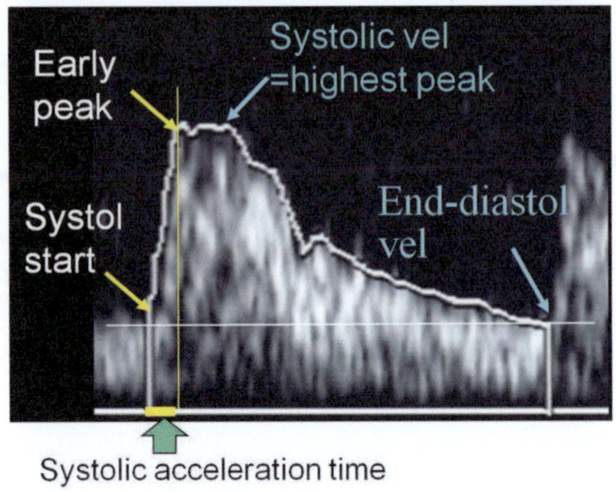

Fig. 10.2 US arterial wave with representation of early and highest peaks. For the measurement of systolic acceleration time, the early peak is to be used. For the measurement of Resistance Index (RI, i.e., systolic velocity minus end-diastolic velocity/systolic velocity), the highest peak is to be used

acceleration time (>0.08 s) is also predictive of stenosis, with a sensitivity/specificity of 53 and 86 %, respectively [3, 4]. A low RI and/or a long acceleration determine the tardus parvus waveform (Figs. 10.4, 10.5, 10.6, 10.7, 10.8). At the site of stenosis, an increased peak systolic velocity (>200 cm/s) can be detected. This is the most specific sign of hepatic arterial stenosis and, if present, is predictive in 96 % of the cases [3, 4].

10.1.1 Thrombosis

Absent arterial flow in all arteries on a technically adequate Doppler imaging study is nearly always indicative of thrombosis. False positives may occur due to severe hepatic edema,

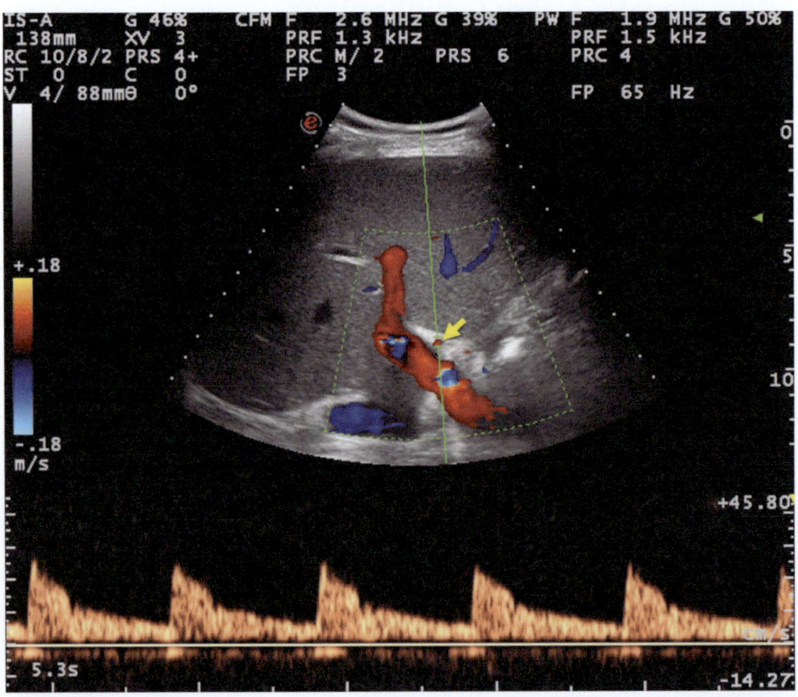

Fig. 10.3 Normal Doppler US waveform of the right hepatic artery detected at its entrance into the right liver lobe, alongside and anteriorly to the right portal branch. The systolic acceleration time is clearly normal (corresponding to a rapid rise of systolic velocity) and the RI is not decreased, namely the end diastolic velocity is relatively low with respect to peak velocity (numeric data not measured in this image)

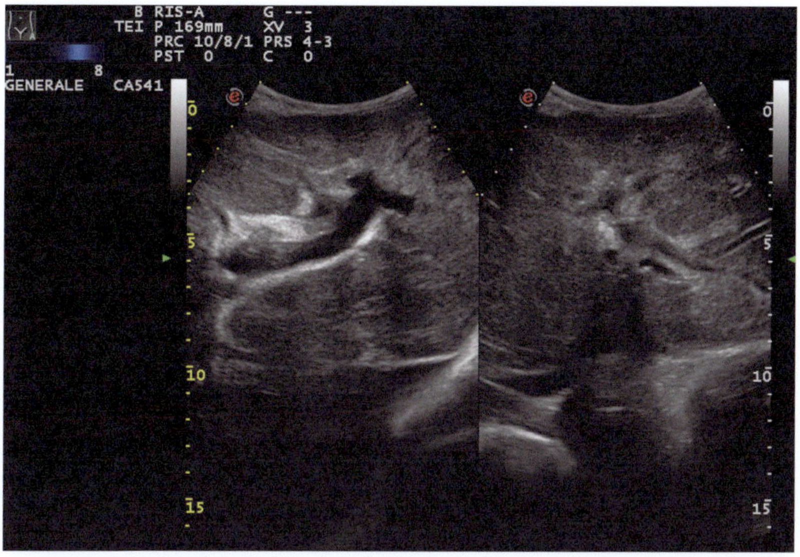

Fig. 10.4 A case of cholangitis with mild bile duct dilatation and inhomogeneous liver echotexture, particularly in the left lobe, visualized through a subcostal epigastric scan. The patient presented with fever and malaise

systemic hypotension, or in a suboptimal ultrasound study. Reduced flow, whether secondary to spasm or to low cardiac output, can also cause non visualization of flow at Doppler US. A loss of diastolic flow or diastolic flow reversal has been suggested as a sign of impending thrombosis [5, 6], especially if it occurs in the main HA.

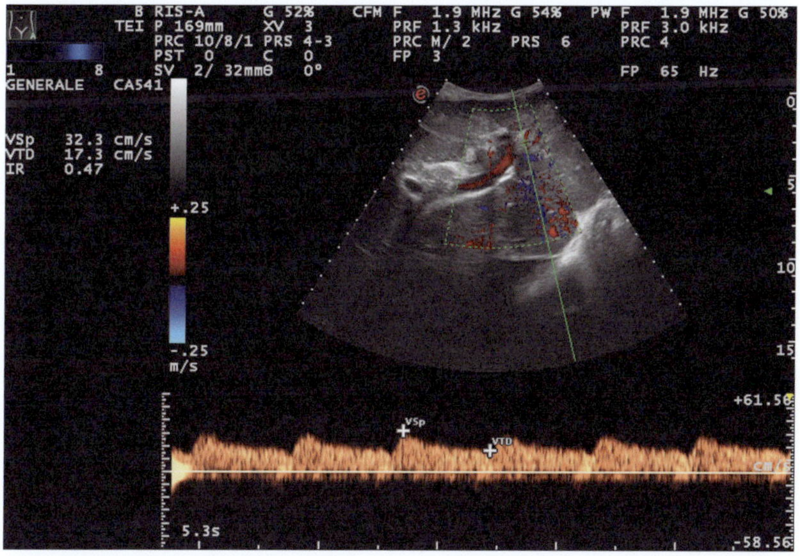

Fig. 10.5 Same case as Fig. 10.4. Right hepatic artery was detectable at both color and pulsed wave Doppler, but showed a ''tardus parvus'' flow trace, corresponding to a low RI (below 0.50, in this instance RI = 0.47) and prolonged systolic acceleration time (over 100 ms, in this instance 128 ms; data not shown)

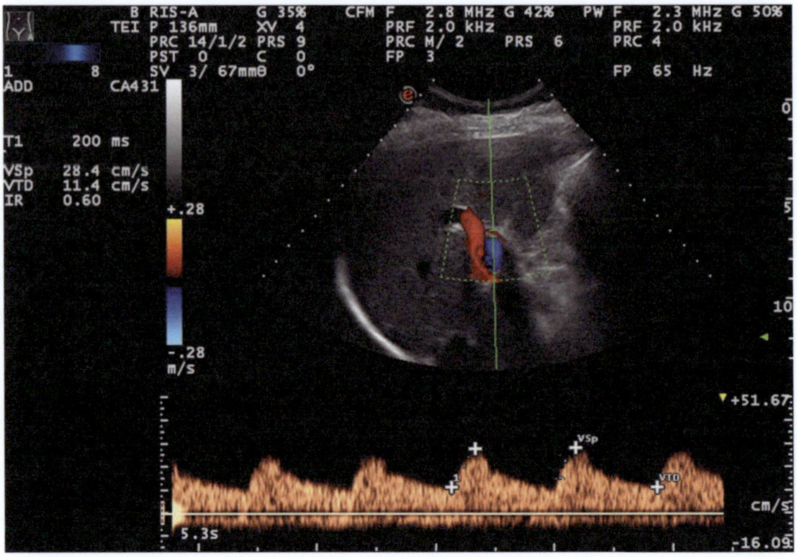

Fig. 10.6 Hepatic artery tracing with normal RI (0.60) but prolonged acceleration time (T1 = 200 ms) detected 12 years after LT

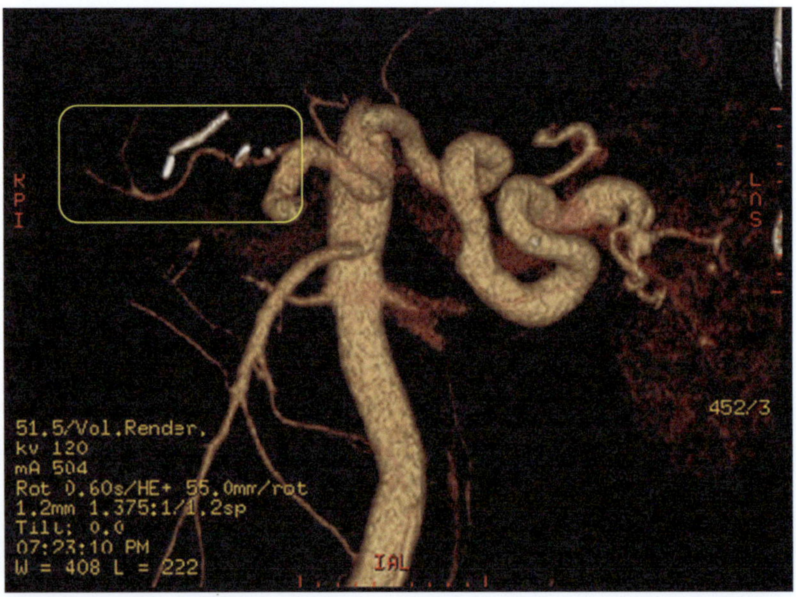

Fig. 10.7 Same case as Fig. 10.6. Angio CT shows elongated narrowing of the proper hepatic artery due to atherosclerosis (*yellow frame*)

Microbubble contrast material-enhanced US may help to improve flow visualization in the HA [7]. In patients in whom no flow is identified in the HA, angiography, computed tomography (CT), or magnetic resonance (MR) angiography are usually required to definitely diagnose

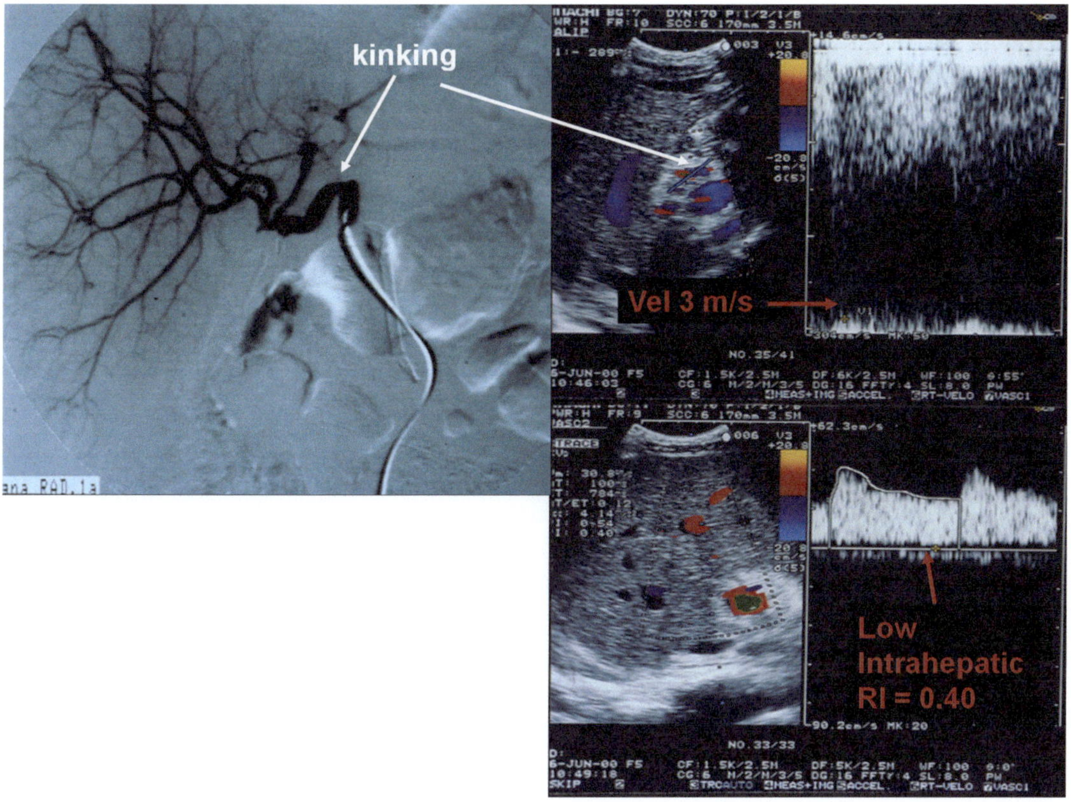

Fig. 10.8 A case of kinking of the hepatic artery shown by angiography (on the *left*) determining a hemodynamic stenosis indicated by Doppler US (on the *right*), with downstream tardus parvus waveform (RI = 0.40), and markedly turbulent and accelerated flow at the site of kinking (peak flow velocity approximately 3 m/s)

thrombosis. The treatment of HA thrombosis usually consists of emergent thrombectomy or retransplantation.

10.1.2 Stenosis

HA stenosis occurs in 2–11 % of transplantations [8, 9]. The most common site of stenosis is the anastomosis, which is often difficult to detect by US, being frequently obscured by bowel. In the very early postoperative period (<72 h after transplantation), increased HA RI (>0.8) is frequently observed, although it usually returns to normal within a few days [10]. Increased RI is associated with fibrotic livers and a prolonged period of ischemia [10]. HA stenosis may be treated with percutaneous angioplasty or surgical intervention [11].

10.1.3 Pseudoaneurysms

HA pseudoaneurysm is an uncommon complication and can be classified as either extrahepatic or intrahepatic. Extrahepatic pseudoaneurysm most commonly occurs at the arterial anastomosis or arises as a complication of angioplasty, whereas intrahepatic pseudoaneurysm may result from percutaneous biopsy, biliary procedures, or infection [12, 13].

A pseudoaneurysm is identified on US as a cystic structure in communication with the HA with a disorganized ''to and fro'' color and spectral Doppler pattern as the arterial blood flows into and out of the pseudoaneurysm (Fig. 10.9).

US detection of a fluid collection near the arterial anastomosis requires further evaluation with pulsed Doppler US to rule out

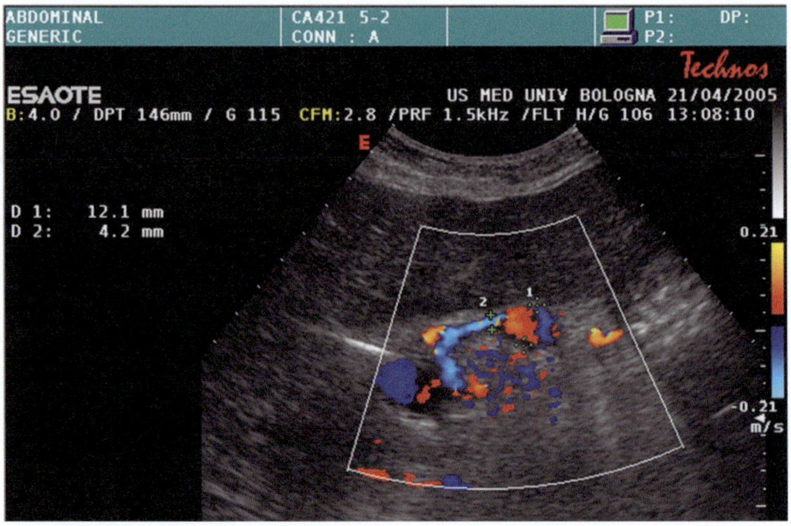

Fig. 10.9 Hepatic artery aneurysm, close to the anastomotic site (diameter of the hepatic artery = 4 mm, maximum diameter of the dilated tract = 12 mm)

pseudoaneurysm. Contrast-enhanced CT demonstrates a focal lesion with central enhancement that follows arterial blood-pool attenuation. Treatment consists of embolization for both types of aneurysms, as well as stent placement or surgical resection for an extrahepatic pseudoaneurysm [13, 14]. A ruptured intrahepatic pseudoaneurysm can lead to a portal or biliary fistula.

10.1.4 Arterioportal Fistula

Intrahepatic arterioportal fistula is usually secondary to liver biopsy of other invasive procedures. On US, the inflowing hepatic arterial RI will be lower than the contralateral normal vessel on the opposite side. In addition, reversed flow in particular portal vein (PV) radicals (considered a rare finding), arterialized PV waveform as well as a focus of turbulence with aliasing at the site of the arterioportal fistula can also be seen [12, 15–17].

10.2 Portal Vein Complications

In orthotopic whole LT, the PV anastomosis is usually performed in an end-to-end fashion between the donor and the recipient portal trunks (Fig. 10.10). In split grafts, the anastomosis is usually performed between the donor and recipient right or left portal branches. In the case of preoperative PV thrombosis and/or portal hypoplasia, PV thrombectomy (Fig. 10.11) and anastomosis on different recipient sites are possible solutions. In this latter case, the anastomosis can be performed on enlarged tributaries of the PV, on the superior mesenteric vein through a donor vascular graft, on the left renal vein or on the recipient inferior vena cava (IVC) (cavoportal hemitransposition). PV complications are less common than arterial complications. They occur in 1–13 % of whole transplantations, and include thrombosis and stenosis [18]. Technical errors, insufficient

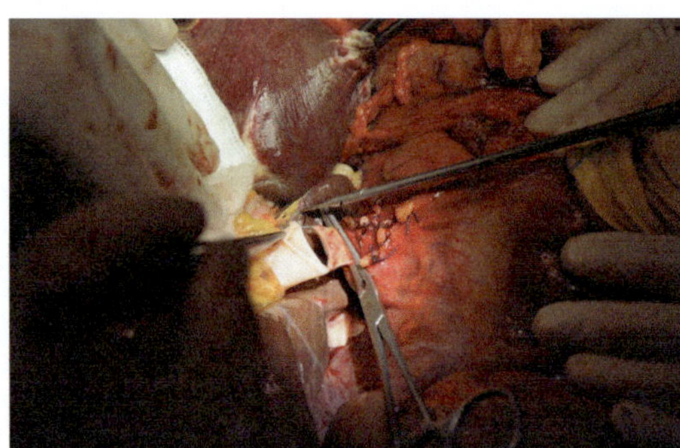

Fig. 10.10 End-to-end portal vein anastomosis in orthotopic whole LT

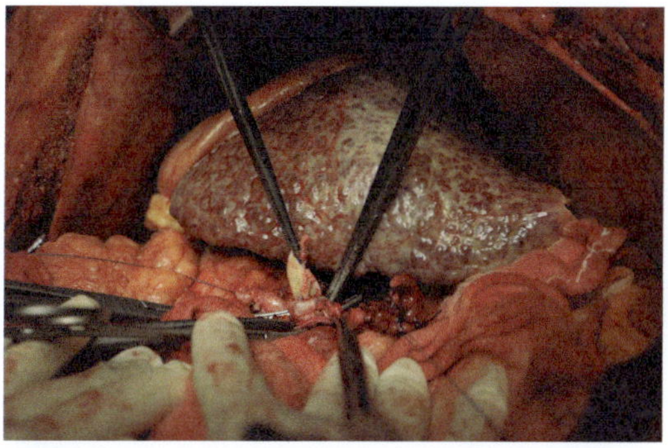

Fig. 10.11 Thrombectomy for partial occlusion of the portal vein during LT

thrombectomy, discrepancy between the sizes of the donor and recipient PVs, hypercoagulable state, and insufficient flow due to spontaneous portosystemic shunts are the main causes of

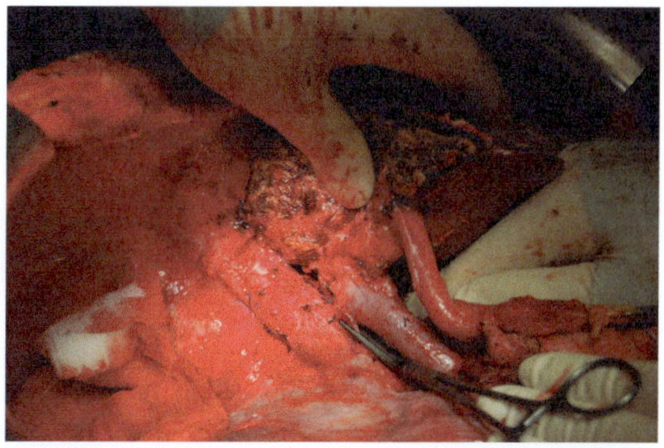

Fig. 10.13 Same case as Fig. 10.12. A hemi-portocaval shunt between the recipient right branch of the portal vein and the inferior vena cava (*IVC*) is shown in this surgical field. The creation of the shunt was mandated following persistence of graft congestion and excessive portal flow not withstanding the attempt to resolve this circulatory abnormality by splenic artery ligation

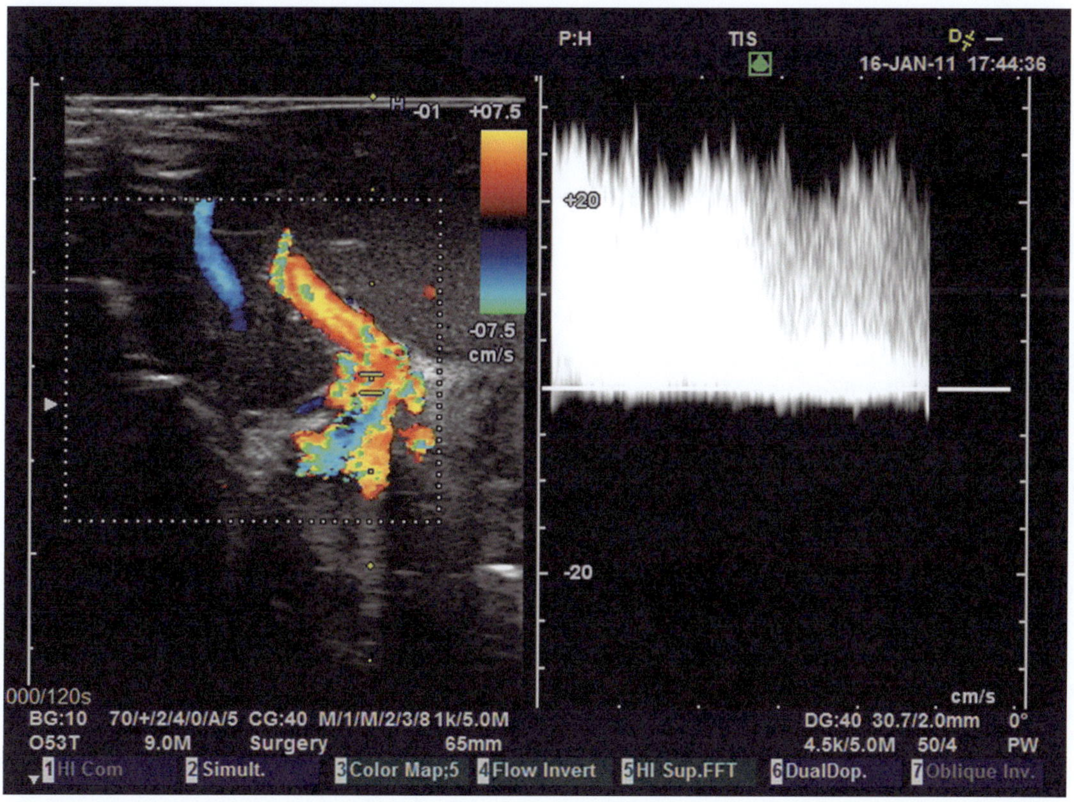

Fig. 10.12 Portal flow of 25 cm/s, associated with congestion of a left lobe graft (segments II–III), a few minutes after portal reperfusion, due to portal hyperflow in a small-for-size graft

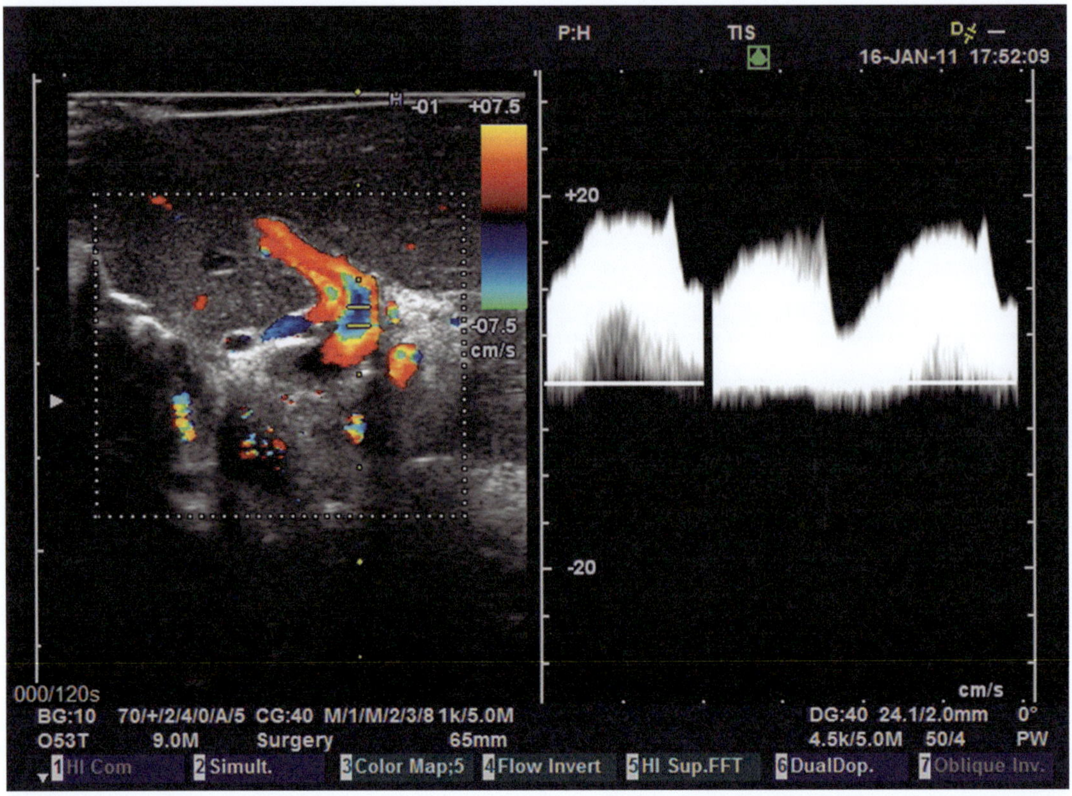

Fig. 10.14 Same case as Figs. 10.12 and 10.13, but after creation of the hemi-portocaval shunt. The portal flow decreased to normal values and became phasic with caval flow changes related to the cardiac cycle

complications [18]. Intraoperatively, a scarce portal flow can be increased with ligation of collaterals of PV or of the left renal vein, in order to reduce the flow through portosystemic shunts. Postoperatively, angioplasty, thrombolysis, thrombectomy, redo anastomosis or re-transplantation can be required.

In split LT, the use of small-for-size grafts (especially left-sided grafts) is often associated with liver congestion and dysfunction. This condition is attributable to excessive portal flow in relationship with the reduced hepatic mass, causing endothelial disruption, and secondarily parenchymal injury with cholestasis. The portal flow can be reduced with splenic artery ligation, splenectomy, or creation of a hemi-portocaval shunt (Figs. 10.12, 10.13, 10.14).

10.2.1 Thrombosis

On US, there is either total absence of flow in the PV on color Doppler, or a mass filling in a portion of the PV and partially occluding it. Contrast-enhanced CT or MR appearance is

Fig. 10.15 Visualization of the end-to-end portal vein anastomosis after LT through an intercostal transcutaneous approach, which appears as white indentations along the main portal trunk at conventional gray-scale US (**a** frame on the *right*), and not producing any change in flow velocity, as depicted by color Doppler US (**b** frame on the *left*). In another case, the portal anastomosis is visualized through a right upper abdominal quadrant subcostal approach (**b**)

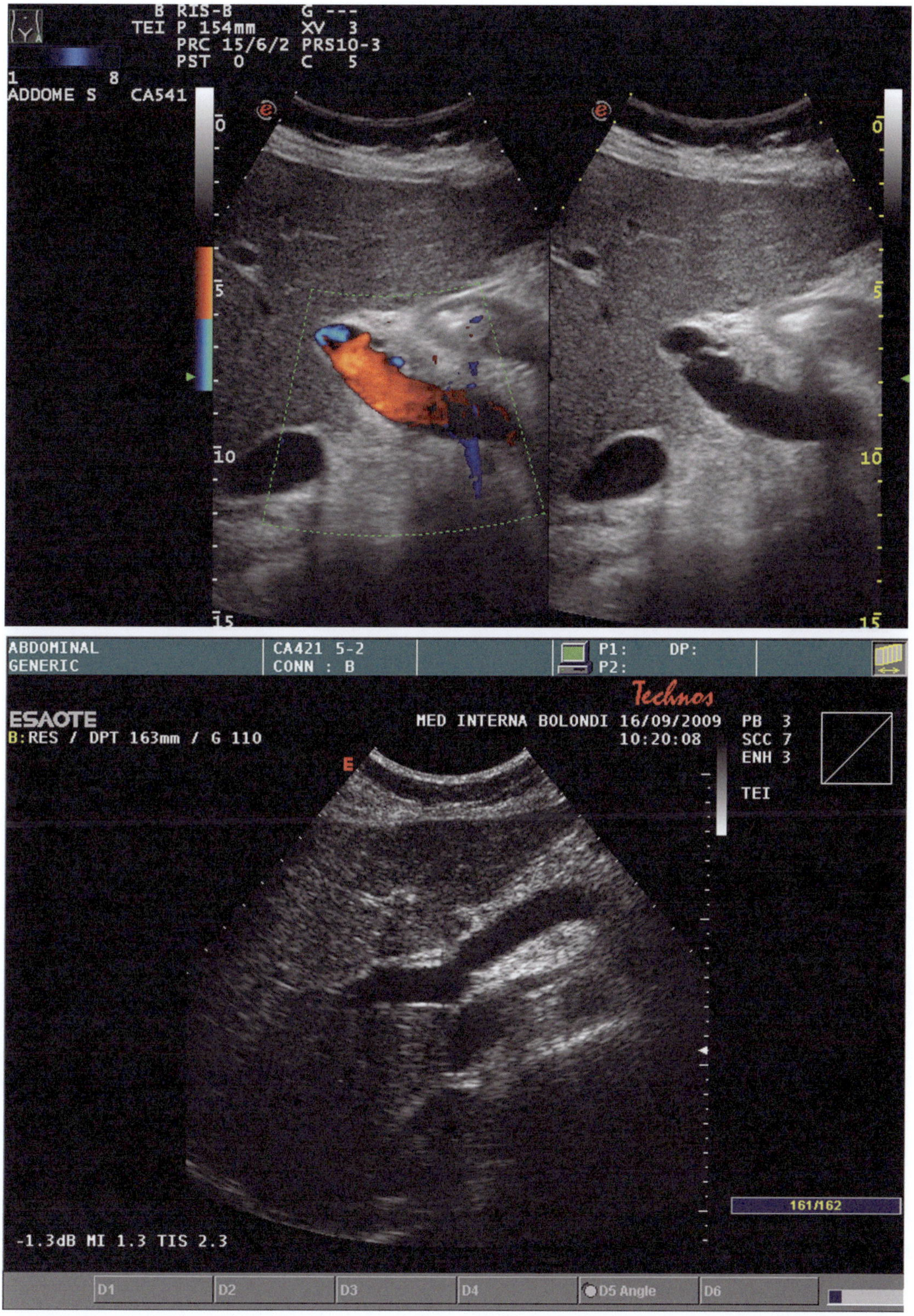
B RIS-B
TEI P 154mm
PRC 15/6/2
PST 0
G ---
XV 3
PRS10-3
C 5
ADDOME S
CA541
ABDOMINAL
GENERIC
CA421 5-2
CONN : B
P1:
DP:
P2:
Technos
ESAOTE
B:RES / DPT 163mm / G 110
MED INTERNA BOLONDI 16/09/2009
10:20:08
PB 3
SCC 7
ENH 3
TEI
161/162
-1.3dB MI 1.3 TIS 2.3
D1
D2
D3
D4
D5 Angle
D6

similar. In the acute phase, the vessel is distended. Subsequently, PV tends to narrow and scar, while the thrombus becomes more echogenic. Hematoma or fluid collections can cause the PV compression, with symptoms similar to thrombosis and absence of PV visualization on US.

10.2.2 Stenosis

PV stenosis usually occurs at the anastomosis [19] (Figs. 10.15, 10.16, 10.17). US findings include peak anastomotic velocity higher than 125 cm/s or an anastomotic-to-preanastomotic velocity ratio of 3:1 [20] (Figs. 10.16, 10.17). Focal narrowing of the PV on US, CT, or MR may represent discrepancy between donor and recipient PV vein size, or may indicate a true stenosis [19].

10.3 Inferior Vena Cava and Hepatic Vein Complications

There are different anastomotic options for the IVC in orthotopic whole LT. With the conventional technique, the recipient retrohepatic IVC is removed with the native liver, and the donor and recipient IVCs are anastomosed superiorly and inferiorly in an end-to-end fashion (Fig. 10.18). Otherwise, the recipient IVC can be preserved. In this case, the so-called ''piggyback'' technique involves the anastomosis of the donor IVC to the stump of the main recipient HVs (left and middle HVs, with or without right HV) (Figs. 10.19, 10.20). Another technique is represented by the end-to-side or side-to-side anastomosis between the donor and the recipient IVC. In split grafts (Figs. 10.21, 10.22), HVs are usually anastomosed to the recipient IVC or to the stump of recipient major HVs. The

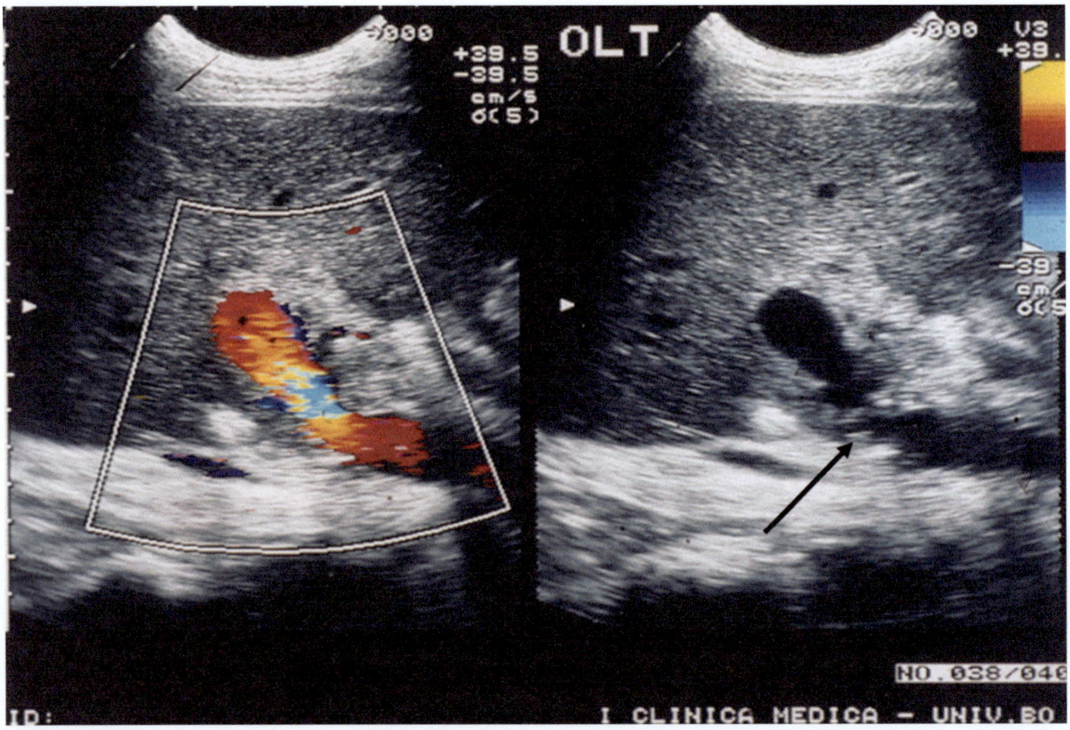

Fig. 10.16 Flow disturbance with turbulences (indicated by the aliasing phenomenon, corresponding to the mixture of *blue*, *yellow*, and *red* colors at color Doppler in the *left* frame) at the site of lumen narrowing at the portal anastomotic site (*black arrow*, *right* frame) and immediately downstream from it. In this instance, a pulse Doppler flow trace sampling is mandatory to ascertain whether a focal acceleration occurs (over × 3–4 the upstream velocities), suggesting a hemodynamic stenosis

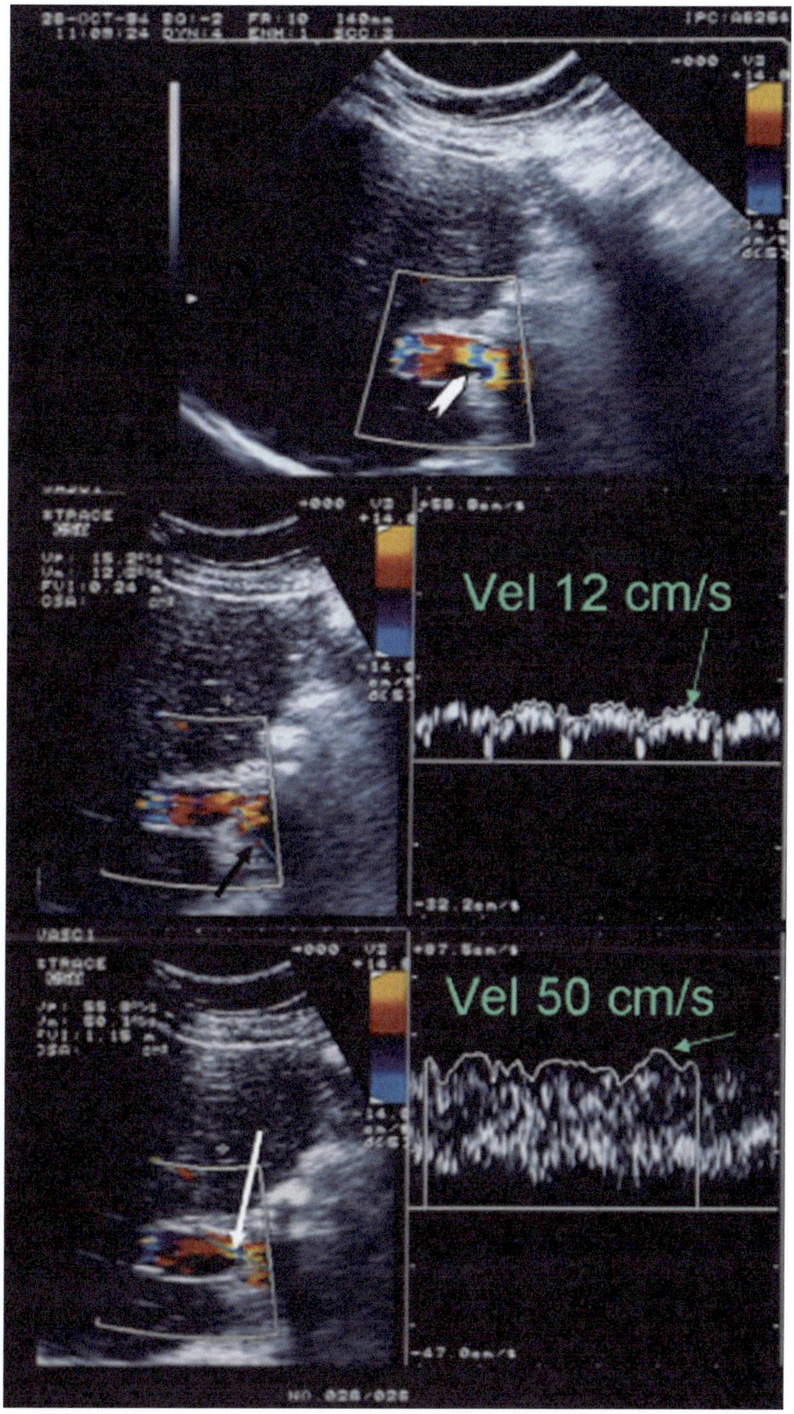

Fig. 10.17 Portal vein flow in the case of hemodynamic stenosis. *White arrow* indicates a color Doppler pattern of aliasing (see legend to Fig. 10.16). Doppler flow trace on the pre-stenotic portal trunk (*black arrow*) shows low velocity, whereas at the site of stenosis a focal aliasing with flow acceleration (over × 4) is demonstrated (*arrowhead*)

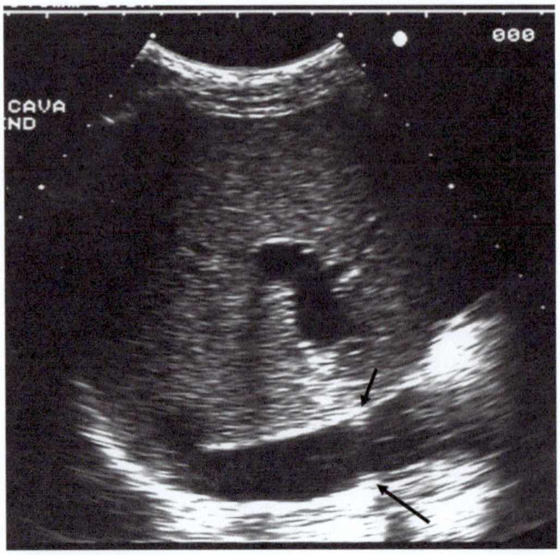

Fig. 10.18 End-to-end inferior IVC anastomosis (*longitudinal view)*

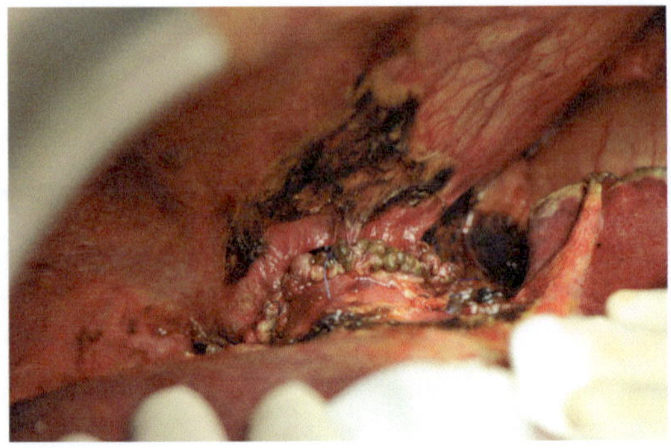

Fig. 10.19 Intraoperative view of piggyback caval anastomosis

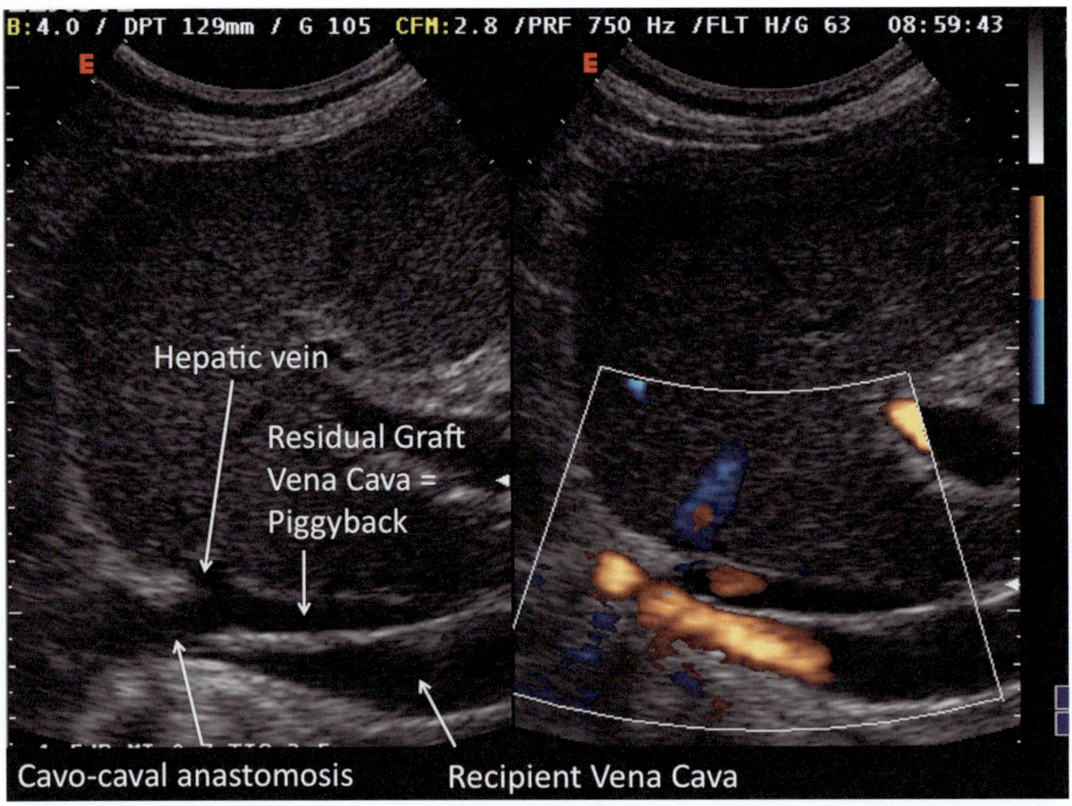

Fig. 10.20 Piggyback anastomosis between the donor suprahepatic IVC and the cuff of recipient major hepatic veins (*lateral view*); hepatic vein (*HV*)

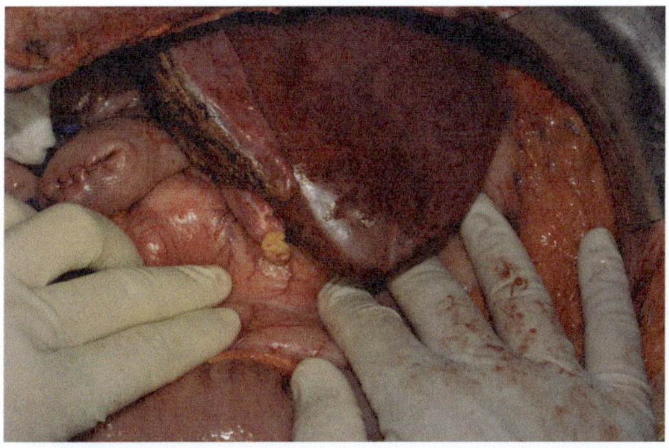

Fig. 10.21 Intraoperative view of a left split graft (including hepatic segments II and III, and the left hepatic vein)

knowledge of the type of anastomosis is essential because stenosis or thrombosis usually occur at the anastomotic site. Complications include IVC and HV stenosis and thrombosis, which occur in 1–2 % of transplantations [21].

10.3.1 HV Stenosis or Thrombosis

The Doppler waveform in a normal HV is typically triphasic, but after transplantation the waveform is often biphasic even without any other signs of flow obstruction [22]. Doppler examinations in a patient with HV stenosis will show decreased mean velocities in both the HVs and PV. Moreover, in the case of outflow obstruction the HV waveform is altered, and when significant stenosis develops it usually shows a monophasic pattern [20] (Figs. 10.23, 10.24). Other findings may include reversal of HV flow, accelerated flow with aliasing just beyond the stenosis, and direct visualization of the stenosis. Direct visualization of the stenosis is often detectable by CT, sometimes with parenchymal perfusion abnormalities. HV thrombosis appears as an intraluminal filling defect and a lack of blood flow. Treatment may be unnecessary in the absence of symptoms; otherwise, balloon angioplasty, reoperation with an additional anastomosis between the inferior stump of the donor IVC and the recipient IVC, or retransplantation can be required.

In split LT, HV flow can lack the phasic pattern due to insufficient size of the venous outflow, inappropriate positioning of the graft, or its postoperative regeneration (Figs. 10.25, 10.26).

10.3.2 IVC Stenosis or Thrombosis

IVC stenosis is caused by anastomotic narrowing [14] or extrinsic compression secondary to graft swelling [19], fluid, or hematoma. US demonstrates a three- to fourfold increase in velocity compared to the prestenotic tract (Fig. 10.27), and associated color Doppler aliasing. Indirect findings include distention of the HVs with dampening and loss of phasicity of the HV waveform when the stenosis is in the suprahepatic IVC. Chong et al. [20] used the venous pulsatility index, defined as the peak venous velocity minus the minimum venous velocity all divided by the peak velocity. Normal vessels had an index of 0.75, while stenoses were associated with a low index, with a mean value of 0.39 [20]. CT and MR venography demonstrate focal narrowing of the IVC, and there may be imaging features of Budd-Chiari syndrome or portal hypertension. The treatment of IVC stenosis usually consists of angioplasty and stenting [18].

The appearance of thrombosis is similar to that in PV, with a space-occupying mass obliterating (in the case of complete thrombosis) or narrowing (in partial thrombosis) either the colorized portion of the vessel on color Doppler, or the contrasted lumen on CT or MR.

10.3.3 Domino Transplantation

Domino transplantation (DT) involves the use of a liver retrieved from recipients of LT with metabolic diseases for a second recipient. It is a

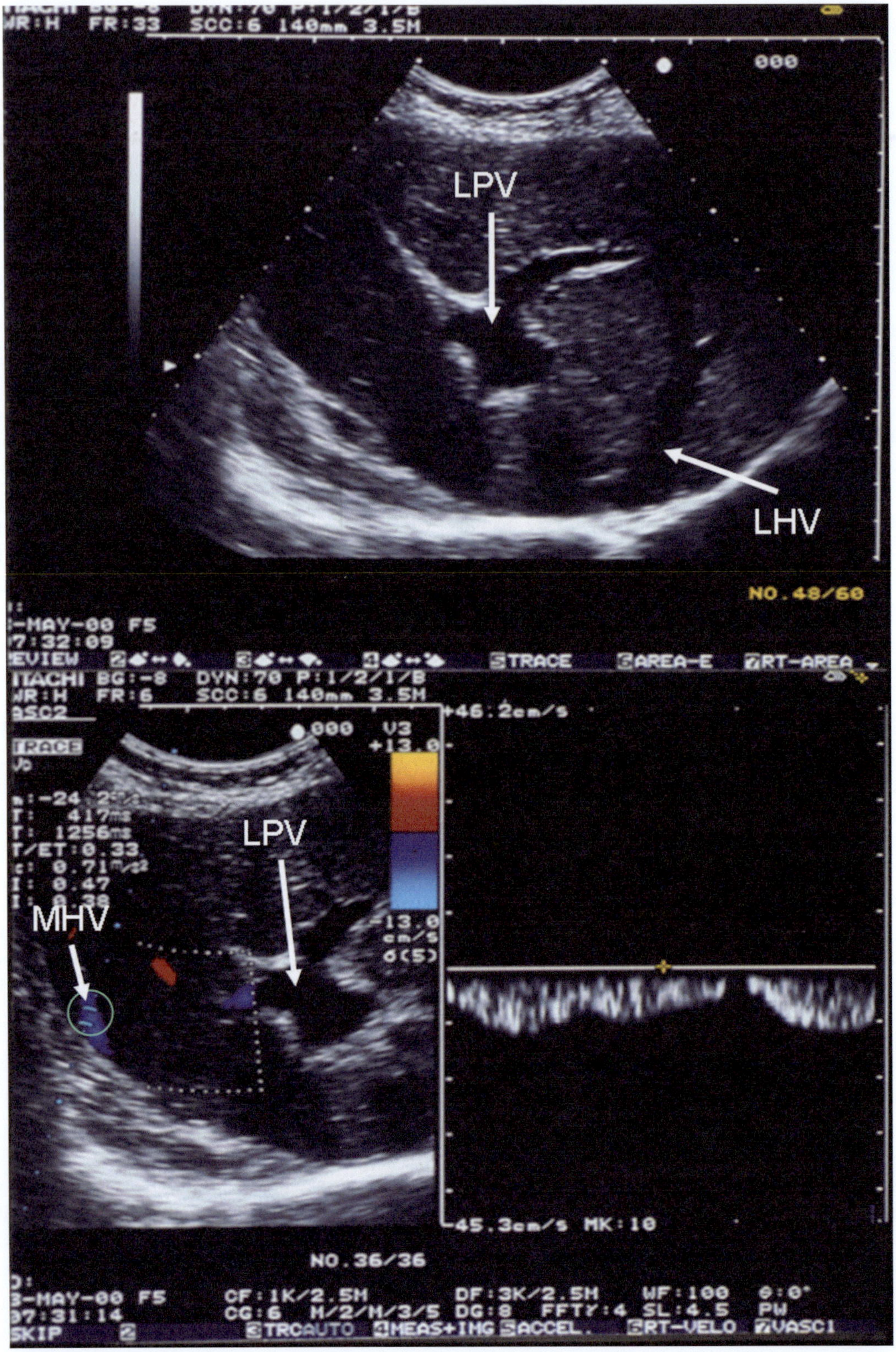

Fig. 10.22 Split liver (left lobe transplantation). Regular triphasic tracing in the middle hepatic vein, which lies along the border of the split graft; left portal vein (*LPV*); left hepatic vein (*LHV*); middle hepatic vein (*MHV*)

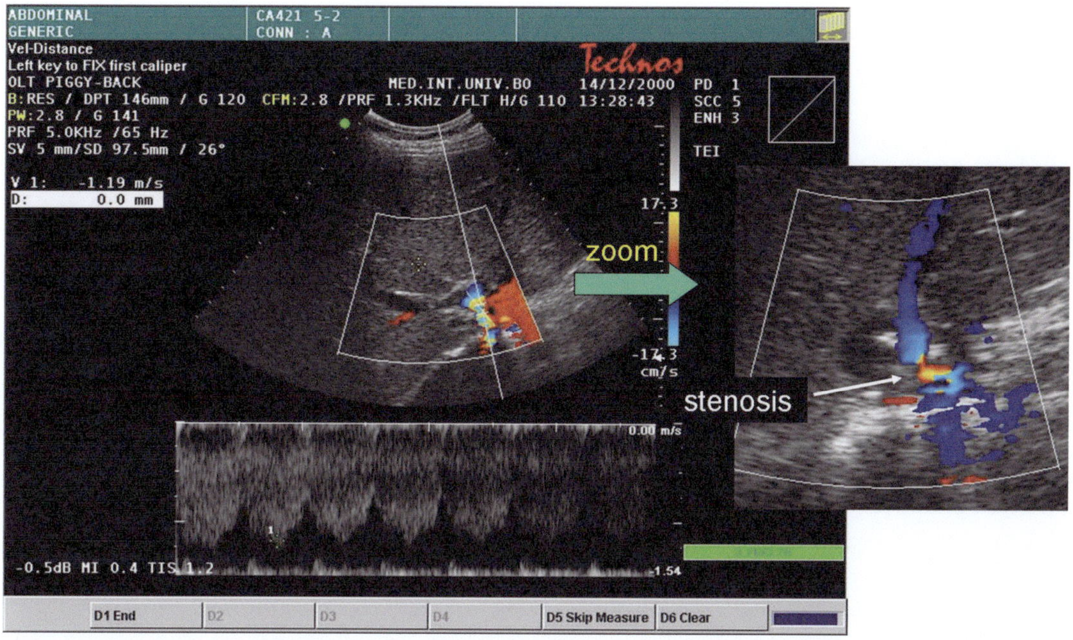

Fig. 10.23 Piggyback caval anastomosis complicated by stenosis (most commonly encountered at the outflow tract of the right hepatic vein) (transversal subcostal view, stenosis outlined by aliasing at color Doppler)

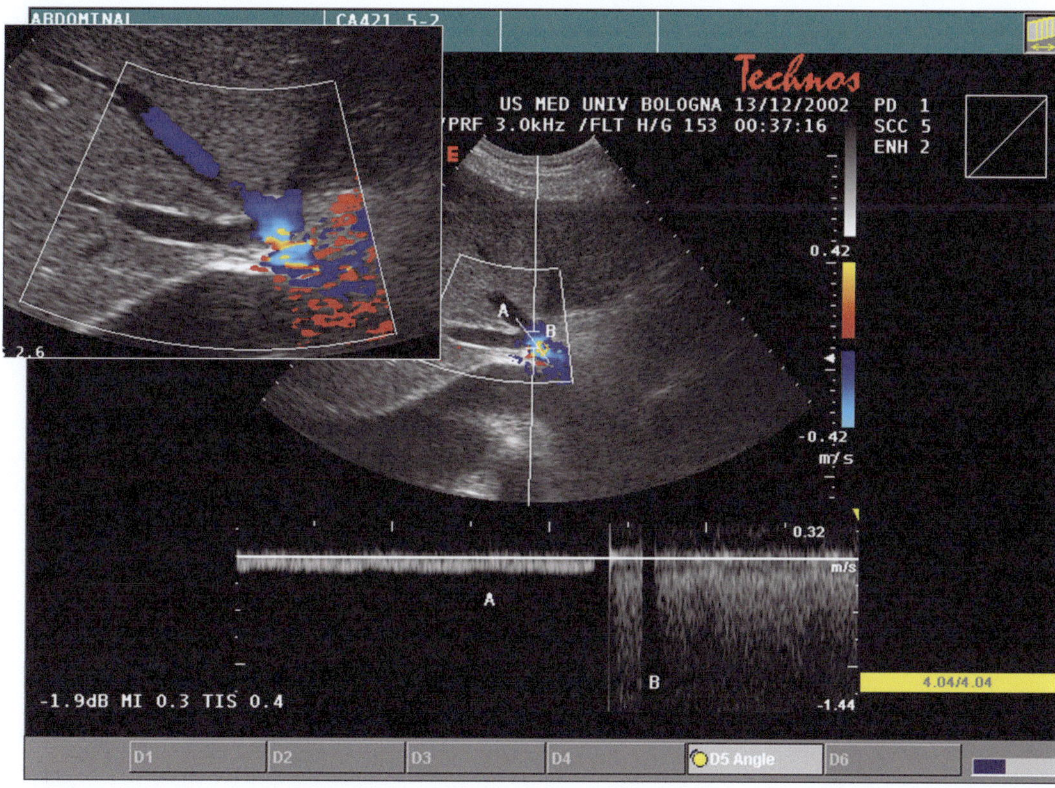

Fig. 10.24 Piggyback caval anastomosis complicated by stenosis (*transversal view*). **a** The flow in the middle hepatic vein (preanastomotic site) is monophasic and rather slow. **b** At the site of stenosis, the flow is turbulent and markedly accelerated

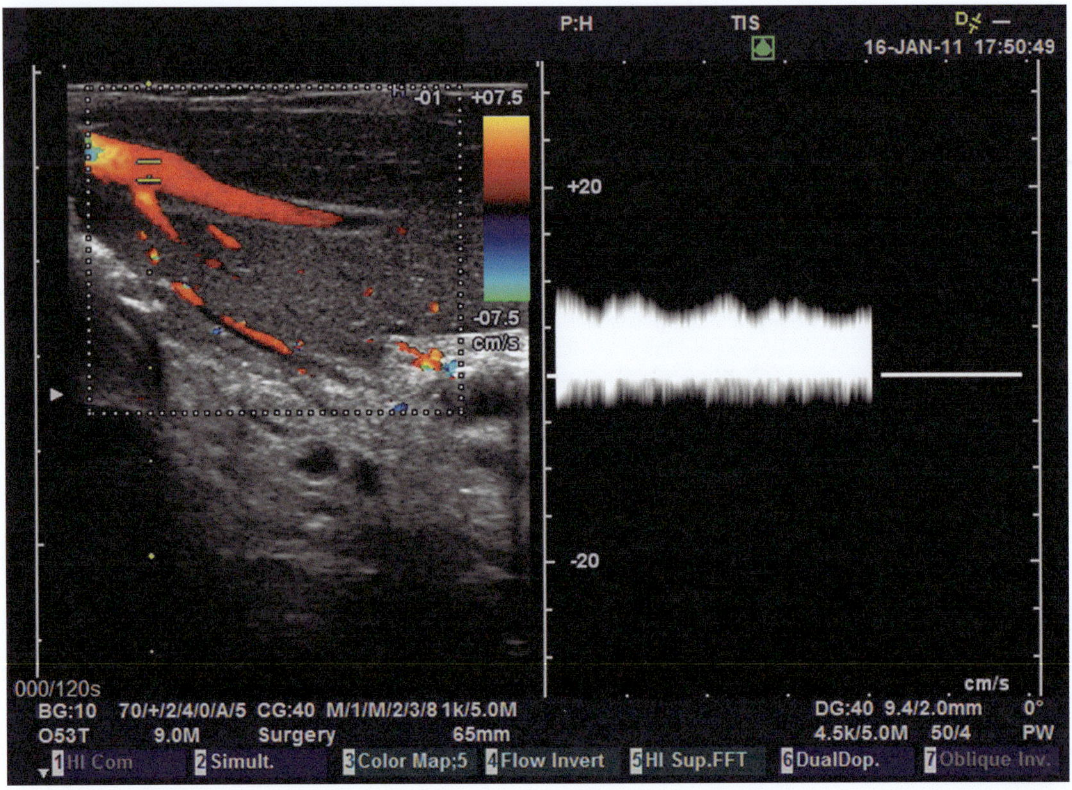

Fig. 10.25 Flattened flow trace in the left hepatic vein in a left lobe graft (segments II–III) after anastomosis between the donor left hepatic vein and the recipient stump of left and middle hepatic veins (intraoperative Doppler US)

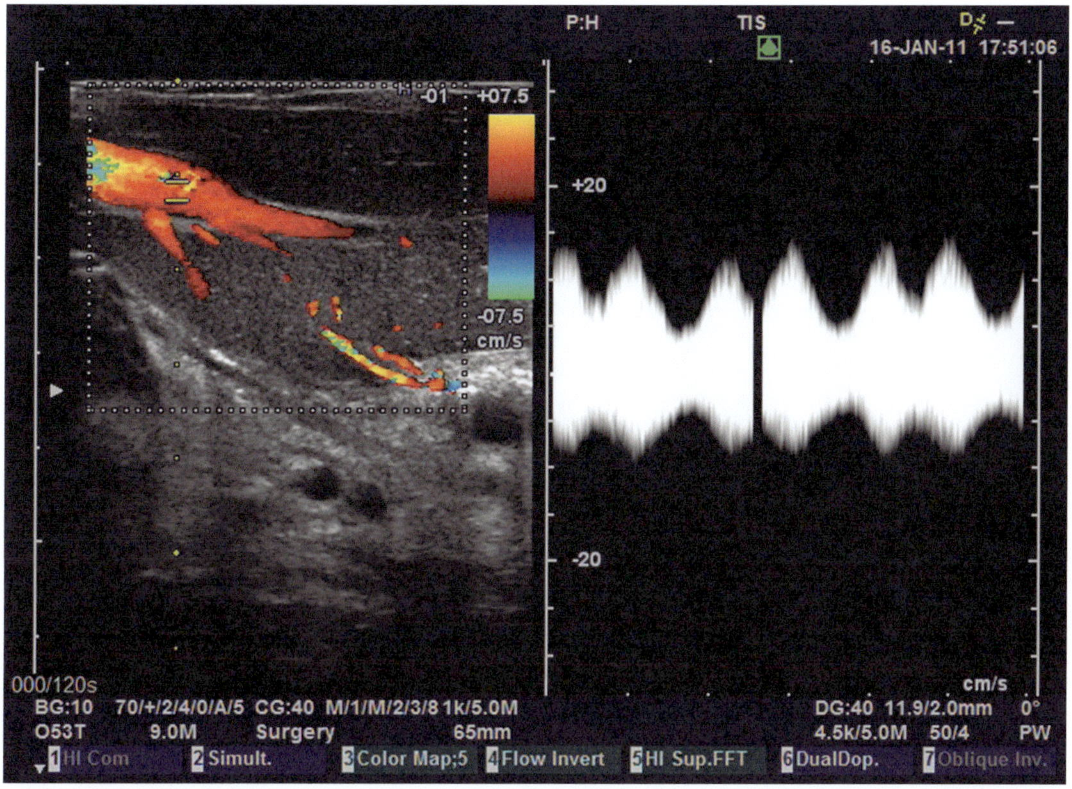

Fig. 10.26 Same case as Fig. 10.25. A better positioning of the graft with its rotation to the left-hand side led to a practically normal phasic flow in the left hepatic vein

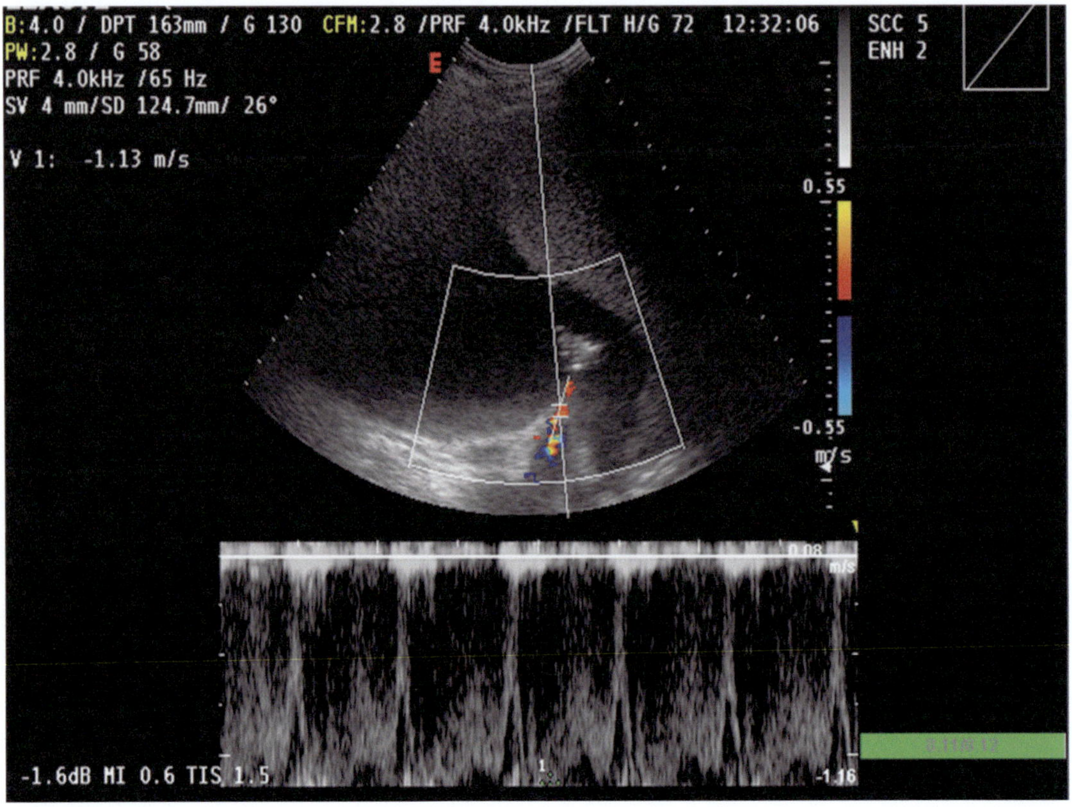

Fig. 10.27 In a patient with abundant right pleural and abdominal effusion, Doppler US shows a narrowed suprahepatic vena cava (end-to-end anastomosis), with limited phasic flow oscillations and high flow velocity (over 1 m/s). Since no focal stenosis is visible, a suspicion of caval stenosis due to graft rotation and caval torsion (consistent with technical surgical situation) is raised

well-recognized tool for expanding organ availability. Since the preservation of the IVC in the donor determines a short stump of main HVs in the domino graft, the caval anastomosis in DT recipients is challenging and its technique is not well defined. We devised a technique for outflow reconstruction, which is now routinely used in our Institution [23].

DT donor hepatectomy is performed with preservation of the IVC. Short veins draining the caudate lobe are sutured or clipped. In order to keep the HV cuff long enough to perform a piggyback reconstruction, no attempt is made to obtain a long caval stump in the native liver, and the orifices of major HVs of the amyloidotic liver do not have sufficient tissue to perform a direct anastomosis with the caval cuff of the DT recipients (Fig. 10.28). At the back table, a vascular graft including the lower portion of the IVC in continuity with the left or right common iliac vein harvested from a deceased donor is used. The conduit is opened longitudinally and placed upon the above-mentioned venous stumps with its inferior wall, which is opened circularly in correspondence and anastomosed with each venous orifice (Fig. 10.29). A venoplasty between the stumps of the amyloidotic graft is performed whenever possible.

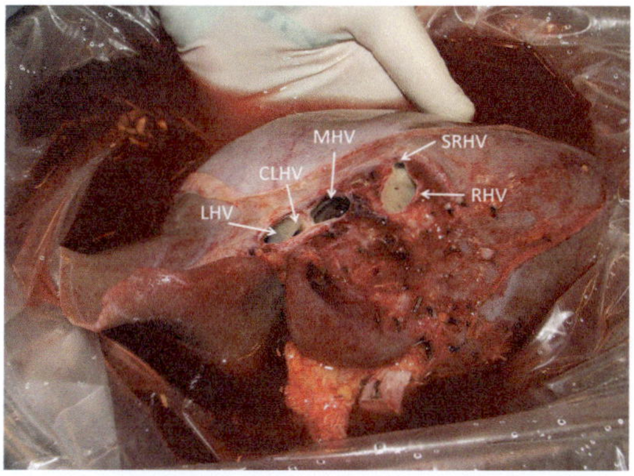

Fig. 10.28 Preparation of the caval anastomosis (piggyback type) in domino transplantation. Amyloidotic liver graft with the orifices of the caudate lobe hepatic vein (*CLHV*), left hepatic vein (*LHV*), middle hepatic vein (*MHV*), right hepatic vein (*RHV*), and superficial right hepatic vein (*SRHV*)

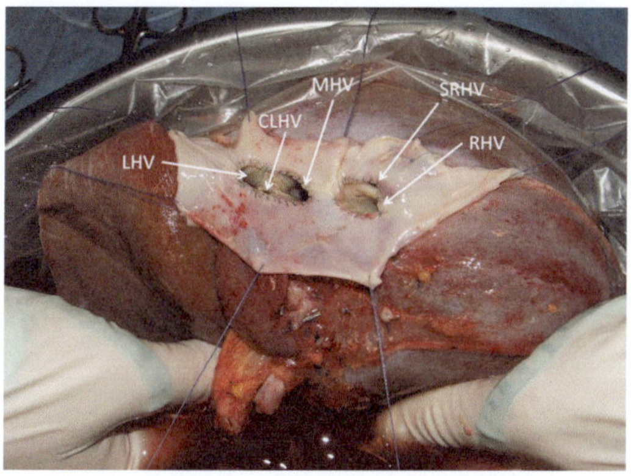

Fig. 10.29 Preparation of the caval anastomosis (piggyback type) in domino transplantation. Venous patch anastomosed to the orifices formed by the caudate lobe hepatic vein (*CLHV*), left hepatic vein (*LHV*) and middle hepatic vein (*MHV*), and by the right hepatic vein (*RHV*) and superficial right hepatic vein (*SRHV*)

The external edge of the vascular graft is trimmed in order to obtain a circular stump, which is anastomosed end-to-end with the recipient cuff formed by the right, middle, and left HVs (Figs. 10.30, 10.31). No venous outflow complications were recorded with this technique in our series (Fig. 10.32).

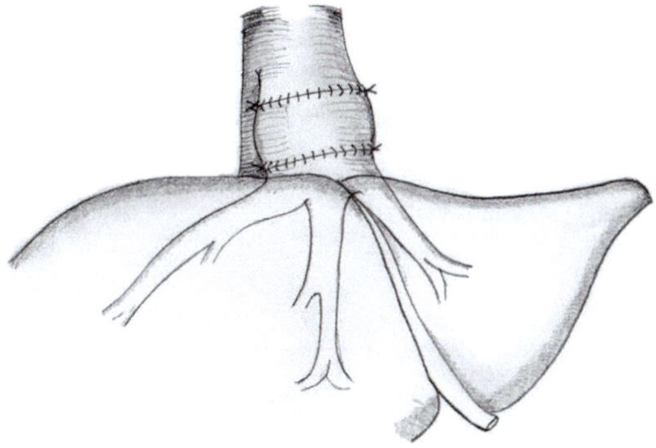

Fig. 10.30 Preparation of the caval anastomosis (piggyback type) in domino transplantation. Scheme of the caval anastomosis with interposition of a venous patch in domino transplantation

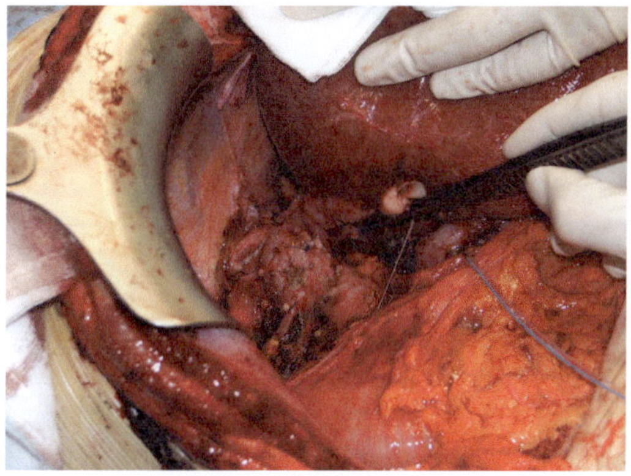

Fig. 10.31 Preparation of the caval anastomosis (piggyback type) in domino transplantation. Intraoperative aspect of the caval anastomosis with interposition of a venous patch in domino transplantation with piggyback technique

10.4 Biliary Complications

The biliary anastomosis is usually performed between the common bile duct of donor and recipient, with or without placement of a T-tube; more rarely, a choledocho-jejunal anastomosis is performed. Biliary complications are the most frequent after LT (up to 25 %) [24], and include anastomotic stenosis, bile duct stricture, stone formation, bile leak, biloma, biliary necrosis,

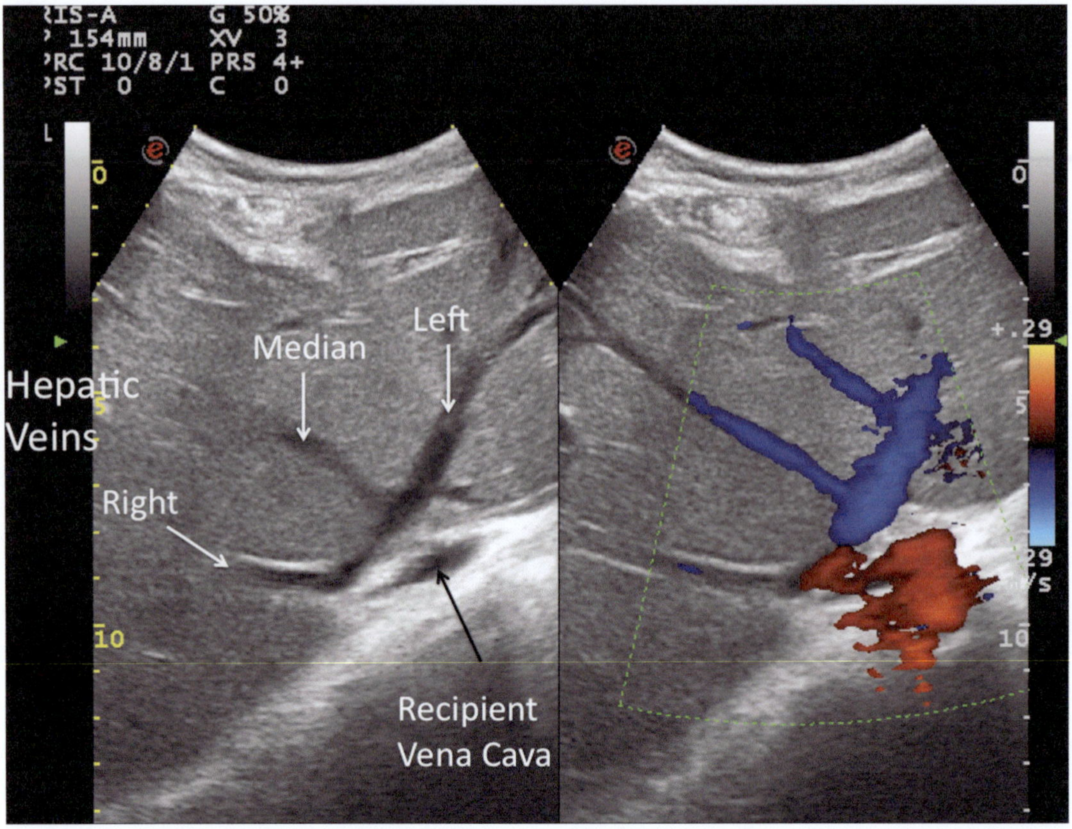

Fig. 10.32 Postoperative color Doppler showing normodirected venous flow in the three major hepatic veins in the domino grafts after caval anastomosis with interposition of a venous patch

abscesses, and cholangitis. In general, US has a lower sensitivity (around 50 %) compared to other imaging techniques for detecting biliary complications [25]. Biliary complications are more common after split LT, which is more technically challenging [26].

Complications can be managed with percutaneous transhepatic cholangiography, endoscopic retrograde cholangiography, surgical correction, or retransplantation [25].

Biliary obstruction can be secondary to anastomotic stricture and choledocolithiasis. US usually demonstrates intrahepatic bile duct dilation. However, nonobstructive dilatation of the extrahepatic donor and recipient ducts can be present without intrahepatic biliary dilatation. Nonobstructive biliary dilatation can be secondary to papillary dyskinesia or to a discrepancy between the size of the donor and recipient ducts, being often clinically insignificant. Conversely, liver grafts may not develop biliary dilatation despite severe stenosis. Nonanastomotic biliary stricture occurs due to ischemia, often as a result of HA thrombosis or stenosis (Fig. 10.4), cholangitis, or recurrent sclerosing cholangitis [24, 25].

Bile leaks are most commonly located at the biliary anastomosis or the T-tube exit site [24, 25], .thus identifiable with cholangiography. Leaks are usually caused by technical errors or dehiscence secondary to ischemia. Persistent, untreated bile leaks can cause bilomas, which appear as rounded and hypoechoic fluid collections at US (Figs. 10.33, 10.34). However, US

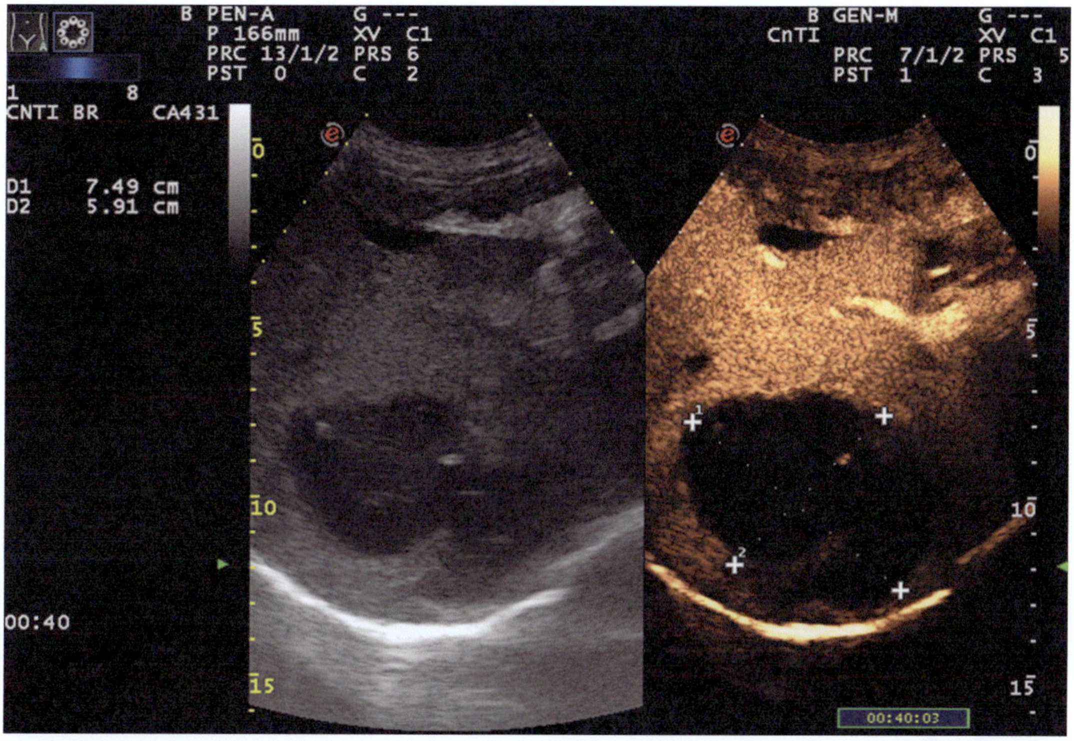

Fig. 10.33 Bile collection (biloma) in a LT patient previously submitted to percutaneous transarterial chemoembolization of recurrent hepatocellular carcinoma (US and contrast-enhanced US images, *left* and *right* frames, respectively). The contrast images better depict the nonperfused areas (corresponding to the biloma, 7.49 and 5.91 cm in cross-sectional diameters), and better distinguish necrotic from vital areas, not well demarcated at conventional US, which apparently shows a smaller size of the lesion

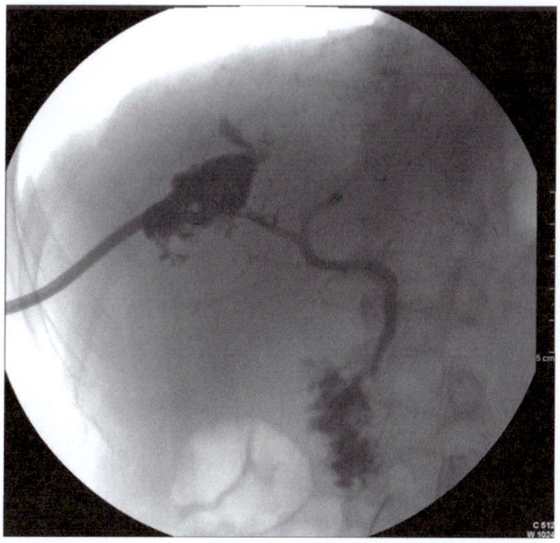

Fig. 10.34 Same case as Fig. 10.33. The contrast medium injection through the abdominal catheter positioned to drain the biloma shows a communication of the biloma with the biliary tree

may not be able to help differentiate bile leaks from non-biliary postoperative fluid collections such as ascites, abscess, hematoma, or from bowel limbs [24, 25].

As mentioned above, liver abscesses consequent to biliary injury may occur due to HA thrombosis or stenosis (Fig. 10.35). Bilomas or abscesses must be differentiated from other lesions with liquid content (Fig. 10.36).

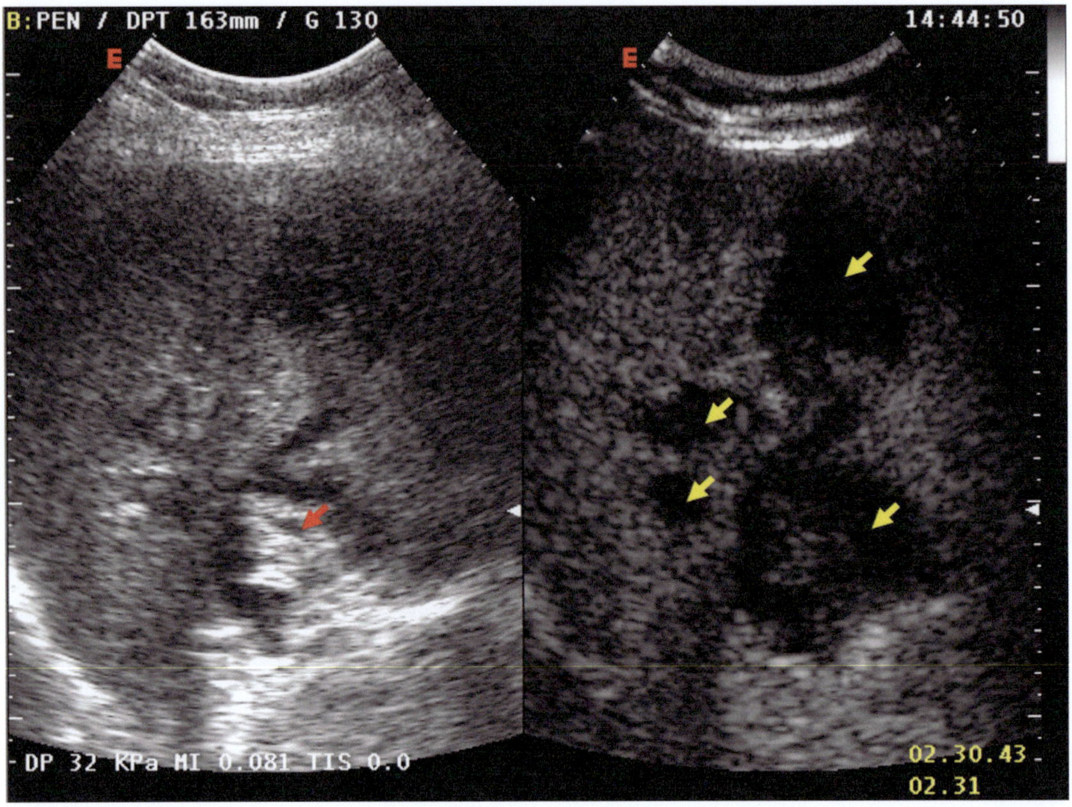

Fig. 10.35 In a patient seen for fever, malaise and right upper abdominal quadrant pain, and tenderness with rapid onset 7 years after transplantation, B-mode gray-scale US shows a rather patchy, inhomogeneous echotexture of the hepatic parenchyma (*left panel*), with possible gas formation (*red arrow*). Contrast-enhanced US (*right panel*) much more clearly demarcates the devascularized (echo-free) necrotic area (*yellow arrows*, no contrast perfusion at all), corresponding to hepatic abscesses and biliary tract damage with bile casts, due to late arterial obstruction

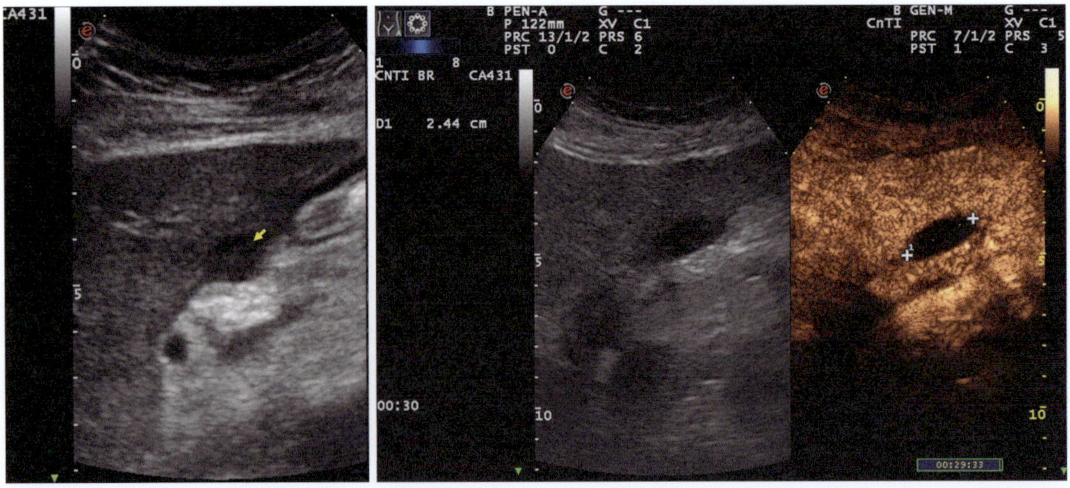

Fig. 10.36 Small subcapsular lesion of the posterior face of the left lobe; **a** longitudinal epigastric scan at gray-scale B-mode US; the lesion is suspected to be a hematoma; **b** a liquid nature is confirmed by contrast enhanced US, which shows the absence of any perfusion (echo-free = black lesion, in the *right frame* of the dual display in **b**)

References

1. Singh AK, Nachiappan AC, Verma HA et al (2010) Postoperative imaging in liver transplantation: what radiologists should know. Radiographics 30:339–351
2. Orons PD, Sheng R, Zajko AB (1995) Hepatic artery stenosis in liver transplant recipients: prevalence and cholangiographic appearance of associated biliary complications. Am J Roentgenol 165:1145–1149
3. Saad WEA, Lin E, Ormanoski M et al (2007) Noninvasive imaging of liver transplant complications. Tech Vasc Interv Rad 10:191–206
4. Dodd GD 3rd, Memel DS, Zajko AB et al (1994) Hepatic artery stenosis and thrombosis in transplant recipients: Doppler diagnosis with resistive index and systolic acceleration time. Radiology 192:657–661
5. Nolten A, Sproat IA (1996) Hepatic artery thrombosis after liver transplantation: temporal accuracy of diagnosis with duplex US and the syndrome of impending thrombosis. Radiology 198:553–559
6. Garcia-Criado A, Gilabert R, Salmeron JM et al (2003) Significance of and contributing factors for a high resistive index on Doppler sonography of the hepatic artery immediately after surgery: prognostic implications for liver transplant recipients. Am J Roentgenol 181:831–838
7. Hom BK, Shrestha R, Palmer SL et al (2006) Prospective evaluation of vascular complications after liver transplantation: comparison of conventional and microbubble contrast-enhanced US. Radiology 241:267–274
8. Wozney P, Zajko AB, Bron KM et al (1986) Vascular complications after liver transplantation: a 5-year experience. Am J Roentgenol 147:657–663
9. Sánchez-Bueno F, Robles R, Ramírez P et al (1994) Hepatic artery complications after liver transplantation. Clin Transplant 8:399–404
10. Caiado AH, Blasbalg R, Marcelino AS et al (2007) Complications of liver transplantation: multimodality imaging approach. Radiographics 27:1401–1417
11. Abbasoglu O, Levy MF, Vodapally MS et al (1997) Hepatic artery stenosis after liver transplantation: incidence, presentation, treatment, and long term outcome. Transplantation 63:250–255
12. Glockner JF, Forauer AR (1999) Vascular or ischemic complications after liver transplantation. Am J Roentgenol 173:1055–1059
13. Sheng R, Orons PD, Ramos HC et al (1995) Dissecting pseudoaneurysm of the hepatic artery: a delayed complication of angioplasty in a liver transplant. Cardiovasc Interv Radiol 18:112–114
14. Nghiem HV, Tran K, Winter TC 3rd et al (1996) Imaging of complications in liver transplantation. Radiographics 16:825–840
15. Saad WEA, Davies MG, Rubens DJ et al (2006) Endoluminal management of arterio-portal fistulae in liver transplant recipients: a single center experience. Vasc Endovasc Surg 40:451–459
16. Chavan A, Harms J, Pichlmayr R et al (1993) Transcatheter coil occlusion of an intrahepatic arterioportal fistula in a transplanted liver. Bildgebung 60:215–218
17. Strodel E, Eckhauser FE, Lemmer JH et al (1987) Presentation and perioperative management of arterioportal fistulas. Arch Surg 122:563–571
18. Nghiem HV (1998) Imaging of hepatic transplantation. Radiol Clin N Am 36:429–443
19. Quiroga S, Sebastià MC, Margarit C et al (2001) Complications of orthotopic liver transplantation: spectrum of findings with helical CT. Radiographics 21:1085–1102
20. Chong WK, Beland JC, Weeks SM (2007) Sonographic evaluation of venous obstruction in liver transplants. Am J Roentgenol 188:W515–W521
21. Uzochukwu LN, Bluth EI, Smetherman DH et al (2005) Early postoperative hepatic sonography as a predictor of vascular and biliary complications in adult orthotopic liver transplant patients. Am J Roentgenol 185:1558–1570
22. Fujimoto M, Moriyasu F, Someda H et al (1995) Recovery of graft circulation following percutaneous transluminal angioplasty for stenotic venous complications in pediatric liver transplantation: assessment with Doppler ultrasound. Transpl Int 8:119–125
23. Cescon M, Grazi GL, Ravaioli M et al (2007) Modified out flow reconstruction with a venous patch in domino liver transplantation. Liver Transpl 13:1756–1757
24. Crossin JD, Muradali D, Wilson SR (2003) US of liver transplants: normal and abnormal. Radiographics 23:1093–1114
25. Zemel G, Zajko AB, Skolnick ML et al (1988) The role of sonography and transhepatic cholangiography in the diagnosis of biliary complications after liver transplantation. Am J Roentgenol 151:943–946
26. Cescon M, Spada M, Colledan M et al (2006) Feasibility and limits of split liver transplantation from pediatric donors: an Italian multicenter experience. Ann Surg 244:805–814

Liver Transplantation from Living Donors

11

Kiyoshi Hasegawa, Yasuhiko Sugawara, and Norihiro Kokudo

Abbreviations

LDLT Living Donor Liver Transplantation

11.1 Introduction

Living donor liver transplantation (LDLT) requires the simultaneous fulfillment of two conflicting demands [1]: (i) ensuring adequate vascular channels and residual liver volume needed to be able to maintain the liver function in the donor, and (ii) in order to facilitate the surgical maneuvers in the recipient and make the postoperative course favorable, ensuring the maximal liver volume and diameter and length of vascular channels within a range that fulfills. Consequently, it is necessary to decide on the plane of the liver transection and where to divide the vascular channels in a way that always maintains a balance between the conditions of the donor and the recipient, and therein lies the difficulty of the LDLT donor operation. Intraoperative ultrasonography is an essential examination method for determining the optimal transection plane and division points. Below we describe the surgical maneuvers and the role of intraoperative ultrasonography by using a right liver graft harvesting operation as an example.

11.2 Intraoperative Ultrasonography Immediately After the Laparotomy

After performing the laparotomy through an upper midline incision and confirming the absence of any findings in the abdominal cavity that would contraindicate surgery in the living donor, a thoracotomy is performed by making an oblique incision toward the right ninth intercostal space (depending on the circumstances in the individual case, we have not performed a thoracotomy in some recent cases). The first intraoperative ultrasonography examination is performed at this point. The absence of any tumor lesions is confirmed, and, first, the course of the right hepatic vein and inferior right hepatic vein is checked, and the diameter of their roots is measured (Fig. 11.1). Attention is then turned to the branching pattern of the middle hepatic vein, and it is examined carefully while drawing a planned line of transection in the surgeon's head. We preoperatively obtain three-dimensional imaging constructed by a computer

K. Hasegawa · Y. Sugawara · N. Kokudo (✉)
Artificial Organ and Transplantation Division, Department of Surgery, Graduate School of Medicine, University of Tokyo, 7-3-1, Hongo, Bunkyo-ku, Tokyo 113-0033, Japan
e-mail: KOKUDO-2SU@h.u-tokyo.ac.jp

K. Hasegawa
e-mail: kihase-tky@umin.ac.jp

Y. Sugawara
e-mail: yasusuga-tky@umin.ac.jp

G. Torzilli (ed.), *Ultrasound-Guided Liver Surgery*,
DOI: 10.1007/978-88-470-5510-0_11, © Springer-Verlag Italia 2014

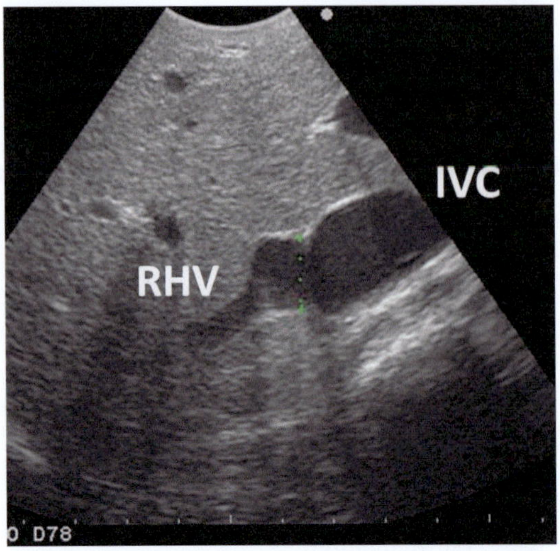

Fig. 11.1 The diameter of the right hepatic vein (*RHV*) is measured (*dotted line*) at its root. IVC, inferior vena cava

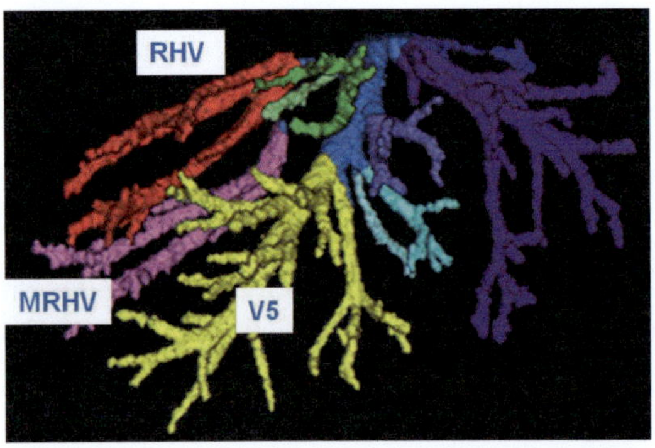

Fig. 11.2 Three-dimensional imaging constructed by a computer software using data of computed tomography. RHV right hepatic vein, MRHV middle right hepatic vein; V5 hepatic vein from the segment 5

software [2], which is useful to understand the anatomic structures as well as the findings of intraoperative ultrasonography (Fig. 11.2).

The diameter of the main branch that flows back to the right liver and the distance from the branch point to the root of the middle hepatic vein (where it joins the inferior vena cava) are measured in advance, especially when reconstructing the branches of the middle hepatic vein branches in the graft liver (Fig. 11.3a, b). The vein graft that is used for reconstruction is ultimately selected on the basis of these data. We often use thawed cryopreserved allogenic veins, but the great saphenous vein of the donor or recipient can also be used.

11.3 Hanging Maneuver and Intraoperative Ultrasonography

Next, the right liver is mobilized, and, in the initial stage, tape is passed between the posterior aspect of the liver and the anterior surface of the inferior vena cava in preparation for the hanging maneuver [3]. First, on the cranial side, the space between the middle hepatic vein and the root of the right hepatic vein is carefully dissected with sharply curved forceps. If even slight resistance is encountered as this is done, the dissection maneuver is stopped [4]. When examined by ultrasonography with the forceps left in the position, air enters the dissection line, and it is visualized as hyperechoic (Fig. 11.4a, b). It is then possible to check the direction of the dissection and avoid injuring the short hepatic veins. On the caudal side, after dissecting the caudate lobe and inferior vena cava and managing the short hepatic veins that come into view to the extent possible, the forceps is gently inserted in the midline and used to dissect craniad. Here, too, the dissection advanced so that it connects with the line of dissection from the cranial side (visualized as hyperechoic), while examining to see whether there are any short hepatic veins in the path of the forceps (Fig. 11.5a, b).

11.4 Hilar Management and Intraoperative Ultrasonography

Cholecystectomy is performed, and the right hepatic artery and right branch of the portal vein are identified in the porta hepatis. In the process of doing so the hepatoduodenal ligament is

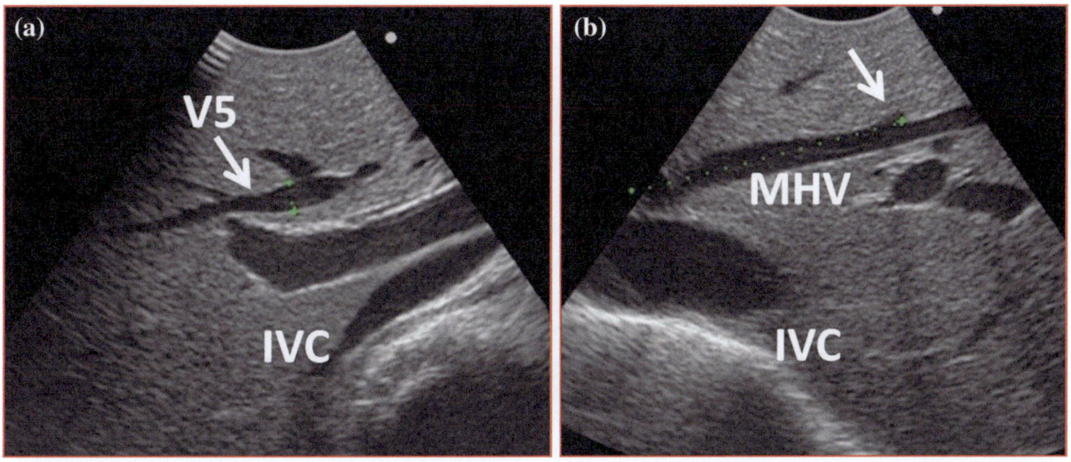

Fig. 11.3 The diameter of the hepatic vein from the segment 5 (*V5*) is measured at its root (**a**), and the length between the root of V5 and IVC (the inferior vena cava) is also measured (**b**; *dotted line*)

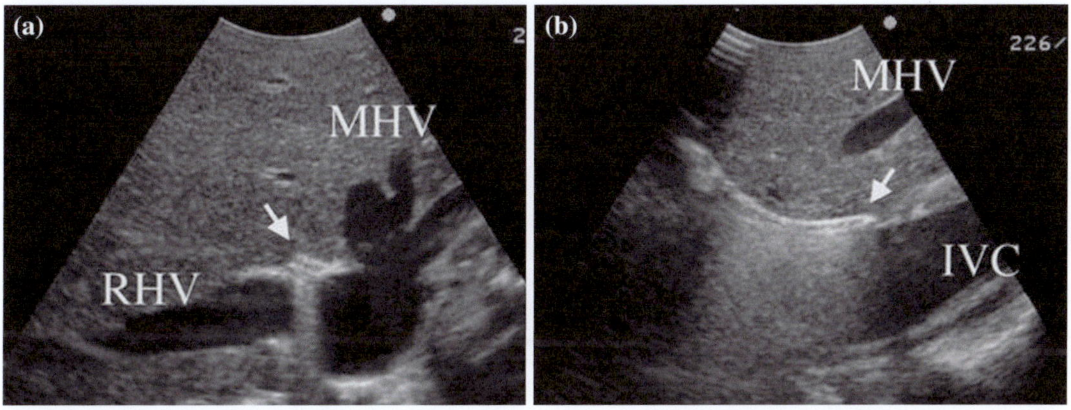

Fig. 11.4 The clamp tip is clearly visualized in the hanging maneuver (**a** transverse view, **b** sagittal view) as a strongly hyperechoic structure with a reverberation artifact (*arrow*). MHV middle hepatic vein, RHV right hepatic vein, IVC inferior vena cava (reproduced from Ref. [4] with permission)

examined by ultrasonography, and if their courses are confirmed in realtime, accidental injury can be avoided.

11.5 Plane of Transection and Ultrasonography

If the right hepatic artery and right branch of the portal vein that have been identified are clamped, since the color of the right liver surface darkens and a demarcation line appears (Fig. 11.6), it can be used as the transection line. If ultrasonography is performed along this planned transection line, it is usually possible to determine the best place to manage (ligate and divide, or secure for reconstruction) the branches of the middle hepatic vein. Unlike anatomical resection, liver dissection for the ultimate aim of liver grafting does not require exposing the surface of the middle hepatic vein. Attaching the liver parenchyma more thinly on the graft side makes it possible to reduce bleeding, however, since graft volume will be lost and the diameter of the middle hepatic vein branch that should be

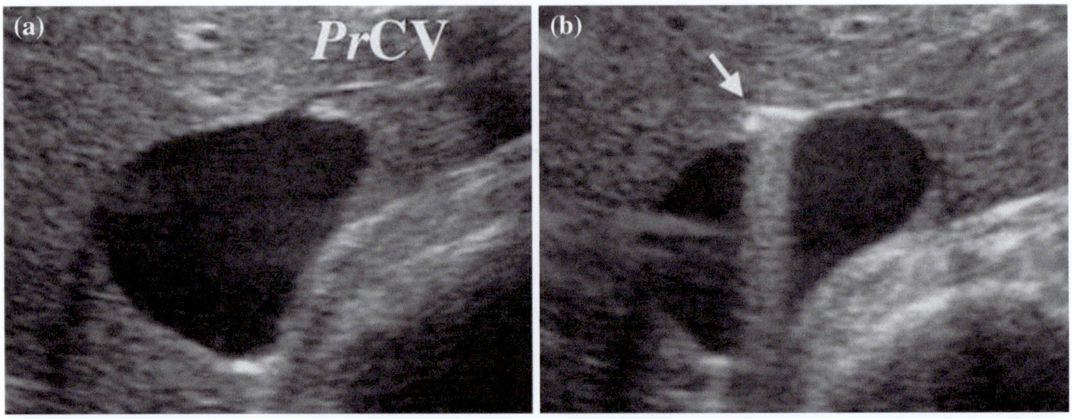

Fig. 11.5 The proper hepatic vein for the caudate lobe (*PrCV*) is visualized (**a**). In the hanging maneuver, the relationship between the dissecting course (*arrow*) and the PrCV can be checked (**b**) (reproduced from Ref. [4] with permission)

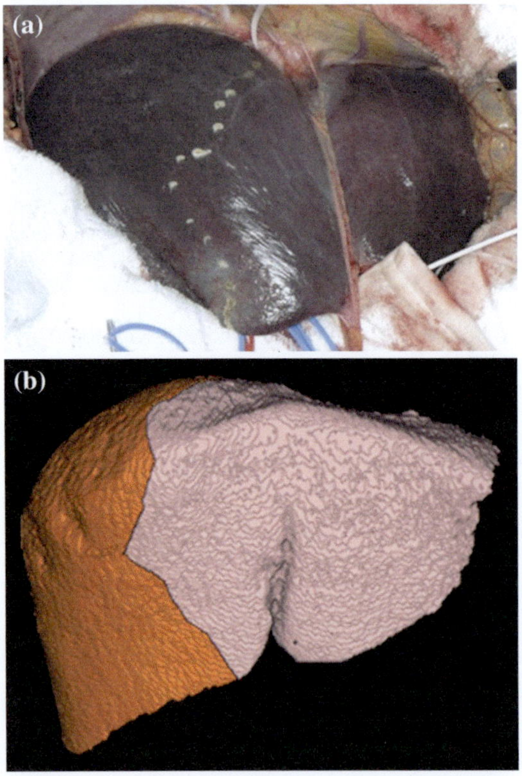

Fig. 11.6 The demarcation line is clearly demonstrated on the liver surface (**a**), which is similar to the line obtained by preoperative simulation (**b**)

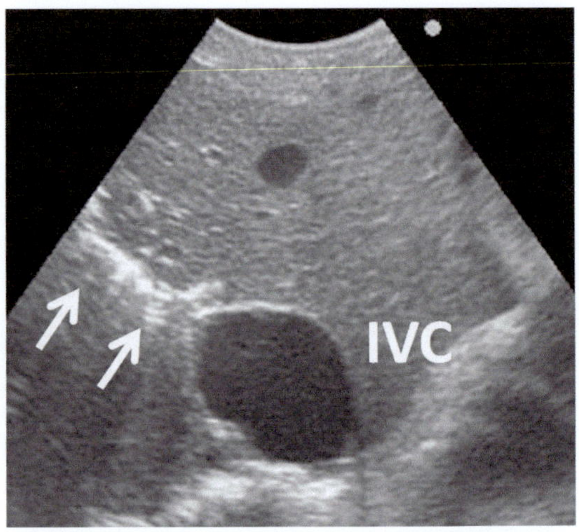

Fig. 11.7 The cutting plane is demonstrated as a hyperechoic line by intraoperative ultrasonography

used for reconstruction will be too small if performed too far from the middle hepatic vein, it should be avoided. Ultrasonography is very useful for checking to see whether the plane of transection is appropriate or not. When doing so, if the ultrasound probe is applied on the remaining liver side (S4), the transection line will be depicted as a hyperechoic line and be easy to identify (Fig. 11.7). If the branches intended for reconstruction are approached, they are carefully divided, and injury is avoided. The distance of the point of division from the main trunk can be checked by ultrasonography so that the main trunk of the middle hepatic vein does not become stenotic.

11.6 Evaluation of the Congested Area and Ultrasonography

If the branches of the middle hepatic vein are divided, the outflow channels of the areas they drain will be interrupted, and depending on the case, (i) blood flow in the portal vein reverses, and it plays the role of an outflow channel (Fig. 11.8), or (ii) the communications that lead to the right hepatic vein (Fig. 11.9) or the right inferior hepatic vein become prominent, etc., and a decrease may occur [5]. If the color Doppler mode is used, images of (i) and (ii) can be observed during the operation. If the right hepatic artery is obstructed after dividing the branches, the liver surface of the region affected by (i) will turn black (Fig. 11.10). No color change occurs in cases in which (ii) has developed.

11.7 Bile Duct Management

Dealing with the right bile duct is one of the important aspects of the graft harvesting procedure. We resect the gallbladder and perform

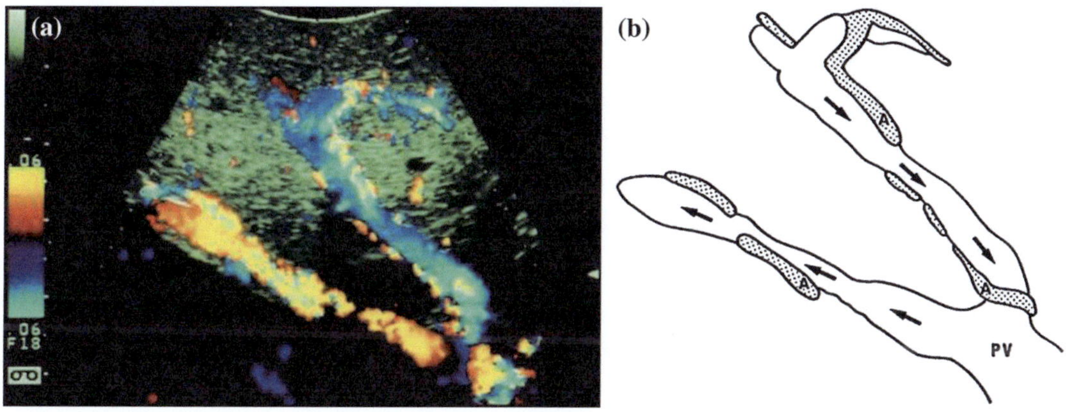

Fig. 11.8 The regurgitation of portal flow in the anterior segment is demonstrated by color Doppler ultrasonography, which is going to the posterior portal vein (reproduced from Ref. [5] with permission)

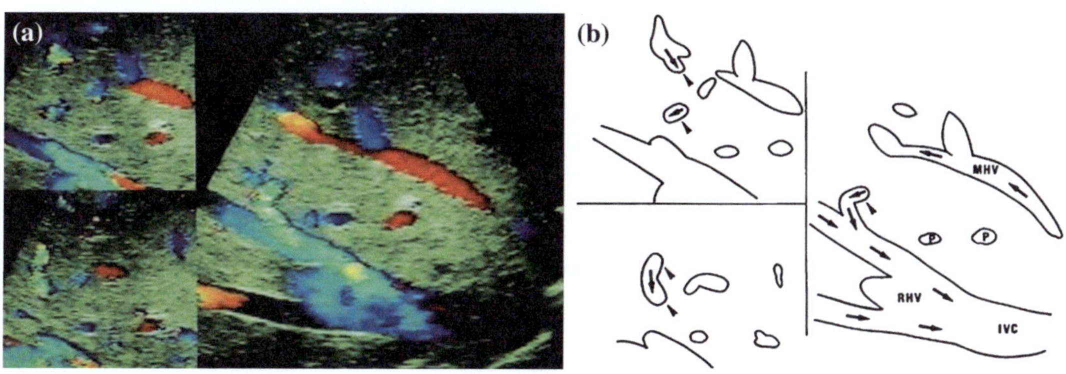

Fig. 11.9 The communication between the middle and the right hepatic veins is visualized by color Doppler ultrasonography (reproduced from Ref. [5] with permission)

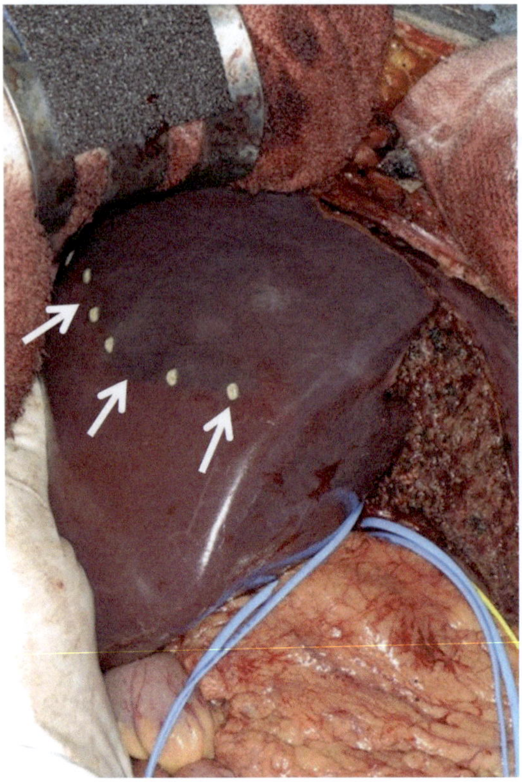

Fig. 11.10 The anterior segment, in which the outflow is obstructed, is demonstrated as discolored area

intraoperative cholangiography via the cystic duct and then decide where to divide it based on the radiographic findings. We do not use intraoperative ultrasonography here.

11.8 After Completing the Transection, and Graft Harvesting

At this point the right liver is connected by just the right hepatic artery, the right branch of the portal vein, and the right hepatic vein (or, when intended for reconstruction, the right inferior hepatic vein). The timing of the division of these vessels is coordinated with the progress of the procedure in the recipient, and the graft liver is removed. The line of division of the right branch of the portal vein is selected so that the branch point is not too close and does not cause stenosis

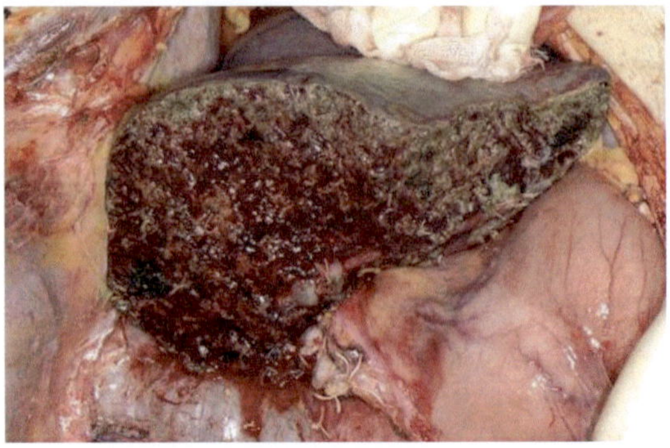

Fig. 11.11 The cutting surface after harvesting the right hemiliver graft is shown

of the left branch. Depending on the circumstances, test clamping can be performed first to confirm that there are no changes in portal blood flow in the remaining liver (left liver). After graft harvesting, the cutting surface of the remaining liver is shown in Fig. 11.11.

11.9 Conclusion

Intraoperative ultrasonography is indispensable to achieving optimal surgery that simultaneously fulfills the demands of both the recipient and the donor.

References

1. Sugawara Y, Makuuchi M, Kaneko J et al (2003) Kokudo. Living-donor liver transplantation in adults: Tokyo University experience. J Hepatobiliary Pancreat Surg 10:1–4
2. Satou S, Sugawara Y, Tamura S et al (2007) Three-dimensional computed tomography for planning donor hepatectomy. Transplant Proc 39(1):145–149
3. Belghiti J, Guevara OA, Noun R et al (2001) Liver hanging maneuver: a safe approach to right hepatectomy without liver mobilization. J Am Coll Surg 193:109–111
4. Kokudo N, Imamura H, Sano K, Sugawara Y, Makuuchi M et al (2005) Ultrasonically assisted retrohepatic dissection for a liver hanging maneuver. Ann Surg 242(5):651–654
5. Sano K, Makuuchi M, Miki K et al (2002) Evaluation of hepatic venous congestion: proposed indication criteria for hepatic vein reconstruction. Ann Surg 236:241–247

Part V
Minimally Invasive Surgery and Interventional Procedures

Laparoscopic Ultrasound: Impact in Liver Surgery

12

Alessandro Ferrero, Luca Viganò, Roberto Lo Tesoriere, and Lorenzo Capussotti

In the recent years laparoscopic liver surgery became more popular, thanks to technical refinements and standardization of technique. Its development relied on the capability to reproduce the same surgical steps of open procedures. Intraoperative liver ultrasonography (IOUS) has a fundamental role in liver surgery to complete disease staging and to guide resection. The same performances have to be expected by laparoscopic ultrasonography (LUS).

LUS use was first reported in 1981 by Fukuda and Nakano [1]. Despite early introduction, it has been poorly developed and studied. Although LUS is reported to increase surgical safety [2], it is currently far from being routinely used: in a recent international survey, LUS use was reported in only 67 % of procedures related to the liver [3].

In this chapter, the performances of LUS and its impact on laparoscopic liver resection will be briefly analyzed by distinguishing staging of liver diseases and guidance to surgical procedures. Both the data of the literature and the potentialities of LUS will be considered.

12.1 Laparoscopic Ultrasonography and Staging

Open IOUS is the most reliable tool for staging liver diseases. In comparison with preoperative imaging, it detects additional nodules in up to 20–30 % of cases [4–6]. These data are still valid even if modern imaging modalities are considered. Few authors analyzed the performances of LUS and reported similar results [7–10]. Foroutani et al. compared LUS with computed tomography [7]: the first one detected additional nodules in 12 % of patients affected by colorectal metastases, in 11 % of those with HCC, and 33 % in those with neuroendocrine metastases. The papers about staging laparoscopies further confirmed these data [11–13]. Jarnagin et al. reported new nodules in 20 % of patients operated for colorectal liver metastases [11]. In Connor et al. series about hilar cholangiocarcinomas, additional hepatic lesions were detected in 7 % of patients and the yield of staging laparoscopy raised from 24–42 % thanks to LUS [12]. In the authors' center, staging laparoscopy and LUS are systematically performed before open hepatectomy in patients affected by biliary tumors. In a series of 71 patients undergoing staging laparoscopy and LUS for biliary cancer, new nodules have been detected in 18 % and the

A. Ferrero (✉) · L. Viganò · R. Lo Tesoriere · L. Capussotti
General and Oncologic Surgery, Ospedale Mauriziano, Largo Turati 62, 10100 Turin, Italy
e-mail: aferrero@mauriziano.it

L. Viganò
e-mail: lvigano@mauriziano.it

R. Lo Tesoriere
e-mail: rlotesoriere@mauriziano.it

L. Capussotti
e-mail: lcapussotti@mauriziano.it

G. Torzilli (ed.), *Ultrasound-Guided Liver Surgery*,
DOI: 10.1007/978-88-470-5510-0_12, © Springer-Verlag Italia 2014

yield of the procedure was 24 %. In patients undergoing explorative laparoscopy, the systematic implementation of LUS is recommended to optimize the yield of the procedure.

LUS staging should be the first surgical procedure during liver surgery. Liver mobilization is not needed, while a complete dissection of adhesions is recommended to have access to the whole liver surface. LUS includes different steps: detection of known lesions and their characterization; disclosure of additional nodules; identification of relationships between lesions and vasculobiliary structures.

First of all, the known lesions have to be identified and characterized. Even after extensive preoperative imaging some nodules are difficult to be classified. LUS helps clarify diagnosis in doubtful cases (Fig. 12.1).

Then, additional lesions have to be excluded (Fig. 12.2). The exploration of the liver must be systematic and visualize all the segments. The authors suggest to perform LUS from left to right (from left lateral to the right posterior segments, including segment 1). Attention should be paid to the visualization of segment 1 and paracaval portion of segment 7 because of deep location. The identification of the posterior glissonean sheath guarantees a complete exploration. Additional neoplastic lesions usually have characteristics similar to those of known nodules. It should be kept in mind to adequately characterize images, especially in patients with nonhomogeneous liver parenchyma (cirrhotic patients or after prolonged chemotherapy) that may have many pseudonodular images.

Once all the lesions have been detected, their relationships with vascular and biliary structures have to be analyzed. This aspect has been almost completely neglected in the literature. In some patients preoperative imaging cannot distinguish if a neoplastic lesion is just contiguous or infiltrates adjacent structures. It can be even more critical in new detected lesions , for which no data other than intraoperative ones are available. Thanks to magnificated images and multiplanar study, LUS may clarify these aspects. The

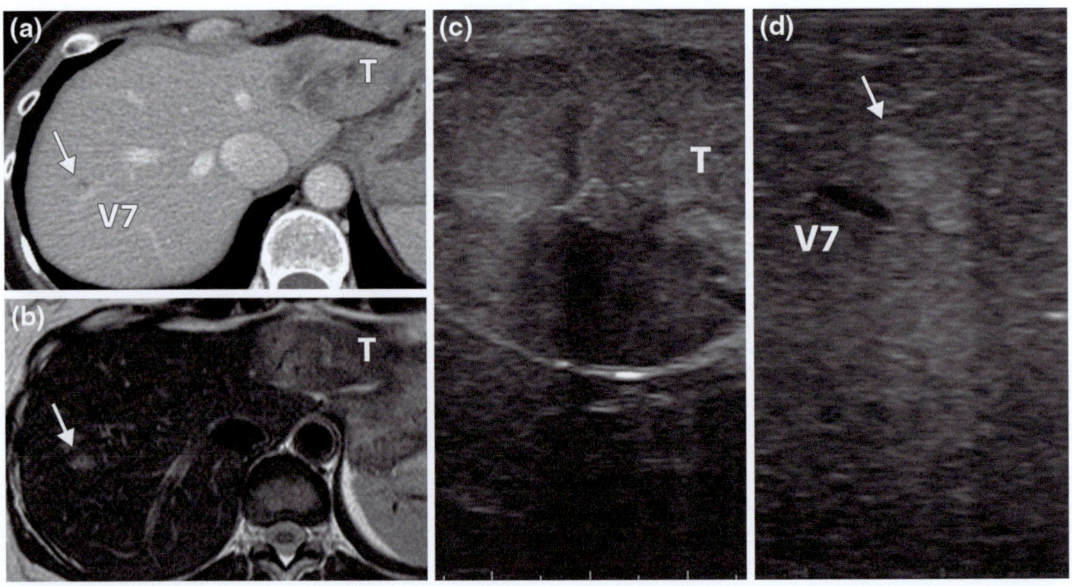

Fig. 12.1 Patient with a 5 cm colorectal liver metastasis in Sg2–3. Preoperative CT (**a**) and MRI (**b**) showing the liver metastasis (*T*) and a 10 mm suspected lesion (*arrow*) in Sg7 close to a branch of the *right* hepatic vein draining Sg7 (*V7*). The suspected lesion shows CT and MRI features similar to the main lesion. **c** Laparoscopic ultrasound of the Sg2-3 metastasis (*T*). **d** The suspected lesion in Sg7 (*arrow*) is clearly identified as a haemangioma showing typical US features (uniform hyperechogenicity, well-defined margins and posterior sonic enhancement)

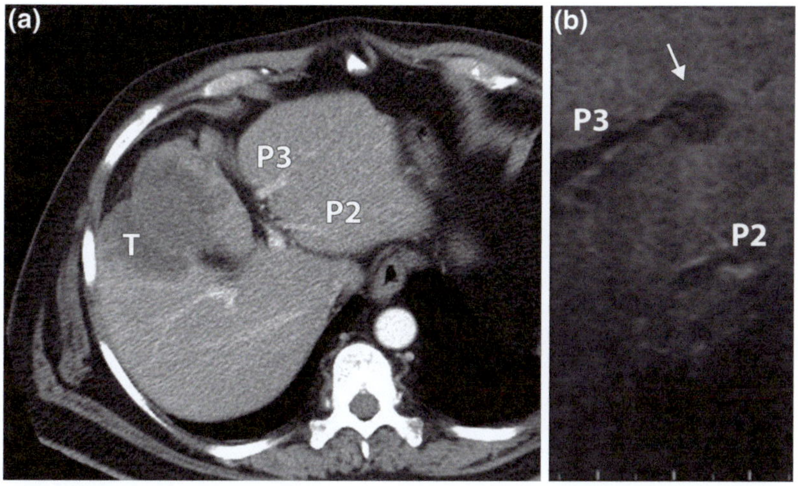

Fig. 12.2 CT scan (**a**) showing a gallbladder cancer (*T*) infiltrating Sg4b-5 without intrahepatic lesions. LUS (**b**) identified an intrahepatic metastasis (*arrow*) missed at CT infiltrating Sg3 portal branch (*P3*). *P2*: Sg2 portal branch

degree of circumferential contact, the loss of hyperechoic peripheral boundary in vessels and an upstream dilatation of biliary ducts may be predictive of infiltration. Some tumors tend to grow into hepatic or portal veins (hepatocellular carcinoma) or biliary ducts (cholangiocarcinoma). LUS can disclose an unknown tumor thrombus (Fig. 12.3) or better characterize a suspected one (Fig. 12.4). The relationships with surrounding structures are even more important in perihilar lesions that grow just beside the main vessels and bile ducts. Not only the intrahepatic extension of the tumor has to be assessed but also it is spread along the hepatic pedicle. Every single anatomic structure has to be identified and studied. LUS is able to confirm an infiltration, reproducing the same images as preoperative ones (Fig. 12.5). The possibility to achieve a conclusive diagnosis in doubtful cases (contact vs. infiltration) can be inferred. Bile ducts can also be accurately evaluated. In hilar cholangiocarcinomas the extension along biliary tree is one of the main determinants of their resectability. LUS can clearly identify the borders of tumor, especially when bile ducts are dilatated (Fig. 12.6). In the authors' opinion,

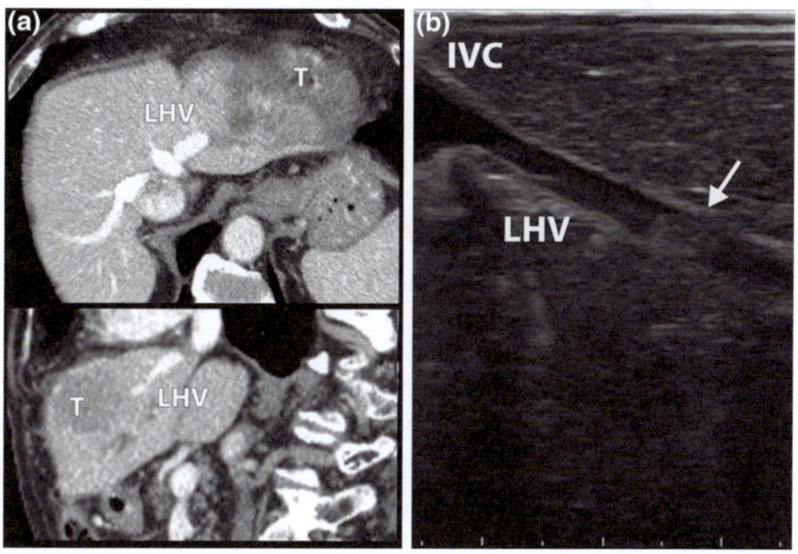

Fig. 12.3 CT scan (**a**) showing a hepatocellular carcinoma (*T*) in Sg2-3. Left hepatic vein (*LHV*) is patent at axial and coronal scans. LUS (**b**) identified a tumor thrombus (*arrow*) in the LHV, 15 mm distally to the confluence into inferior vena cava (*IVC*)

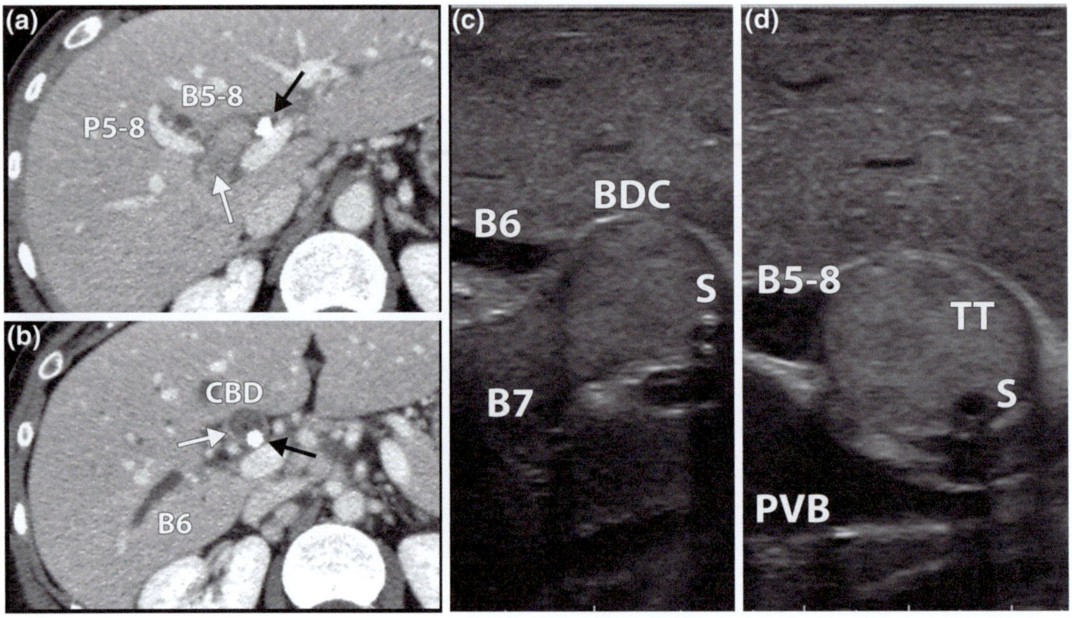

Fig. 12.4 Patient with a peripheral cholangiocarcinoma in Sg7. **a** CT scan showing a suspected tumor thrombus (*white arrow*) in Sg7 bile duct. Right anterior sector bile duct is dilated (*B5-8*). A biliary stent (*black arrow*) is visible at the bile duct confluence. **b** The thrombus (*white arrow*) reaches the common bile duct (*CBD*) where the biliary stent is visible (*black arrow*). Sg6 bile duct (*B6*) is dilated. **c** LUS longitudinal scan of right posterior bile duct bifurcation. Sg7 bile duct (*B7*) is filled with the tumor thrombus occluding the confluence with Sg6 bile duct. The biliary stent (*S*) can be seen in the bile duct confluence (*BDC*). **d** LUS cross section of the BDC. The tumor thrombus (*TT*) occludes *B5-8*. *PVB* portal vein bifurcation

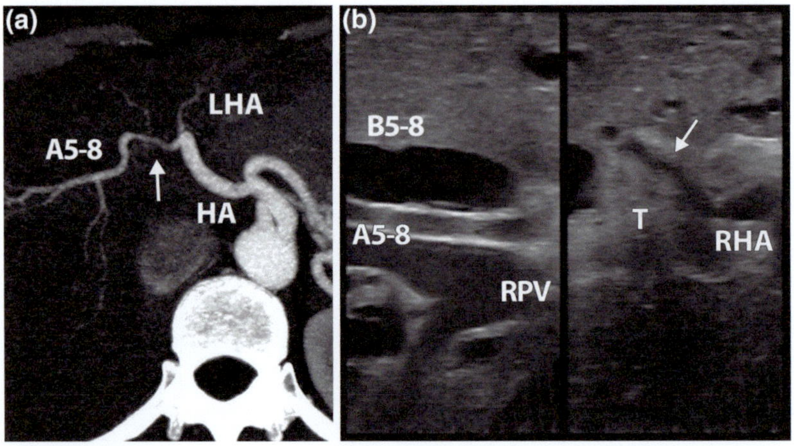

Fig. 12.5 Perihilar cholangiocarcinoma. **a** CT arterial reconstruction. Right hepatic artery is encased by the tumor (*arrow*) just before the second order division. *HA* hepatic artery, *LHA* left hepatic artery, *A5-8* right anterior hepatic artery. **b** LUS confirmed the presence and the extension of right hepatic artery (*RHA*) infiltration (*arrow*). *A5-8* is free from tumor (*T*). *RPV* right portal vein. *B5-8* dilated Sg5-8 bile duct

LUS can accomplish a complete staging even for these complex diseases (Fig. 12.7). To date, no study confirmed these hypotheses and surgical exploration with direct dissection remains the standard. Prospective analyses are needed to confirm potentialities of LUS.

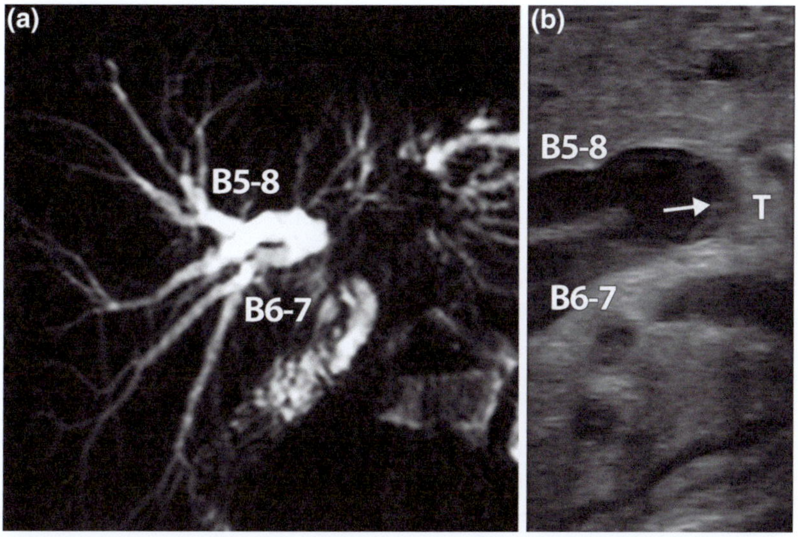

Fig. 12.6 Hilar cholangiocarcinoma. **a** MR cholangiography showing bilateral biliary dilatation without separation of the right anterior (*B5-8*) and posterior (*B6-7*) bile ducts. **b** LUS showing the tumor (*T*) and the distance between biliary infiltration (*arrow*) and B5-8 and B6-7 confluence

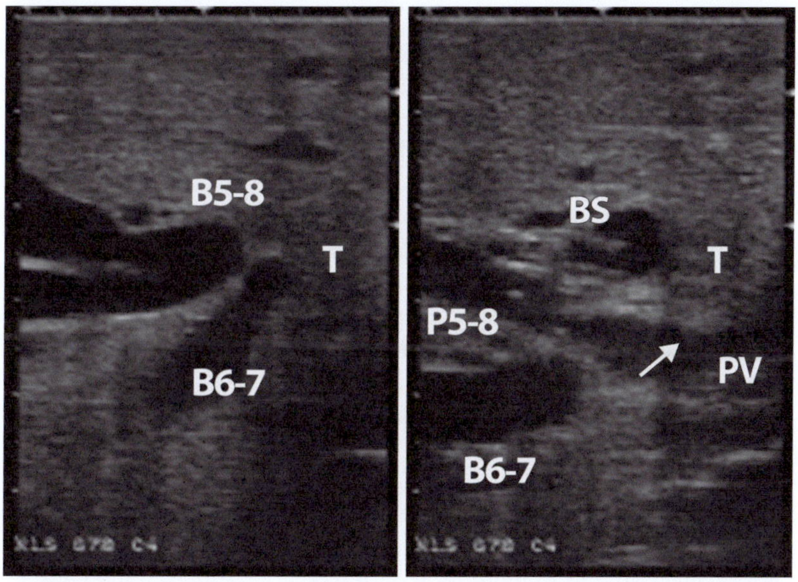

Fig. 12.7 LUS of a patient with type IIIA hilar cholangiocarcinoma (*T*) separating the *right* anterior (*B5-8*) and posterior (*B6-7*) bile ducts. The biliary stent (*BS*) is visualized in B5-8. The tumor infiltrates (*arrow*) the portal vein bifurcation (*PV*). *P5-8* portal branch to Sg5-8

12.2 Performance of Laparoscopic Ultrasonography Compared to Intraoperative Open Ultrasonography

Even if encouraging data about LUS has been reported, its reliability in comparison with open IOUS can be assessed only by a direct comparison between the two. In the literature few data are available. In 1996 Cozzi et al. reported a similar sensitivity of the two procedures in detecting hypoechoic artificial lesions in fresh pig livers [14]. In 1997 Tandan et al. analyzed a small series of patients undergoing both laparoscopic and open IOUS before liver resection [15]. Sensitivity and specificity of LUS were good (93 and 100 %, respectively). So far, no further analyses have been published. Recently, the authors conducted a prospective study to clarify these issues [16]. Between September 2009 and March 2011, 65 consecutive patients scheduled for open hepatectomy underwent both laparoscopic and open IOUS. Patients with hilar or gallbladder cholangiocarcinoma were excluded. 119 lesions were diagnosed at preoperative imaging. Despite the high number of preoperative imaging modalities (CT-scan in 100 % of cases, MRI in 67 % and PET-CT in 54 %), laparoscopic IOUS detected 22 additional lesions (+18.5 %) in 14 patients (21.5 %) having a median diameter of 7 mm (2–15). Open IOUS detected two additional lesions (both beside additional nodules detected by LUS), whereas did not confirm four lesions detected by LUS: overall 20 new lesions (+16.8 %) in 10 patients (15.4 %). In comparison with open IOUS, per-lesion LUS sensitivity was 98.6 % and per-patient accuracy was 93.8 %. Agreement between the two procedures for new malignant nodules detection was 99.3 % in per-lesion analysis and 100 % in per-patient one. Considering the detection of vascular and biliary infiltrations similar results have been observed. In comparison with preoperative imaging, new infiltrations were detected by both laparoscopic and open IOUS in six (9.2 %) patients. One additional patient had an infiltration of the left hepatic duct demonstrated by open IOUS, while preoperative imaging and LUS depicted a contact only. Per-lesion sensitivity of laparoscopic versus open IOUS was 96.9 %. Agreement between the two was 99.3 %.

In conclusion, the reliability of LUS for staging liver diseases was demonstrated by its performances similar to those of open IOUS.

12.3 Laparoscopic Ultrasonography and Liver Resection

Indeed, LUS has several roles during liver surgery: it is the only way to understand the precise liver anatomy and to recognize the presence of vasculobiliary anomalies. Furthermore it has an important role for the intraoperative planning of the operation, identifying the exact site of the lesion and eventual new nodules within the liver. Moreover, probably the most important role of LUS is to assist the surgeon during the resection.

12.3.1 Identification of Liver Anatomy

Liver surgeon should be aware of possible anomalies of patient's liver anatomy. Preoperative imaging can give information about vasculo-biliary anatomy, but only LUS can precisely identify the pattern of glissonian and vein anatomy. The ultrasound study of the liver should represent the first step of any liver surgery and does not require any previous mobilization. LUS exploration should be performed before any other maneuver on the liver, because surgical dissection during pneumoperitoneum causes gas spread into the anatomic planes, giving some artifacts. Since the most frequently performed anatomical laparoscopic liver resection is the left lateral sectionectomy, LUS can easily identify the actual anatomy of the left liver. The portal branches of Sg2 and Sg3 arise from the umbilical portion of the left portal vein. Usually a single branch for each segment can be visualized (Fig. 12.8), but sometimes two or three branches are identified. Both segmental arterial branch and biliary duct can be recognized on the left side of the umbilical fissure. This information is very useful if an extrahepatic dissection of Sg2–3 pedicles is preferred. Hepatic veins confluence in the inferior vena cava can be visualized by LUS, too. During left hepatectomy or left lateral sectionectomy left hepatic vein is usually transected at its confluence in the vena cava. Identifying the presence of a common trunk and knowing its length can facilitate the extrahepatic dissection of the left hepatic vein (Fig. 12.9a). The parenchymal transection during the left lateral sectionectomy is performed along the umbilical scissure where the scissural vein runs. Even the confluence pattern of the scissural vein into the left or middle hepatic vein can be visualized (Fig. 12.9b), in order to avoid a lesion of the scissural vein during the transection, that can be difficult to manage.

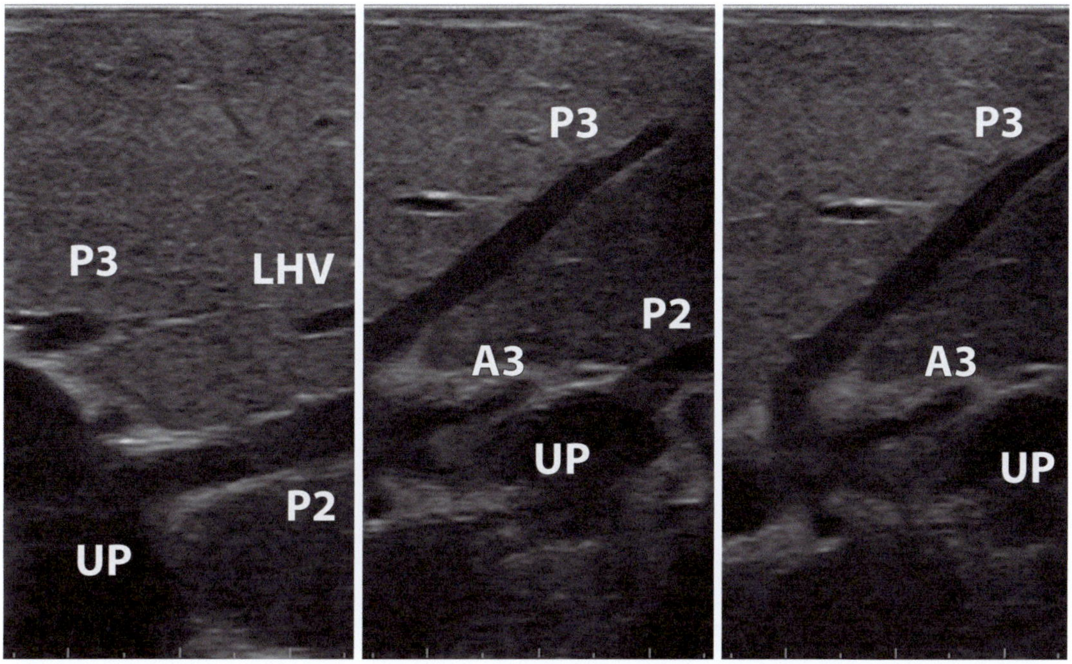

Fig. 12.8 LUS identification of the origin of segment 3 (*P3*) and segment 2 (*P2*) portal branches from the *left* side of the umbilical portion of the left portal vein (*UP*). *A3* segment 3 hepatic artery, *LHV* left hepatic vein

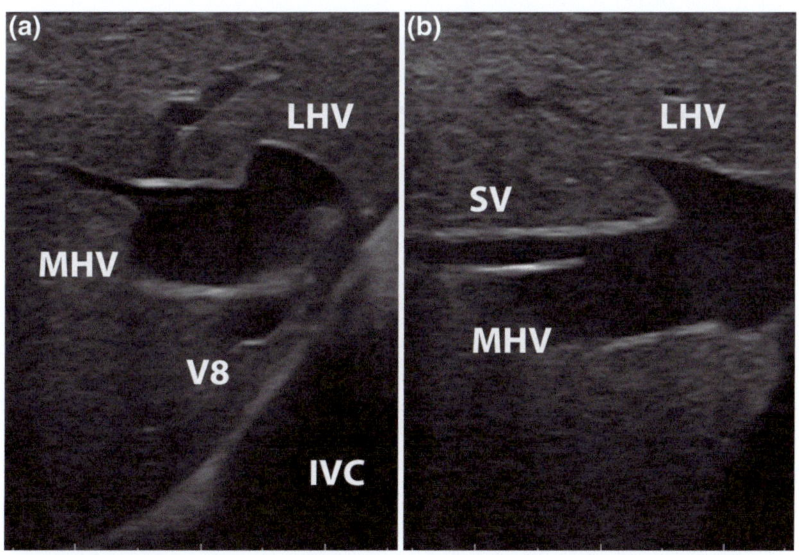

Fig. 12.9 Hepatic vein common trunk. **a** LUS identification of a short common trunk. *MHV* middle hepatic vein, *LHV* left hepatic vein, *V8* hepatic vein draining Sg8, *IVC* inferior vena cava. **b** LUS identification of the scissural hepatic vein (*SV*) confluence in the MHV

12.3.2 Planning the Liver Resection

Unfortunately laparoscopic surgery presents some inherent limitations, such as the lack of tactile sensation, impairing the planning of the operation: ultrasound can compensate these limits by allowing the surgeon to see beyond the surface of the liver. During the first step of the operation, relationships between tumor and intrahepatic vasculobiliary pedicles can be

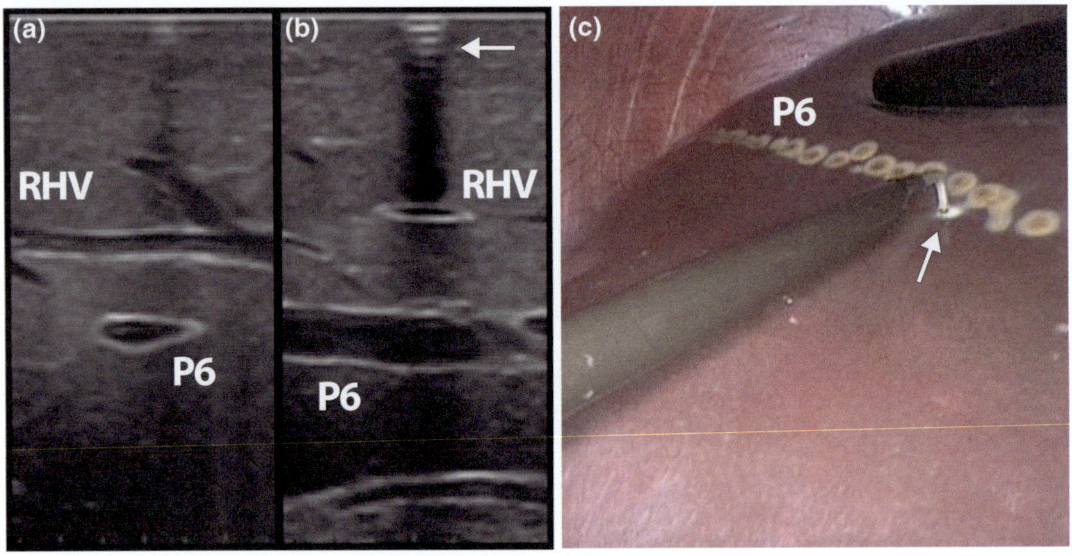

Fig. 12.10 Laparoscopic wedge resection of Sg5-6 for HCC. **a** Right hepatic vein (*RHV*) is visualized in the longitudinal scan. Cross section image of segment 6 portal branch (*P6*) is visible posterior to RHV. **b** A 90° rotation of the probe allows the longitudinal scan of P6 and the cross section of RHV. The liver surface projection of *P6* crossing RHV is marked with electrocautery (*arrow*). **c** Intraoperative image. The intersection of RHV and P6 is marked on the liver surface (*arrow*)

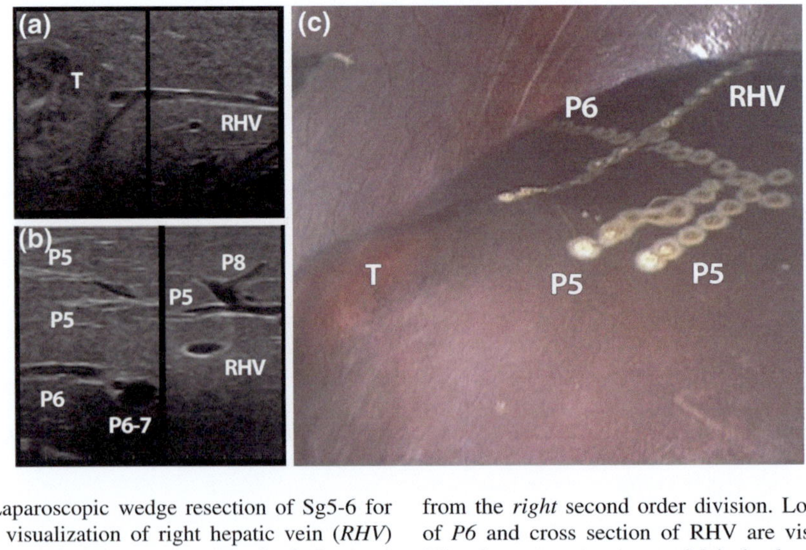

Fig. 12.11 Laparoscopic wedge resection of Sg5-6 for HCC. **a** LUS visualization of right hepatic vein (*RHV*) distally infiltrated by the tumor (*T*). **b** Sg5 portal branches (*P5*) reaching the tumor are identified arising from the *right* second order division. Longitudinal scan of *P6* and cross section of RHV are visualized behind *P5*. **c** Intraoperative image. Main landmarks are marked on liver surface: two *P5*, *P6*, and *RHV*

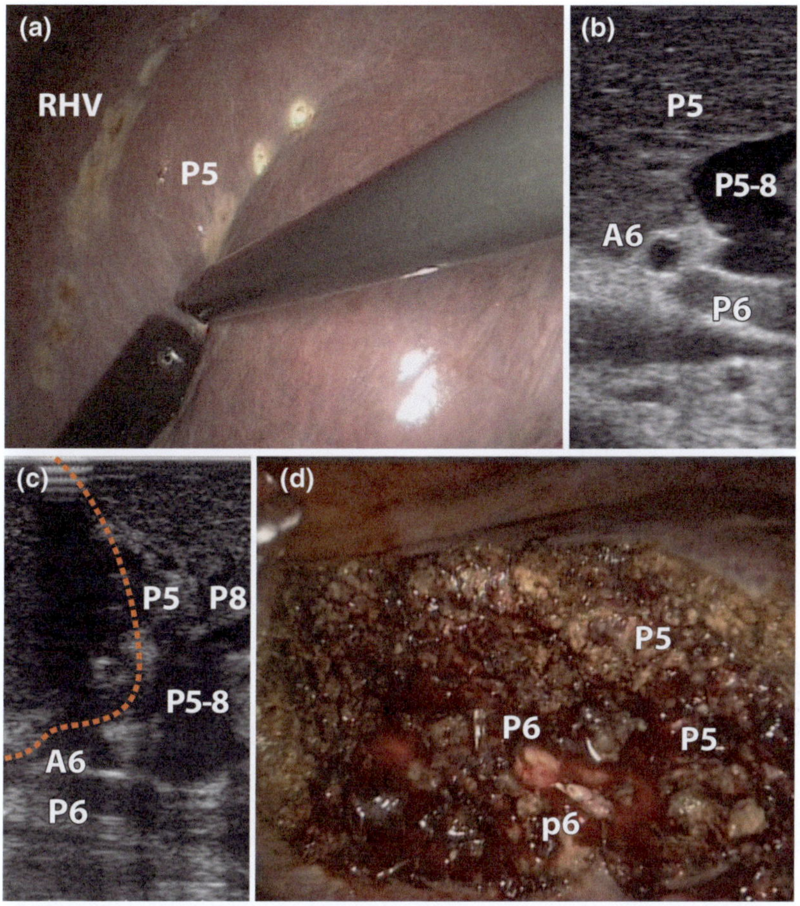

Fig. 12.12 Laparoscopic segmentectomy of Sg5. **a** The liver surface projections of right hepatic vein (*RHV*) and one Sg5 portal pedicle (*P5*) are marked. **b** LUS scan showing the origin of P5. P5-8 anterior right portal pedicle, A6 Sg6 artery, P6 Sg6 portal branch. **c** The section plane (*dotted line*) is checked on the left side of the cut surface. It runs across P5 and along A6 and P6. **d** Intraoperative image of the cut surface of the liver at the end of Sg5 segmentectomy. Sg6 portal branch (*P6*) is exposed on the cut surface. Stumps of two Sg5 pedicles (*P5*) and of a small P6 branch (*p6*) are visible

precisely visualized. In order to try to be always aware of the liver anatomy, both in planning the resection and during liver transection, we strongly suggest to mark the planes where the main vascular structures run with the electrocautery on the liver surface. This procedure is even more useful in case of nonanatomical resection, mainly of the right liver (Figs. 12.10 and 12.11). Nevertheless, drawing on the liver surface the lines corresponding to intrahepatic vessels can facilitate the plan of an anatomical resection, too (Fig. 12.12). Sometimes even the left lateral sectionectomy can be tailored to the site of the lesion, according to the relationships between tumor and the left hepatic vein (Fig. 12.13). When all the vessels are identified and marked, the resection lines are safely designed on the liver surface with the electrocautery and the liver transection can start.

12.3.3 Assessing the Transection Plane

During laparoscopic liver resection the scheduled transection plane is not always easily recognized, because the view of the operative field is limited and can be worsened by the bleeding.

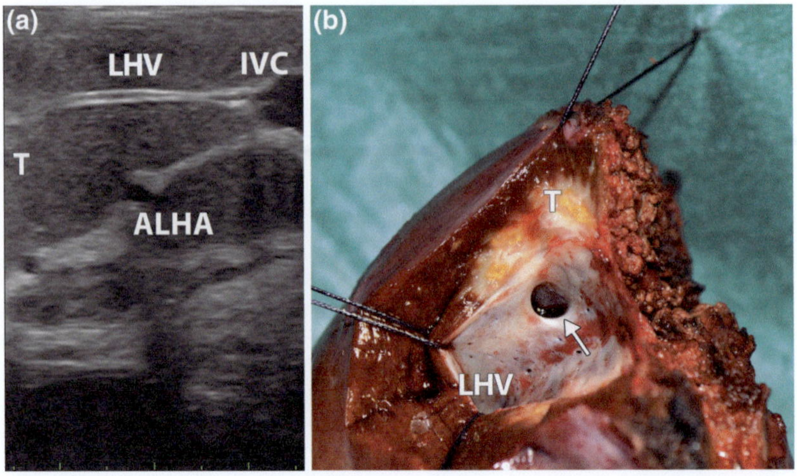

Fig. 12.13 Laparoscopic left lateral sectionectomy for colorectal metastasis. **a** Tumor (*T*) infiltrates left hepatic vein (*LHV*) close to inferior vena cava (*IVC*) confluence. A cross section of an accessory left hepatic artery (*ALHA*) originating from left gastric artery can be seen in the lesser omentum. **b** Surgical specimen. The metastasis, fibrotic after chemotherapy, infiltrates the LHV, close to its confluence with the scissural vein (*arrow*)

Moreover, the correct distance between tumor and resection plane is sometimes difficult to be maintained, leading the surgeon to stay too close to the tumor. In order to increase the orientation and to maintain an adequate surgical margin, during the parenchymal transection the resection plane is repeatedly checked by ultrasound. LUS can provide the surgeon with immediate feedback of possible changes of the dissection plane. Any glissonian pedicle or vein encountered during liver transection can be checked and recognized by LUS before ligature and section (Fig. 12.14). Color Doppler ultrasound allows the user to visualize blood flow and can assess the flow in and near the area of interest, thus avoiding injury to important vessels during dissection. When an anatomical segmentectomy is scheduled, LUS can precisely visualized that the section of the segmental pedicles is performed at their origin from the sectorial branches (Fig. 12.12c). During right or left hepatectomy, the plane of transection is usually guided by the hemiliver ischemic demarcation obtained after the hilar dissection. Nevertheless we suggest always to check the relationships between the section plane and the plane where the middle hepatic vein runs, in order to correctly expose it on the cut surface and not to include it in the specimen (Fig. 12.15). The possibility to guide interstitial treatments associated to the hepatectomy, such as radiofrequency or microwave ablation, gives an added value to the procedure, mainly in hepatocellular carcinoma management.

LUS has also some drawbacks and limitations. The hand–eye coordination of the probe visualized through the video laparoscope can be difficult. The orientation and following interpretation of the images can be complicated. Some ultrasound-specific drawbacks add to the difficulties of interpretation such as shadowing, multiple reflections, variable contrast depending from liver parenchyma status and the fact that the quality of the images also may be somewhat operator dependent. Nevertheless, despite these difficulties, LUS remains an indispensable tool for surgeons dealing with laparoscopic liver resections.

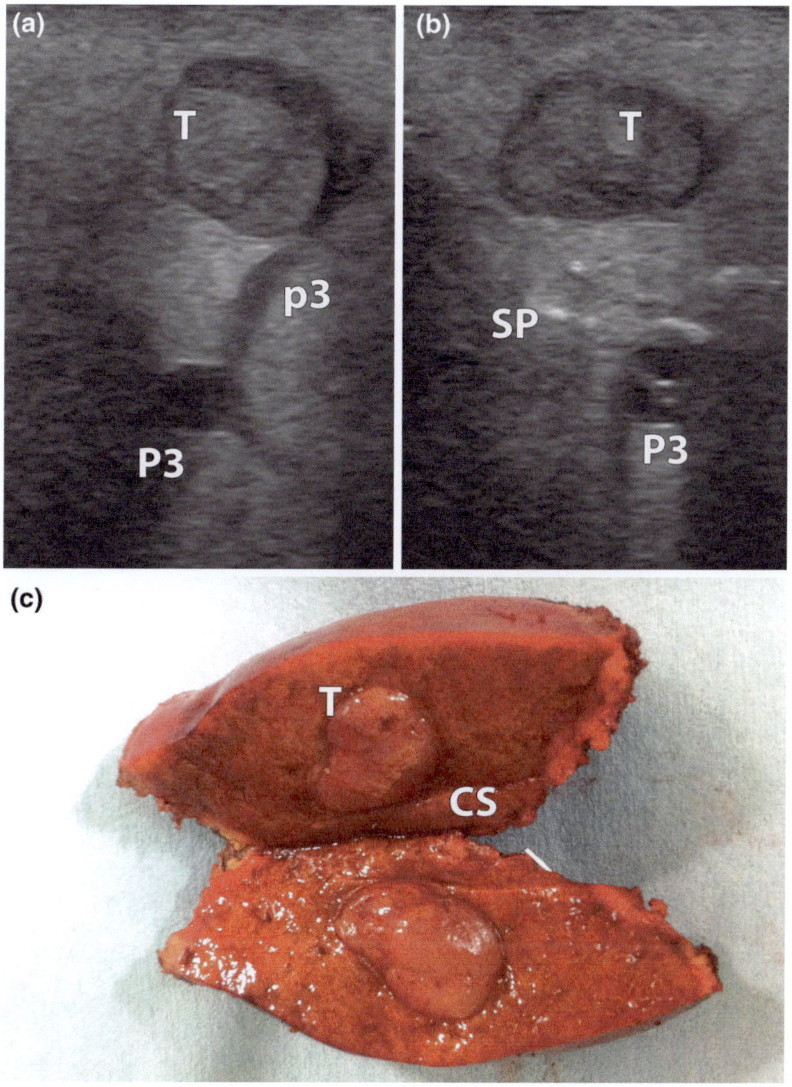

Fig. 12.14 Laparoscopic wedge resection of Sg3 for HCC. **a** LUS shows a tumor (*T*) with hypoechoic heterogeneous pattern and hypoechoic rim. Sg3 portal branch (*P3*) and the tumor feeding branch (*p3*) are identified. **b** LUS guidance to resection. The correct section plane (*SP*), running between tumor and P3, is checked. **c** Surgical specimen with adequate margin. *T* tumor, *CS* cut surface

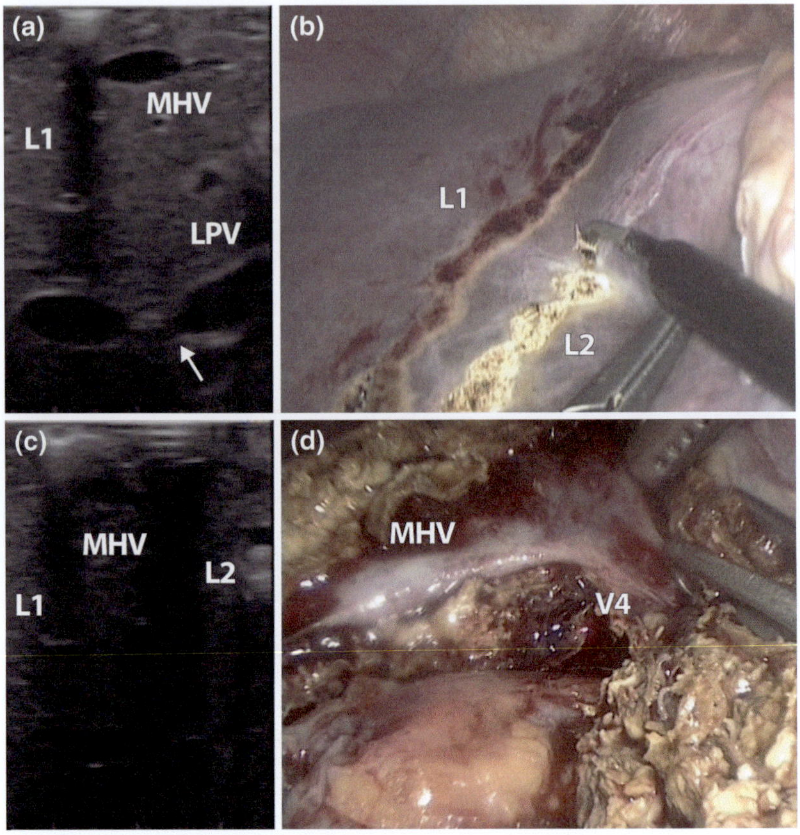

Fig. 12.15 Laparoscopic left hepatectomy. **a** LUS checking of the transection line. After left portal vein (*LPV*) ligation (*arrow*) the transection line based on the ischemic demarcation (*L1*) is checked: L1 is wrongly *right* to the middle hepatic vein (*MHV*), which has to be preserved. **b** A new section line (*L2*) is marked on the liver surface left to the *MHV* under ultrasonographic guidance. **c** The correct new transection line (*L2*) is checked. **d** Parenchymal transection. MHV is correctly exposed on the cut surface. A branch draining Sg4 (*V4*) in the MHV is isolated before division

References

1. Fukuda MMF, Nakano Y (1982) Studies on echolaparoscopy. Scan J Gastroenterol 17:186
2. Machi J, Johnson JO, Deziel DJ et al (2009) The routine use of laparoscopic ultrasound decreases bile duct injury: a multicenter study. Surg Endosc 23:384–388
3. Vapenstad C, Rethy A, Langø T et al (2010) Laparoscopic ultrasound: a survey of its current and future use, requirements, and integration with navigation technology. Surg Endosc 24:2944–2953
4. Sietses C, Meijerink MR, Meijer S et al (2010) The impact of intraoperative ultrasonography on the surgical treatment of patients with colorectal liver metastases. Surg Endosc 24(8):1917–1922
5. van Vledder MG, Pawlik TM, Munireddy S et al (2010) Factors determining the sensitivity of intraoperative ultrasonography in detecting colorectal liver metastases in the modern era. Ann Surg Oncol 17(10):2756–2763
6. D'Hondt M, Vandenbroucke-Menu F, Préville-Ratelle S et al (2011) Is intra-operative ultrasound still useful for the detection of a hepatic tumour in the era of modern pre-operative imaging? HPB 13(9):665–669
7. Foroutani A, Garland AM, Berber E et al (2000) Laparoscopic ultrasound vs triphasic computed tomography for detecting liver tumors. Arch Surg 135(8):933–938
8. Milsom JW, Jerby BL, Kessler H et al (2000) Prospective, blinded comparison of laparoscopic ultrasonography vs. contrast-enhanced computerized tomography for liver assessment in patients undergoing colorectal carcinoma surgery. Dis Colon Rectum 43(1):44–49
9. John TG, Greig JD, Crosbie JL et al (1994) Superior staging of liver tumors with laparoscopy and laparoscopic ultrasound. Ann Surg 220(6):711–719
10. Cuesta MA, Meijer S, Borgstein PJ et al (1993) Laparoscopic ultrasonography for hepatobiliary and pancreatic malignancy. Br J Surg 80(12):1571–1574
11. Jarnagin WR, Bodniewicz J, Dougherty E et al (2000) A prospective analysis of staging laparoscopy in patients with primary and secondary hepatobiliary malignancies. J Gastrointest Surg 4(1):34–43
12. Connor S, Barron E, Wigmore SJ et al (2005) The utility of laparoscopic assessment in the preoperative staging of suspected hilar cholangiocarcinoma. J Gastrointest Surg 9(4):476–480

13. Callery MP, Strasberg SM, Doherty GM et al (1997) Staging laparoscopy with laparoscopic ultrasonography: optimizing resectability in hepatobiliary and pancreatic malignancy. J Am Coll Surg 185(1):33–39
14. Cozzi PJ, McCall JL, Jorgensen JO, Morris DL (1996) Laparoscopic vs open ultrasound of the liver: an in vitro study. HPB Surg 10(2):87–89
15. Tandan VR, Asch M, Margolis M et al (1997) Laparoscopic vs. open intraoperative ultrasound examination of the liver: a controlled study. J Gastrointest Surg 1(2):146–150
16. Viganò L, Ferrero A, Amisano M et al (2013) Comparison of laparoscopic and open intraoperative ultrasonography for staging of liver tumours. Br J Surg 100(4):535–542

13 Ultrasound-Guided Intraoperative Ablation Therapies

Roberto Santambrogio, Matteo Barabino,
and Enrico Opocher

13.1 Introduction

The increased application of laparoscopy in the field of abdominal oncology has led to an increased use of laparoscopic ultrasound (LUS) as a valuable tool for staging of neoplastic diseases [1]. In regard to liver surgery, LUS provides, in experienced hands, a wealth of information for resectability assessment by detecting nonpalpable lesions and visualizing sharp relationships between tumors and vascular structures [2, 3]. Moreover, LUS can serve as guidance for any interventional procedure such as biopsy or thermal ablation of a lesions in radiofrequency (RFA) or microwave (MWA) ablation [4]. LUS-guided thermal ablation of liver tumors can be mastered relatively quickly by a surgeon already familiar with laparoscopic and ultrasound techniques. The learning curve mainly relates to the interpretation of the ultrasonographic images and to the technical tricks of interventional maneuvers [4].

R. Santambrogio (✉) · M. Barabino · E. Opocher
Hepato-Biliary-Pancreatic and Digestive Surgery,
San Paolo Hospital, University of Milan,
Via di Rudinì 8, 20142 Milan, MI, Italy
e-mail: rsantambrogio@mclink.it

M. Barabino
e-mail: matteo.barabino@ao-sanpaolo.it

E. Opocher
e-mail: enrico.opocher@unimi.it

13.2 Indications

An appropriate multidisciplinary selection of the patient is accomplished according to the tumor's features, liver function, and comorbidities. Relative contraindications for LRFA ablation are:

- tumor located adjacent to main biliary duct (due to risk of delayed stenosis of the main biliary tract)
- intrahepatic bile duct dilation
- bilioenteric anastomosis
- untreatable/unmanageable coagulopathy

13.2.1 Hepatocellular Carcinoma

The Barcelona Clinic Liver Cancer (BCLC) group (and further AASLD updates) proposed a staging/treatment classification, based on the authors' synthesis of several studies including variables relating to the tumor, liver function, and physical status [5, 6]. Thus, RFA is now proposes as the treatment of choice for patients with a single HCC smaller than 2 or 3 cm in diameter, even when surgical resection is possible [7]. Indications for RFA of larger HCCs (more than 3 cm) are less clear. In this setting, the risk of an incomplete ablation increases with the increment of the HCC diameter [8]. A percutaneous approach is not indicated and, in our center we use LRFA instead, if the patient has at least one of the following criteria [9]:

G. Torzilli (ed.), *Ultrasound-Guided Liver Surgery*,
DOI: 10.1007/978-88-470-5510-0_13, © Springer-Verlag Italia 2014

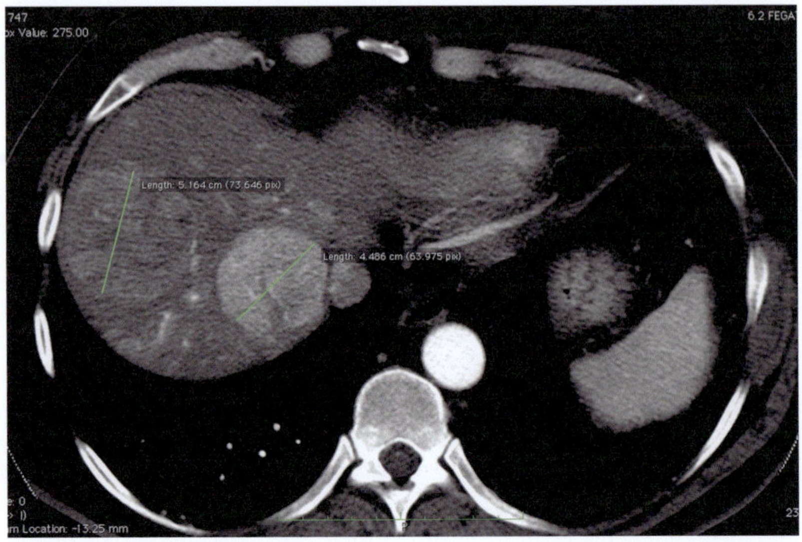

Fig. 13.1 CT scan showing two large tumors in the right lobe of the liver

(a) severe impairment of the coagulation tests (platelets <40.000 and/or International Normalized Ratio (INR) >1.20);
(b) large tumors (but with a diameter of less than 5 cm) or multiple lesions requiring repeated punctures (Fig. 13.1);
(c) superficial lesions adjacent to visceral structures which can be displaced by laparoscopic maneuvers: colon appears to be at greater risk (Fig. 13.2a) than the stomach (Fig. 13.2b) or small bowel for thermally mediated perforation;
(d) lesions close to intrahepatic structures (Fig. 13.3): the laparoscopic approach guarantees a lower risk of biliary thermal injuries either performing a "cooling technique" for these lesions or associating a cholecystectomy for lesions close to the gallbladder (Fig. 13.4);
(e) deep-sited lesions with a very difficult or impossible percutaneous approach (Fig. 13.5);
(f) short-term recurrence of HCC following liver surgery, ethanol injection or TACE.

Table 13.1 shows the different reasons to propose an LRFA rejecting a percutaneous approach or a hepatic resection.

13.2.2 Liver Metastases

Surgical resection represents the gold standard for the management of LM [10]. Unfortunately, only 10–25 % of patients are amenable to liver resection due to the characteristics of either hepatic lesions (location, number, remnant liver volume) or patients (comorbidities, chemotherapic toxicity, performance status) [11]. The

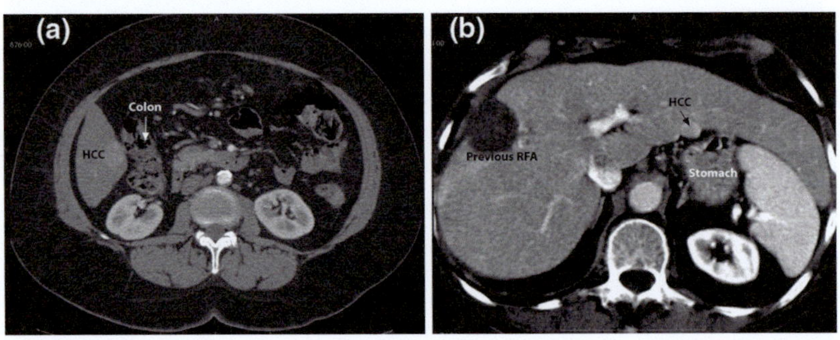

Fig. 13.2 CT scan showing superficial lesions adjacent to visceral structures: colon (**a**) or stomach (**b**)

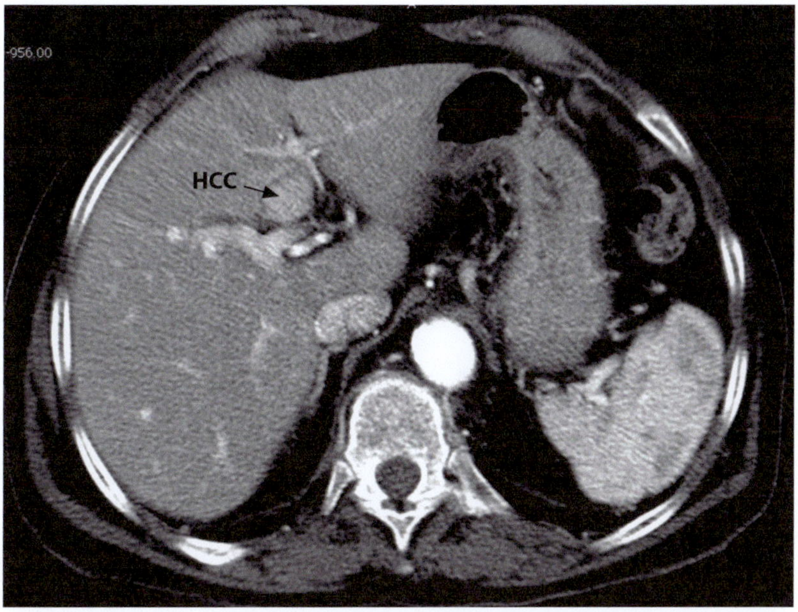

Fig. 13.3 CT scan showing a HCC nodule contiguous to intrahepatic biliary convergence

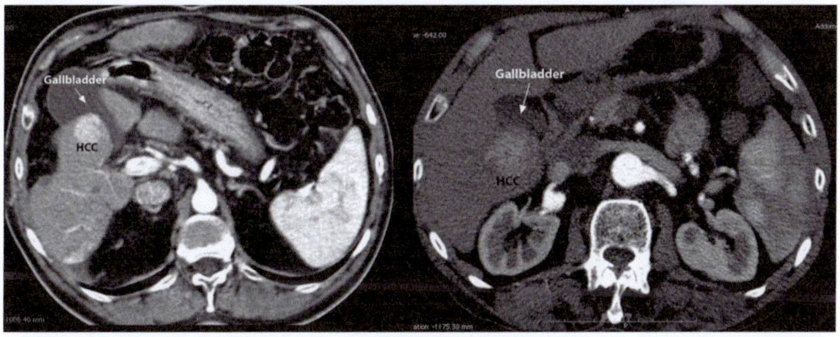

Fig. 13.4 CT scans showing HCC nodules contiguous to gallbladder

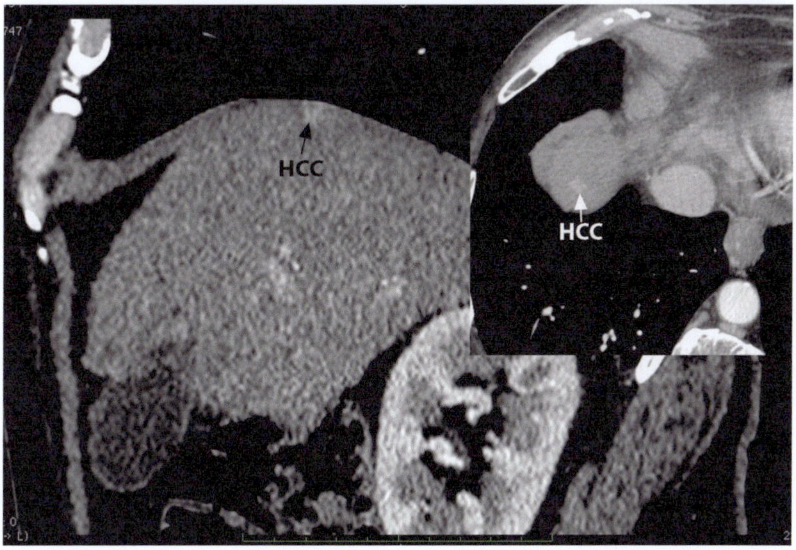

Fig. 13.5 CT scan showing a deep HCC nodule of the hepatic dome not visible upon percutaneous ultrasound examination

Table 13.1 Reasons to reject percutaneous RFA or hepatic resection (HR) for 379 patients submitted to LRFA (more than 1 reason for each patient)

Percutaneous RFA	N (%)	Hepatic resection (HR)	N (%)
HCC contiguous to visceral structures	113 (30 %)	HR > 2 segments	161 (42 %)
Superficial lesion	74 (19 %)	Patients > BCLC A2 stage	226 (60 %)
Lesion difficult or impossible to percutaneous US visualization	230 (61 %)	Local recurrence post-TACE	37 (10 %)
LUS staging (for suspected other nodule)	344 (91 %)	Other concomitant severe disease	95 (25 %)
Pts at risk of bleeding (plts < 50,000 and/or INR > 1.2)	154 (41 %)	Patient refusal	95 (25 %)
		Age > 78 years	52 (14 %)

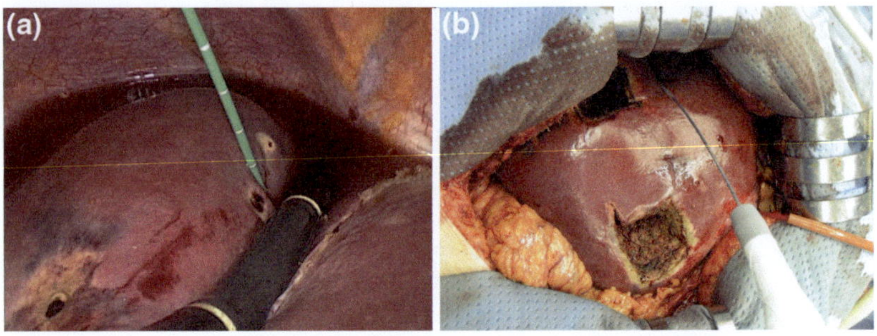

Fig. 13.6 Laparoscopic MWA of two liver metastases in segment 4 during hemicolectomy (**a**) and in a second time multiple hepatic resections associated to RFA in the right lobe (**b**)

rationale for choosing RFA versus surgical resection in patients with LM has been multifactorial. A large percentage of patients were thought to have disease that was technically unresectable. Most of the remaining patients were poor surgical candidates for a combination of reasons, including clinically important medical comorbidities, advanced age, and aggressive disease. In this setting of unresectable patients, RFA could represent an acceptable indication [12]. The number of lesions should not be considered an absolute contraindication to RFA: nevertheless, most centers preferentially treat patients with five or fewer lesions. The target tumor should not exceed 3 cm in longest axis to achieve best rates of complete ablation with most of the currently available devices.

A particular scenario is if a colorectal cancer patient undergoes laparoscopic surgery for primary disease with synchronous LM. LRFA may be safely used concomitantly with colon resection in patients who may have resectable LM, but liver resection in a synchronous manner would be risky or, if the patient has an unresectable LM; in this case, LRFA could represent the first stage in a two-stage treatment (Fig. 13.6).

13.3 Which "Weapon"? RFA or MWA

Both radiofrequency and microwave technology are effective. In RFA, high-frequency alternating current causes thermal coagulation and protein denaturation; as the temperature is increased above 45 °C, cellular proteins denature and cell structure is lost. RF ablation can be performed by either monopolar or bipolar techniques;

monopolar techniques are more commonly used for tumor ablation [13]. When a monopolar technique is used, a large dispersive electrode (grounding pad) is usually placed on the patient's thigh. Current passing through tissue from the active electrode leads to ion agitation, which is converted by means of friction into heat. The process of cellular heating induces almost immediate and irrepairable cellular damage, which leads to coagulation necrosis. The nature of the thermal damage caused by RF heating depends on both the tissue temperature achieved and the duration of heating. The diameter of coagulation necrosis was also found to be influenced by electrode diameter [14]. Currently, two RF technologies are commercially marketed (Fig. 13.7): one of these devices consists of a needle with a movable hub that deploys a variable number of curved electrodes into the adjacent tissue in a radial manner. The configurations of the multiple electrodes are designed to produce large spherical thermal injuries. The second device consists of a straight, internally cooled needle electrode. The internal cooling is designed to prevent charring of the adjacent tissues and thus any larger thermal injury. In our experience, for the particular indications in the laparoscopic approach, the "cooled" needle is preferred [4]. The major factor limiting the size of the thermal injury produced by all two devices is hepatic perfusion. Normal blood flow through the liver produces perfusion-mediated tissue cooling, above all if the lesion is near to a larger vessel (heat sink effect) [15].

MWA is another local ablation therapy, which has been used for more than 20 years [16]. It has recently attracted considerable

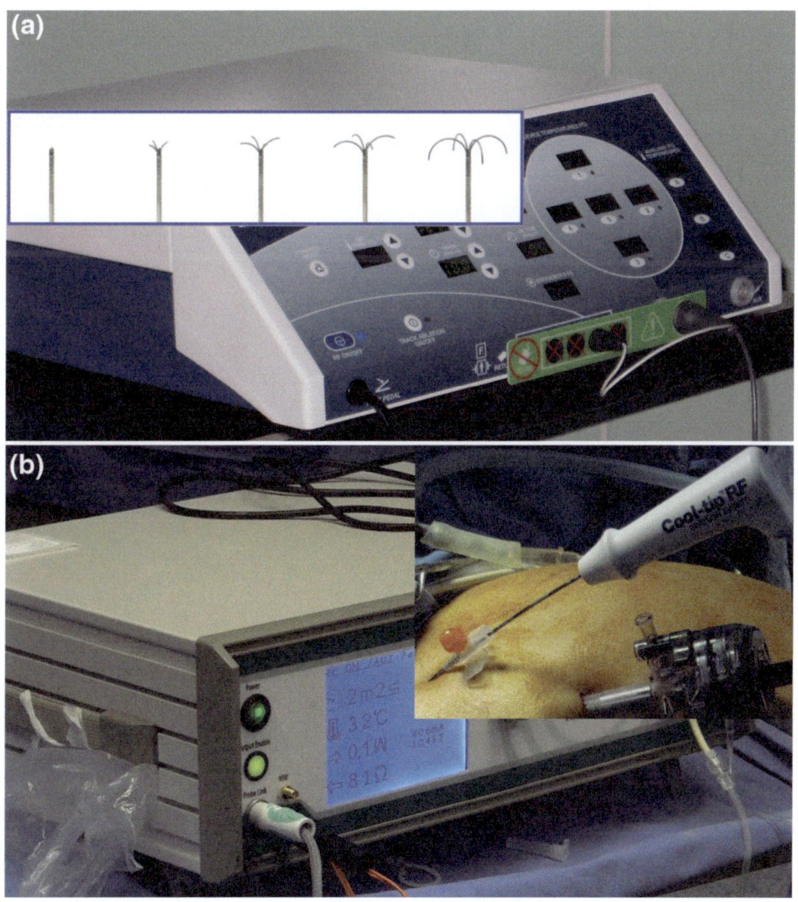

Fig. 13.7 RF technologies: one of these devices consists of a needle with a movable hub that deploys a variable number of curved electrodes (**a**) and the second device consists of a straight, internally cooled needle electrode (**b**)

attention because of the tremendous progress in microwave technology [17]. Microwaves generate heat by oscillation of dipole water molecules within tissues. Frequencies of 915 MHz and 2.45 GHz are currently used for tissue ablation, with a single, dual, or triple antenna (Fig. 13.8). The advantage of MWA is that the heating is primarily active, and the transmission of microwaves in living tissue is not limited by tissue desiccation and charring. In addition, MWA does not require use of earth plates on the patient's body, thus avoiding potential earth plate burn injury that can occur with RFA. With a single application of a 2.45 GHz system, it can create a 4 × 6 cm ablation in 4 min and a 5 × 7 cm ablation in 8 min. MWs offer all of the same benefits as RFA energy for thermal ablation but they are not as dependent on tissue properties and have the ability to heat faster in a larger volume. Thus, MWs are less susceptible to perfusion or heat sinks and may be able to penetrate deeper into low-conductivity materials [18]. On the other hand, the MW antenna usually has a larger diameter (14 G) and the lack of heat

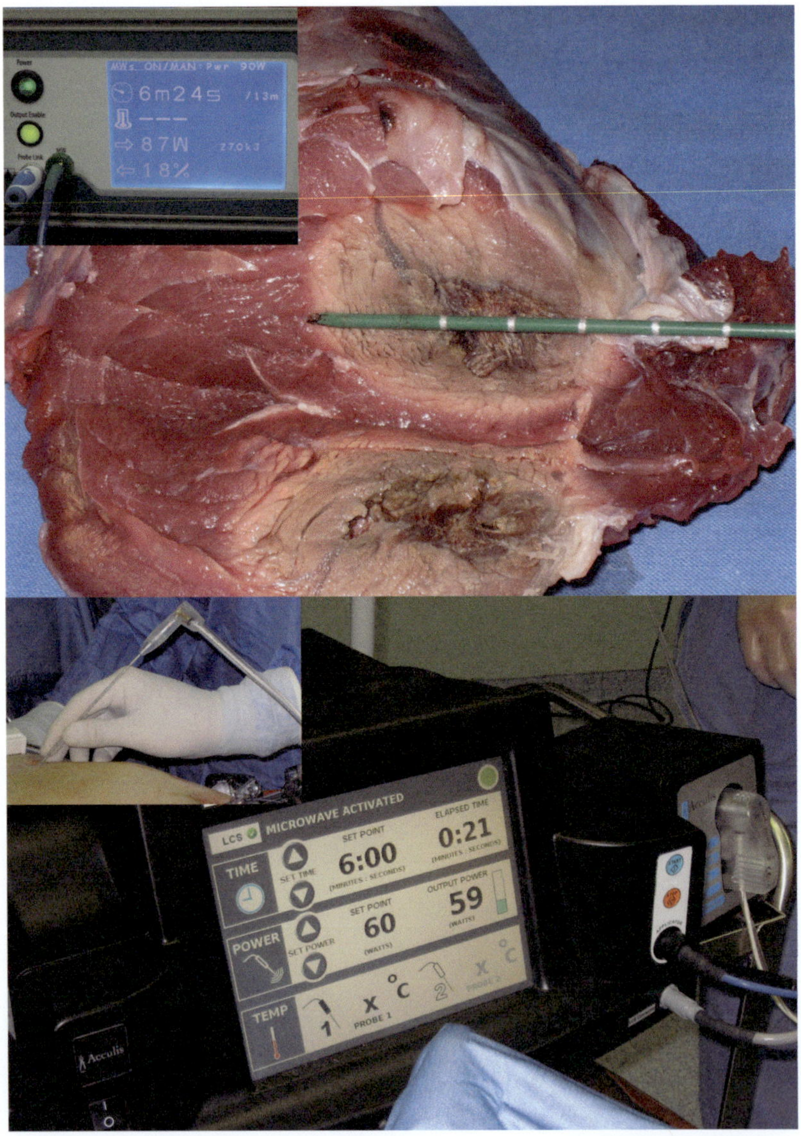

Fig. 13.8 MW technologies

sink effect increases the risk of vascular and biliary injuries. So, it's impossible to establish which tool is better: it's recommended to have the possibility to choose which technology depending on size and location of the tumor.

13.4 Thermal Ablation: The Procedure

13.4.1 Operative Room

An efficiently operating room setup for LRFA/MWA is critical for success. A proper table that allows the patient to be placed in both full Trendelemburg and reverse Trendelemburg positions during operation is essential. The optimal situation is to have the ultrasound monitor in the same line of vision as the monitor for the laparoscopic telescope. A convenient way to visualize both laparoscopic and ultrasound images simultaneously is to employ a screen-splitting device for a single monitor: a picture-in-picture visualization is particularly helpful in the LRFA procedure (Fig. 13.9). Generally, the ultrasound unit is located on the right side of the patient adjacent to the armboard with the laparoscopic equipment off the right shoulder of the patient: the surgeon stands at the right side of the patient (Fig. 13.10). Also the RFA/MWA machine is positioned on the patient's right side. An equipment checklist is necessary to ensure that all items are available:

- laparoscopic equipment (generally housed in a cart on wheels):
  - monitor: flat panel monitor has better resolution and it is more mobile than the than traditional monitor;
  - insufflator: we recommend a high-flow insufflator capable of delivering flow rates up to 30 l/min;
  - camera–processor unit: the laparoscopic camera can be either single chip or three chip; these provide high-quality color reproduction and highest degree of fidelity;
  - light source: a high-intensity light source is a prerequisite for a satisfactorily bright laparoscopic image;
- laparoscopic optics: a 30 or 45° laparoscope is preferable for closeup viewing of the surface architecture of the liver and for providing

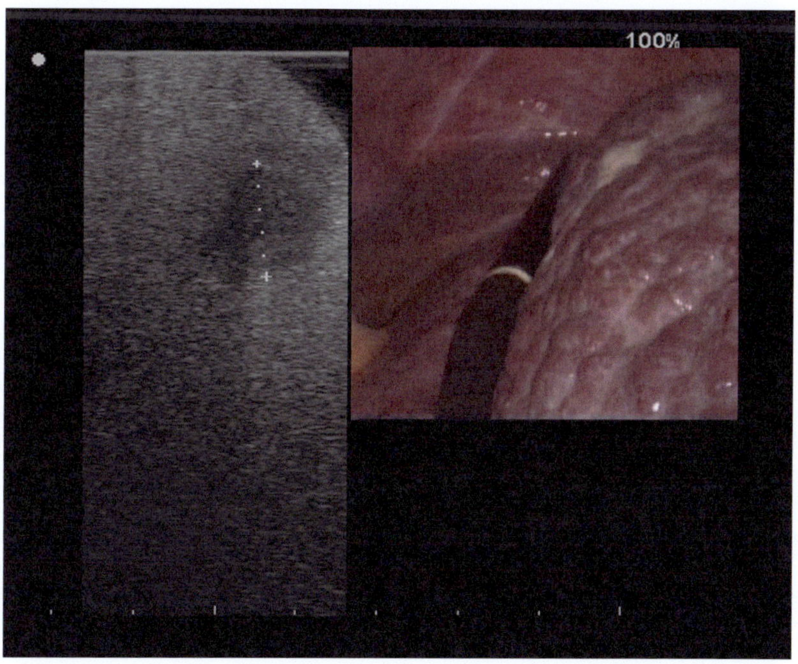

Fig. 13.9 A screen-splitting device for a single monitor in order to visualize both laparoscopic and ultrasound images simultaneously

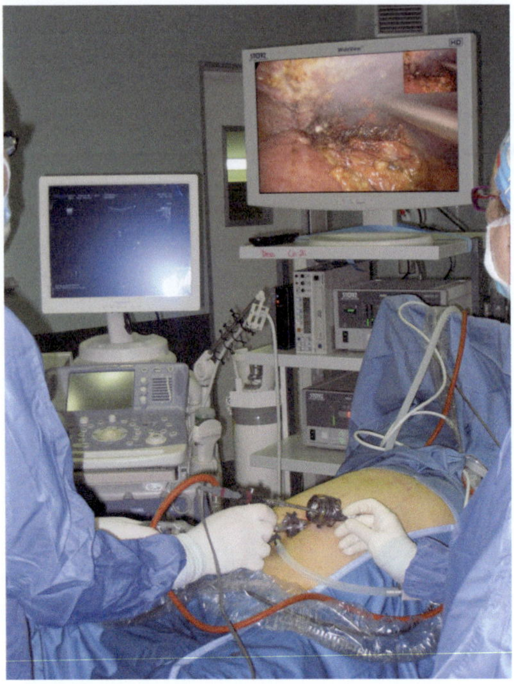

Fig. 13.10 The ultrasound unit is located on the right side of the patient with the laparoscopic equipment off the right shoulder of the patient

guidance to the electrode under direct vision. In addition, by rotation of the telescope, it allows different angles of inspection during the electrode infission;

- energy sources for coagulation and cutting: standard unipolar or bipolar electrocautery can be used for hemostasis and dividing tissue. For cirrhotic patients with extremely vascular tissue such as adhesions, alternative energy sources such as ultrasonic coagulation may be more suitable.
- ultrasound equipment: we used an ultrasound machine connected to a laparoscopic ultrasound (LUS) probe with a flexible tip, 10 mm in diameter and 50 cm in length. A 5–7.5 MHz linear-array transducer was side-mounted near the tip of the shaft. The length of the transducer surface was 38 mm, which produced an image footprint of approximately 4 cm in length and 6 cm in depth. Recently, we also used a microconvex probe that permits the application of intravenous ultrasound contrast agents during LUS of the liver: the addition of contrast enhancement during the intraoperative ultrasound will improve image conspicuity, correct diagnosis of new malignant nodules, ablation efficacy in hepatic tumors, and oncologic margin outcomes (Fig. 13.3);
- suction irrigator;
- table with small retractors for umbilical incision, trocar cannulae (size and number depend on the planned operation), and laparoscopic instruments (atraumatic graspers, bowel grasping forceps, coagulated hook and scissors);
- 18 G tru-cut biopsy needle: it is useful to use a cutting needle with an automatic trigger mechanism in order to hold the probe with one hand and the needle with the other. Because of the presence of pneumoperitoneum which separates the surface of the liver from the abdominal wall, the use of longer needles (25–27 cm) can be necessary for lesions localized in the posterior segments or in the highest part of the liver (segments 4a and 8);
- RFA/MWA machine and electrode/antenna: actually we used a dual ablation system which in the same hardware has both a MWA and an RFA energy generator. For RFA technology, we prefer a 17 G internally cooled electrode with an exposed tip length of 3 cm and shaft length of 250 mm. For MW technology, we use a 14-G interstitial antenna with a shaft length of 270 mm.

13.4.2 Laparoscopic Technique

LRFA/MWA is performed under general endotracheal anesthesia. A Foley catheter is useful only for cirrhotic patients for monitoring postoperative urinary output. A nasogastric tube is sometimes useful to deflate the stomach before the procedure. If RFA equipment is used, at least two large surface area grounding pads must be used.

Patient positioning is dependent on the location of the hepatic lesions to be treated. Generally, position of the patient is supine on the operating room with the left arm extended: the surgeon stands either on the right side (Fig. 13.11) or between the legs of the patient (Fig. 13.12). Patients with tumors in segments 6 and 7 can be placed in either an oblique position with the right side elevated up to 45° or left decubitus position with the right arm elevated and across the chest and the surgeon standing at either the right or the left side of the patient (Fig. 13.13).

The location for introducing the LUS probe is limited by the location of the trocars: first, the umbilical port can be made for laparoscopic exploration, and the second trocar site for LUS can be selected depending on both the preoperative imaging evaluation and the intraoperative conditions as determined by laparoscopy. Exploration of the liver parenchyma can be usually performed with a direct contact technique thanks to the natural humidity of the liver surface, which allows a good acoustic contact with the transducer. However, the dome of the liver may be difficult to examine because of the lack of adequate contact between the probe and the convex liver surface: this can be overcome by instilling saline solution and scanning the highest part of the organ through the fluid (water-immersion method) (Fig. 13.14). Furthermore, in some instances, it may be useful to reduce to 6–8 mmHg the pneumoperitoneum favoring a correct angle of transducer contact with the liver surface.

The whole liver is initially screened and each tumor is measured in size by LUS and described according to the Couinaud classification of liver anatomy. After the lesions have been identified, the therapeutic electrode can be accurately inserted into the tumor.

When dealing with lesions localized in segment 1 or in the posterior segments of an enlarged liver, a longer laparoscopic electrode could be necessary (27 cm). The electrode has to pass the abdominal wall and the pneumoperitoneum space prior to reaching the liver surface

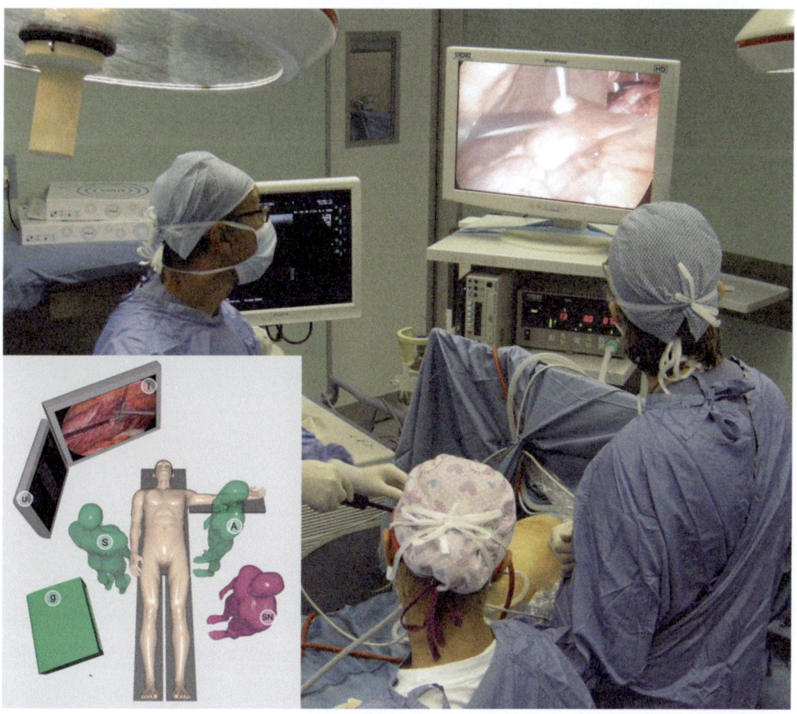

Fig. 13.11 Patient and operating room positions for LRFA: supine position with legs adducted (surgeon stands on the patient's *right side*) for lesions in segments 4, 5, and 8

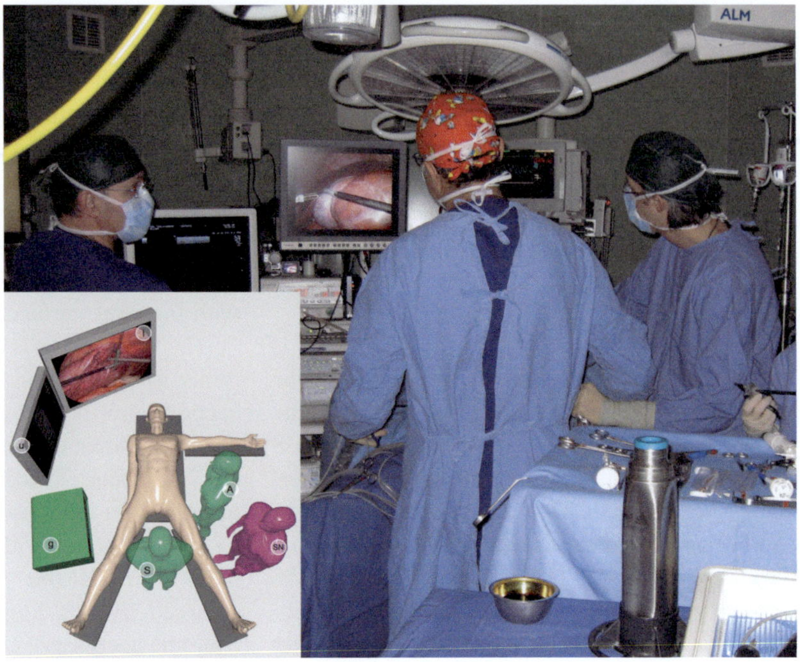

Fig. 13.12 Patient and operating room positions for LRFA: supine position with legs abducted (surgeon stands between the legs) for lesions in segments 1, 2, 3, and 4

meeting a fulcrum, which complicates the movements of the tip of the electrode. This problem can be coped with by the aid of either a 2-mm trocar or a 14-G cannula needle placed through the abdominal wall and the electrode is then placed through this sheath.

A LUS-guided interventional procedure can be successfully performed if the following ideal working conditions are fulfilled: (1) the lesion has to be well visible: the ultrasound probe must be oriented on the liver surface to display the largest diameter of the entire lesion; (2) the

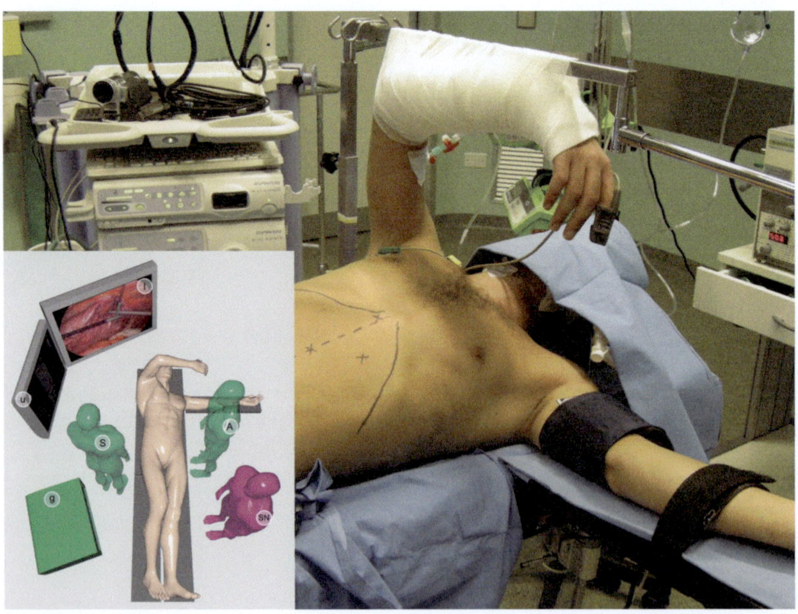

Fig. 13.13 Patient and operating room positions for LRFA: oblique position with the right side elevated up to 45° or left decubitis position with the right arm elevated and across the chest (surgeon stands at the *left side* of the patient) for lesions in segments 6 and 7

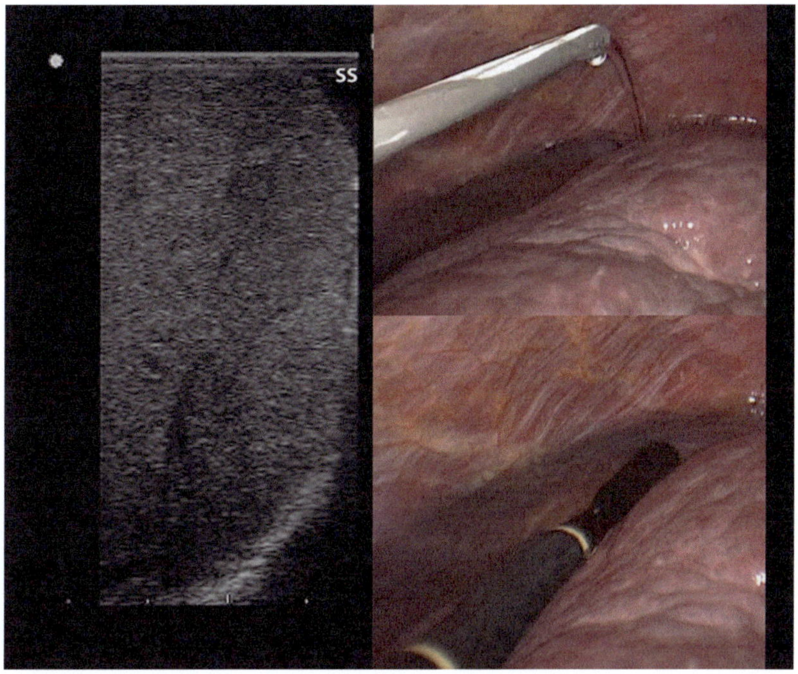

Fig. 13.14 The dome of the liver may be more easily examined by instilling saline solution (*SS*) and scanning this part of the organ through the fluid which creates an acoustic window

electrode must be positioned near the transducer of the LUS probe in order to introduce it slightly oblique to the transducer and with an acute angle to the axis of the LUS probe (Fig. 13.15).

In fact, after inserting the electrode into the liver parenchyma, slight rotation of the probe can identify the mark of the electrode and guide its tip into the lesion. If the access of the electrode is too acute in respect to the surface of the liver, it is well possible that the electrode remains superficial and parallel to the long axis of the probe without reaching the lesion. For lesions located at posterior segments, it is necessary to insert the electrode on the liver surface further than the lesion: in this case, the transducer can not simultaneously visualize the tumor and the electrode tip (Fig. 13.16). On the other hand, because any LUS-guided interventional procedure is totally free-hand, a puncture adapter has been proposed: the incorporation of the biopsy channel into the shaft of the ultrasound probe permits accurate placement of the electrode only in lesions seated in some areas of the liver. For lesions that required multiple overlapping ablations, the zones farthest from the LUS transducer were ablated first so that the ultrasound artifacts of dissolved nitrogen did not obscure electrode placement for subsequent ablations.

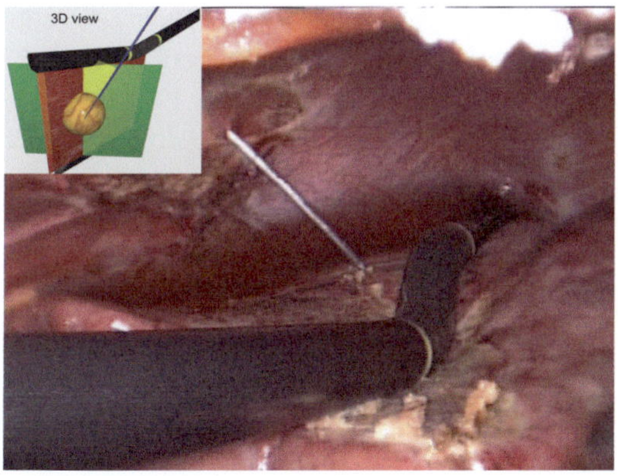

Fig. 13.15 In order to exactly center the lesion, it is important to evaluate both the angles of the electrode incidence respect to the LUS image of the lesion

13.4.3 Technical Variants: Intrahepatic Vascular Occlusion

This approach determines an ischemic area surrounding the lesion increasing the necrosis volume [19]. This effect can reduce the risk of

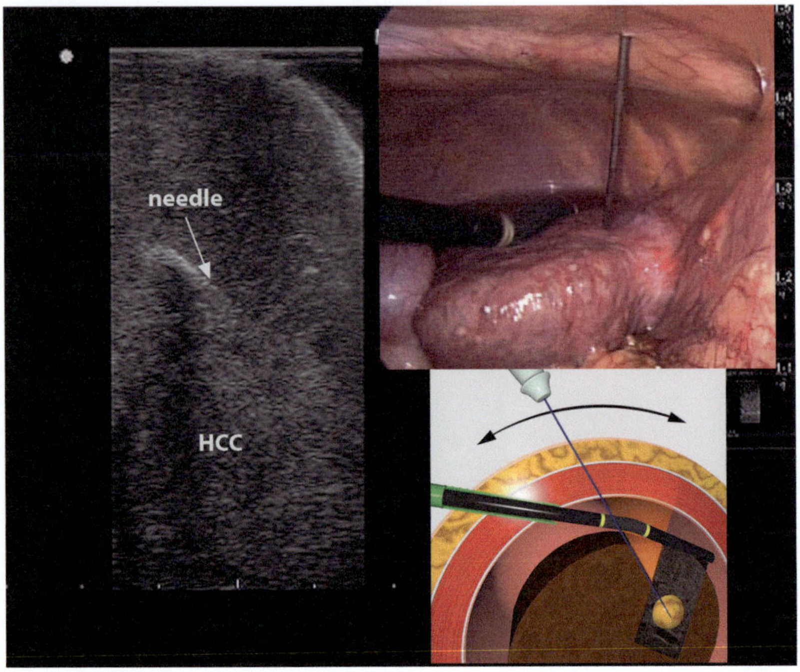

Fig. 13.16 If the lesion is situated inside the posterior segments, the electrode must be inserted more fore into the liver (blind zone of insertion) to reach a deeply located tumor

immediate therapy failure (partial ablation) and of local recurrences. In order to obtain a selective intrahepatic portal venous occlusion, the primary vessel of the lesion was identified by color Doppler imaging: using ultrasonographic guidance, the electrode was directed toward this area with direct puncture of the nearby blood vessel and the ablation cycle lasted either 2–4 min using RFA or 60–90 s using MWA. Another evaluation with color Doppler imaging was performed to confirm a coagulative ablation of the vascular area: a discolored area on the liver surface could also be visualized (Fig. 13.17). Then, the lesion was treated with the insertion of the electrode in the usual way.

13.4.4 Technical Variants: Cooling Technique

If the tumor is located in the hepatic hilar region, RFA/MWA may cause bile duct stenosis due to physical or heat damage to the bile duct.

It is possible to prevent this biliary damage inserting preoperatively an endoscopic nasobiliary drainage tube and then percutaneous RFA/MWA is performed with intraductal perfusion of cold 5 % glucose isotonic solution [20]. It is possible to perform the same cooling technique through a percutaneous transhepatic biliary drainage, but it is more demanding because intrahepatic biliary ducts are usually thin. Another technique is the intraductal cooling of the main bile ducts during laparoscopic RFA/MWA. The tube can be inserted in the main biliary duct either through the cystic duct (cholecystectomy must be performed) or through a direct incision of the main bile duct (choledochotomy). However, these procedures can be very difficult in cirrhotic patients [21].

Another less invasive but effective approach is to insert some gauzes in the peritoneal cavity and then place them around the hepatoduodenal ligament. Then, an irrigator with cold saline solution infuses them: cold vascular flow in the portal and arterial systems protects the bile ducts from the thermal effects of RFA/MWA by dissipating the heat generated in the ablated area (Fig. 13.18).

The possible "heat sink" effect of central bile duct cooling might also affect the efficacy of RFA/MWA in terms of local recurrences, thus in

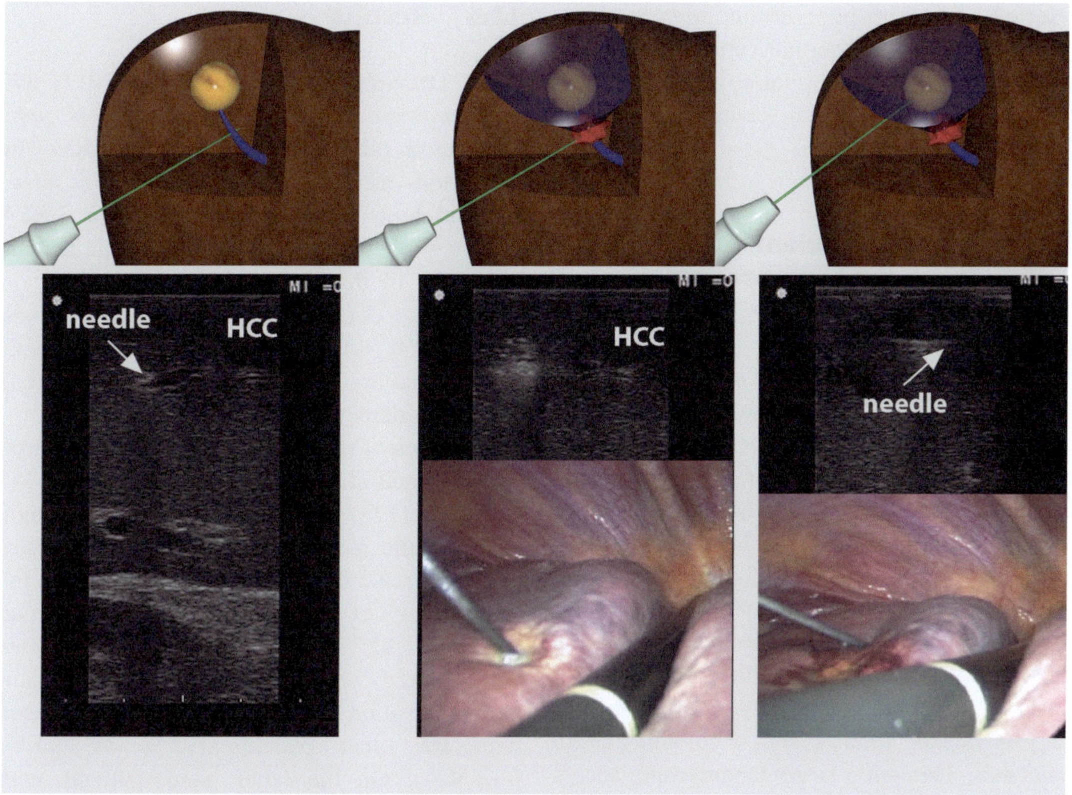

Fig. 13.17 Intrahepatic vascular occlusion: the primary vessel of the lesion was identified by color Doppler imaging: using LUS guidance, the electrode was directed toward this area with direct puncture of the nearby blood vessel and the ablation cycle lasted 2–4 min: a discolored area on the liver surface is seen. Then, the lesion was treated with the insertion of the electrode in the usual way

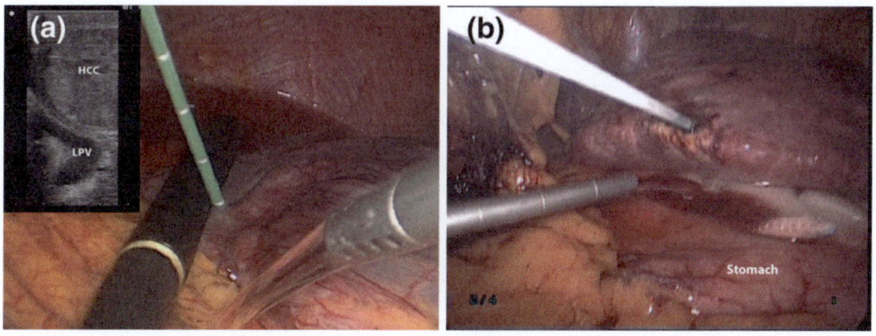

Fig. 13.18 **a** Lesion (*HCC*) located near the left glissonian pedicles (*LPV*); **b** lesion (*HCC*) located on the inferior surface of the liver, contiguous to gastric wall: cold saline solution is injected on some gauzes positioned around the hepatoduodenal ligament (**a**) or under the left lobe (**b**)

selected cases with huge lesions next to carrefour structures, a thermal ablation can be scheduled a priori via cooling technique followed by a transarterial chemoembolization (TACE) one month later.

13.4.5 Technical Variants: Contrast-Enhanced Laparoscopic Ultrasound

Some HCC nodules show an isoechoic pattern and also during LUS examination they can be difficult to discern. The application of intravenous ultrasound contrast agents during transcutaneous ultrasonography of the liver has been shown to improve nodule characterization in comparison with unenhanced ultrasound. The addition of contrast enhancement of intraoperative ultrasound in the evaluation of liver tumors will improve image conspicuity, correct diagnosis of new malignant nodules, ablation efficacy in hepatic tumors, and oncologic margin outcomes. Through a larger laparoscopic access (about 35 mm diameter), a microconvex ultrasound probe (model UST-9146T, Aloka®) can be introduced maintaining the pneumoperitoneum with a purse string suture (Fig. 13.19). In this way it is possible to perform a contrast-enhanced laparoscopic ultrasound, identifying the HCC nodule and checking the necrosis result following RFA (Fig. 13.20).

13.5 Results

From December 1997 to August 2012, 379 patients with HCC and liver cirrhosis were considered eligible for LRFA according the indications mentioned above. Table 13.1 shows the different reasons to propose an LRFA rejecting a percutaneous approach or an hepatic resection. In this series, 360 patients were in BCLC stage A (A1: 103 pts; A2: 50 pts; A3: 38 pts; A4: 169 pts), 14 in stage B, and 5 in stage C. For the analysis, only patients in BCLC stage A were considered (360 pts).

Complete ablation (technique effectiveness) was obtained at 1 month in 330 out of the 355 patients (93 %): 94 % of patients with single HCC nodule and 92 % with multiple nodules (p = N.S.). No differences were found when the RFA group was compared with the MWA group (93 % vs. 92 %; p = N.S.) or when patients were treated with cooling technique for dangerous position of the lesions in comparison with the other patients (92 % vs. 93 %; p = N.S.). On the other hand, patients with intrahepatic vascular occlusion had no incomplete ablation while the other patients had 91 % complete ablation ($p = 0.010$). Table 13.2 shows the immediate postoperative complications according the Clavien's classification [22]. Only four patients had grade IIIb complications requiring surgical reintervention (two hemorrhages from trocar access, one from liver surface

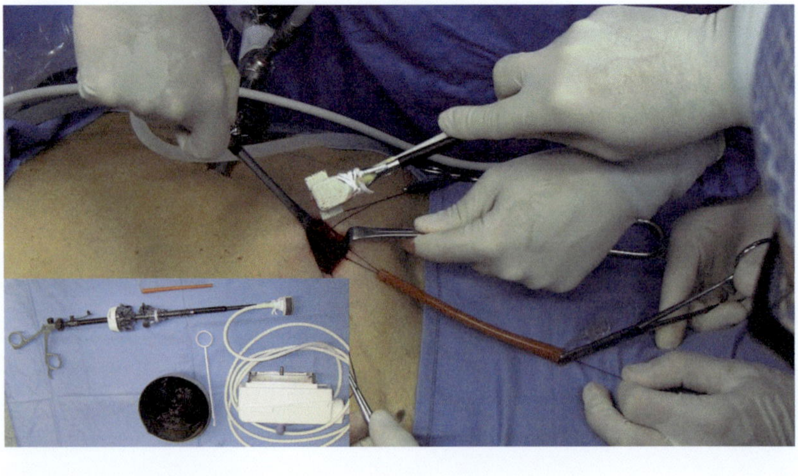

Fig. 13.19 A microconvex transducer is introduced in the peritoneal cavity through a 3 cm access

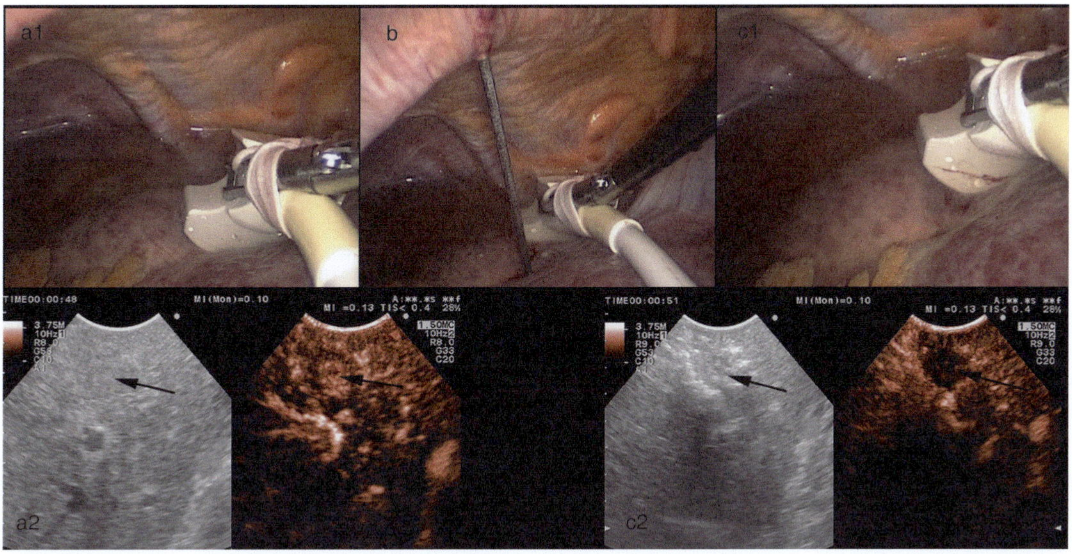

Fig. 13.20 CELU permits the application of intravenous ultrasound contrast agent to improve nodule characterization in comparison with unenhanced ultrasound (*a1* and *a2*). After the RFA (*b*) CELU shows the necrosis effect of RFA (*c1* and *c2*)

Table 13.2 Postoperative complications (more than 1 complication for each patient)

	N (%)	Clavien classification
Ascites	22 (6 %)	Grade I: 13
		Grade II: 8
		Grade IIIa: 1
Encephalopathy	14 (4 %)	Grade I: 11
		Grade II: 3
Jaundice (>3 mg/dl)	33 (9 %)	Grade I: 30
		Grade II: 3
Wall wound hematoma	32 (9 %)	Grade I: 29
		Grade II: 2
		Grade IIIb: 1
Peritoneal hemorrhage	3 (0.8 %)	Grade IIIb: 3
Upper digestive bleeding	0	
Visceral perforation	0	
Biliary fistula	1 (0.6 %)	Grade IIIa: 1
Hepatic abscess	0	
Pleural effusion	2 (1.2 %)	Grade I: 1
		Grade IIIa: 1
Skin burn	1 (0.6 %)	Grade II: 1
No complication	266 (74 %)	

Table 13.3 HCC recurrences

	Total HCC recurrences	P	Local recurrences	P	Early recurrences (<12 m.)	p
Total pts. (355)	205 (58 %)		83 (23 %)		117 (33 %)	
RFA (49)[a]	17 (35 %)	NS	11 (22 %)	NS	16 (33 %)	NS
MWA (62)[a]	20 (32 %)		10 (16 %)		11 (18 %)	
Cooling technique (49)	20 (41 %)	0.010	7 (14 %)	NS	11 (22 %)	NS
Others (306)	185 (60 %)		76 (25 %)		106 (35 %)	
Vascular occlusion (71)[b]	41 (58 %)	NS	12 (17 %)	NS	19 (27 %)	NS
Others (174)[b]	88 (51 %)		45 (26 %)		59 (34 %)	

[a] From December 2009 when MWA has been used first
[b] From May 2004 when Vascular occlusion was used first

for insertion of ethanol injection needle, and one from a diaphragmatic vein) and only three had grade IIIa complications (one paracentesis, one thoracentesis, and one endoscopic nasobiliary drainage).

During followup (28.4 ± 28.9 months), 205 patients (58 %) had intrahepatic recurrences. Table 13.3 shows the different patterns of HCC recurrences and the behavior for each group of different techniques. The treatment of superficial lesions or contiguous to other structures is very effective using the cooling technique, without severe complications: no biliary stenosis, no visceral damages, no portal thrombosis. The other techniques (MWA or vascular occlusion) tend to reduce local and early recurrences without reaching a statistical significance: further followup and patients are necessary to evaluate these findings.

References

1. Vapenstad C, Rethy A, Lango T et al (2010) Laparoscopic ultrasound: a survey of its current and future use, requirements and integration with navigation technology. Surg Endosc 24:2944–2953
2. Montorsi M, Santambrogio R, Bianchi P et al (2001) Laparoscopy with laparoscopic ultrasound (L-LUS) for the pre-treatment staging of hepatocellular carcinoma: a prospective study. J Gastrointest Surg 5:312–315
3. Santambrogio R, Opocher E, Pisani Ceretti A et al (2007) Impact of intraoperative ultrasonography in laparoscopic liver surgery. Surg Endosc 21:181–188
4. Santambrogio R, Bianchi P, Pasta A et al (2002) Ultrasound-guided interventional procedures of the liver during laparoscopy: technical considerations. Surg Endosc 16:349–354
5. Bruix J, Sherman M (2005) Management of hepatocellular carcinoma. Hepatology 42:1208–1236
6. Bruix J, Sherman M (2011) Management of hepatocellular carcinoma: an update. Hepatology 53:1020–1022
7. Livraghi T, Meloni F, Di Stasi M et al (2008) Sustained complete response and complications rates after radiofrequency ablation of very early hepatocellular carcinoma in cirrhosis: is resection still the treatment of choice? Hepatology 47:82–89
8. Livraghi T, Goldberg SN, Lazzaroni S et al (2000) Hepatocellular carcinoma: radiofrequency ablation of medium and large lesions. Radiology 214:761–768
9. Santambrogio R, Opocher E, Costa M et al (2005) Survival and intrahepatic recurrences after laparoscopic radiofrequency of hepatocellular carcinoma in patients with liver cirrhosis. J Surg Oncol 89:218–226
10. Jones RP, Jackson R, Dunne DFJ et al (2012) Systematic review and meta-analysis of follow-up after hepatectomy for colorectal liver metastases. Br J Surg 99:477–486
11. Quan D, Gallinger S, Nhan C et al (2012) The role of liver resection for colorectal cancer metastases in anera of multimodality treatment: a systematic review. Surgery 151:860–870
12. Wong SL, Mangu PB, Choti MA et al (2010) American Society of Clinical Oncology 2009 clinical evidence review on radiofrequency ablation of hepatic metastases from colorectal cancer. J Clin Oncol 28:493–508

13. Gazelle GS, Goldberg SN, Solbiati L, Livraghi T (2000) Tumor ablation with radio-frequency energy. Radiology 217:633–646
14. Goldberg SN, Dupuy DE (2001) Image-guided radiofrequency tumor ablation: challenges and opportunities, Part I. J Vasc Interv Radiol 12:1021–1032
15. Rossi S, Garbagnati F, Lencioni R et al (2000) Percutaneous radiofrequency thermal ablation of nonresectable hepatocellular carcinoma after occlusion of tumor blood supply. Radiology 217:119–126
16. Saitsu H, Yoshida T, Taniwaki T et al (1991) Laparoscopic coagulonecrotic therapy using microtase for small hepatocellular carcinoma (in Japanese). Nippon Shokakibyo Gakkai Zasshi (JPN J Gastroenterol) 88:2727
17. Lee KF, Hui JWY, Cheung YS et al (2012) Surgical ablation of hepatocellular carcinoma with 2.45 GHz microwave: a critical appraisal of treatment outcomes. Hong Kong Med J 18:85–91
18. Qian GJ, Wang N, Shen Q et al (2012) Efficacy of microwave versus radiofrequency ablation for treatment of small hepatocellular carcinoma: experimental and clinical studies. Eur Radiol 22:1983–1990
19. Santambrogio R, Costa M, Barabino M, Opocher E (2008) Laparoscopic radiofrequency of hepatocellular carcinoma using ultrasound-guided selective intrahepatic vascular occlusion. Surg Endosc 22:2051–2055
20. Elias D, El Otmany A, Goharin A et al (2001) Intraductal cooling of the main bile ducts during intraoperative radiofrequency ablation. J Surg Oncol 76:297–300
21. Lam VWT, Ng KKC, Chok KSH et al (2008) Safety and efficacy of radiofrequency ablation for periductal hepatocellular carcinoma with intraductal cooling of the central bile duct. J Am Coll Surg 207:e1–e5
22. Clavien PA, Barkun J, De Oliveira ML et al (2009) The Clavien-Dindo classification of surgical complications: five-year experience. Ann Surg 250:187–196

14 Robotic Ultrasound-Guided Liver Resections

Alberto Patriti, Marco Carlani, and Luciano Casciola

14.1 Introduction

Advances in intraoperative ultrasound are reducing the need for major hepatectomies irrespective of tumor number and location and even in demanding conditions such as tumor invasion of the hepatic veins [1]. This trend is based on the evidence that a parenchyma-sparing resection can be considered as oncologically effective as major hepatectomy for both colorectal liver metastases (CRLM) and hepatocellular carcinoma (HCC), even though the different nature of the diseases impinge on technical aspects of liver resection for HCC [2]. The impaired liver function secondary to the underlying cirrhosis requires a balance between oncologic requirements and parenchyma preservation. HCC spreads along portal veins and can give rise to satellite nodules up to 2 cm from the primary tumor. Therefore, anatomic resection of parenchyma involved by the tumor along with its feeding portal branch is considered the gold standard treatment for HCC [3]. Furthermore, parenchyma preservation has the additional advantage of reducing morbidity without changes in long-term results and offers the possibility of repeated hepatectomies in case of liver recurrence [4]. Whether laparoscopic surgery is following the advances in open ultrasound-guided liver surgery is still questionable especially for lesions in contact with liver vessels and located in the posterosuperior (PS) segments. In studies investigating the role of laparoscopy to approach PS liver malignancies, a major resection is still the procedure of choice in contrast to minor liver resections for lesions of the anterior segments [5]. This discrepancy can be relied to two main reasons. Laparoscopic intraoperative ultrasound (LIOUS) exploration and ultrasound-guided liver resection results challenging for deeply located, small lesions, and the rigid laparoscopic tools do not allow to perform the curved or angulated resection lines necessary for a parenchyma-preserving resection in the posterior area of the liver [5]. Robotics (da Vinci Robotic System Intuitive Surgical Inc., Sunnyvale, CA), introducing the possibility of image integration and the "wrist-like" movements of the robotic tools, promises to overcome these limitations extending indications for a minimally invasive parenchyma-sparing surgery even to lesions located in the PS segments or in contact with liver vessels.

A. Patriti (✉) · L. Casciola
Department of Surgery, Division of General Minimally Invasive and Robotic Surgery, Local Healthcare Unit 2 Umbria, San Matteo degli Infermi Hospital, Via Loreto, 06049 Spoleto, PG, Italy
e-mail: albertopatriti@gmail.com

L. Casciola
e-mail: lucianocasciola@gmail.com

M. Carlani
Department of Radiology and Radiotherapy, Local Healthcare Unit 2 Umbria, San Matteo degli Infermi Hospital, Via Loreto, 06049 Spoleto, PG, Italy
e-mail: marco.carlani@gmail.com

G. Torzilli (ed.), *Ultrasound-Guided Liver Surgery*,
DOI: 10.1007/978-88-470-5510-0_14, © Springer-Verlag Italia 2014

In this chapter, technical and technological features to carry out robotic ultrasound-guided liver resections (RUGLR) are discussed.

14.2 The da Vinci Robotic System

The da Vinci robotic system has been gradually upgraded from the first three-arm system to the current lightweight da Vinci Si with four arms and a high-definition (HD) 3D camera. The robotic system is designed to detect, filter, and translate electromechanically the surgeon's finger movements into precise and scaled micro-movements of the instruments. Basically, three modules compose the da Vinci: the *surgeon console*, the *robotic cart*, and the *endoscopic column* or *vision cart*. The *robotic instruments*, connected to the robotic arms, are articulated with seven degrees of freedom [6].

14.2.1 Surgeon Console

The console contains hardware, software, and the human interfaces of the system. The latter are the binocular viewer, the master control, control panels for system setup, and the foot control pedals. The surgeon operates sitting in front of the console viewing the operating field in a high-definition 3D viewing screen. Two master controllers allow the surgeon to move robotic instruments using the thumb and index finger of each hand. The system translates the surgeon's wrist and finger movements into real-time movements to the surgical instruments. There are five foot pedals in the da Vinci S model: clutch pedal that disengages the instruments from the controllers, camera, and focus pedals allowing adjustment of the surgical view, bipolar and monopolar coagulation pedals. Two panels are positioned on each side, on the left we have camera and endoscopic calibration and motion scaling; on the right, the system start control, emergency stop control, and standby buttons. In case of need, the system can be rapidly disengaged into standby mode.

14.2.2 Patient-side Cart

The console is connected to the cart by a cable carrying bidirectional information. The cart consists of four robotic arms; one for the camera and three for the instruments. Plastic drapes are necessary to cover the arms for sterility because these are the sole components of the robot reaching the surgical field. The robotic arms work into the patient's abdominal cavity through dedicated 8-mm trocars. Each arm moves likewise the human arm through a series of multiple joints and a terminal pivot joint, corresponding to the 8-mm trocar.

The endoscopic column and camera system has all the features of a standard laparoscopic column with a monitor, a CO_2 insufflator, a dual high-intensity light source, and a camera unit. The camera system, with a 10× magnification, has a dual lens system with two three-chip cameras. The spatial separation of these images projected to the surgeon's eyes in the binocular viewer allows true 3D imaging at the console.

EndoWrist instruments. A wide range of dedicated instruments is available (forceps, hook, bipolar, grasper, etc.). Almost all the instruments have an articulated tip with seven degrees of freedom; the only exception is the ultrasonic dissector. Position sensing abolishes the human tremors. Almost all the instruments may be used 10 times.

14.3 Image Integration in Robotic Surgery

Both open and minimally invasive liver surgery largely depend on preoperative imaging (computer tomography and magnetic resonance) and intraoperative ultrasonography (IOUS) for the evaluation of vascular and biliary anatomy, identification of known and occult intrahepatic lesions, and operative planning. This aspect is particularly important in minimally invasive surgery where tactile feedback is not afforded. Despite the rapid evolution of technology behind medical robotics there are still a whole host of issues that make robot-assisted liver surgery suboptimal and that are probably going to be fixed in the near future. Traditionally, several LCD monitors are used to deliver the surgical view, the ultrasound view, and the preoperative imaging. Further screens are needed to deliver anesthesia information. When translating laparoscopic liver resection to the robotic approach, the issue of multiple data sources on multiple monitors becomes cumbersome, as it requires that the surgeon disengage from the robotic console to glance at critical information sources. By disengaging, the surgeon may find difficult to integrate critical information on tumor location during resection of the tumor. Actually, there are different solutions for this issue. The simplest way is to connect the video out channel of the laparoscopic ultrasound to the robot video in. As shown in Fig. 14.1, the s-video cable connects the Aloka ProSound Alpha-7 video out to the video in of the laparoscopic column of the da Vinci S. The ecographic view can be observed by the console surgeon on the 3D screen in a "split screen" display mode and by the assistant on the monitor of the column (Fig. 14.2). The disadvantage of this method is the impossibility to manage multiple data sources. In order to compare the LIOUS with preoperative images, the surgeon needs a computer at the console side. TilePro software (Intuitive Surgical Inc., Sunnyvale, CA), working with the da Vinci Si platform , has troubleshooted this problem. TilePro may show multiple data sources into the robotic operative view giving the surgeon a more reliable system to integrate all the anatomical information. TilePro delivers information from up to two data sources simultaneously. Data are superimposed on the surgical view and can be delivered via s-video or digital visual interface (DVI) input into the console. There can be a total of six data sources, which may be

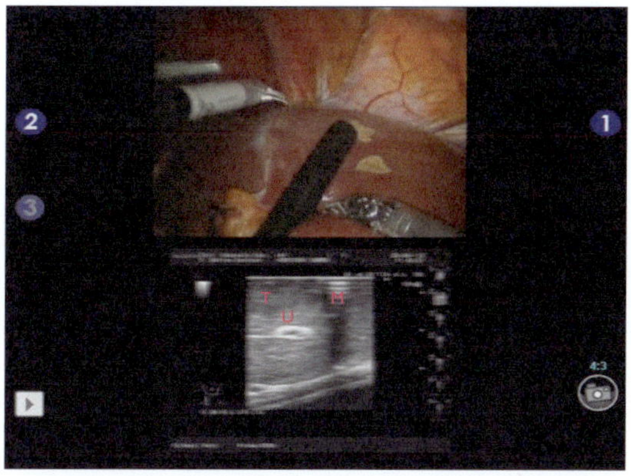

Fig. 14.2 Split-screen display mode using a traditional laparoscopic transducer; tumor (*T*); umbilical portion (*U*); resection margin marked with the bipolar forceps (*M*)

Fig. 14.1 Connections via s-video cable between Aloka ProSound Alpha-7 and da Vinci S

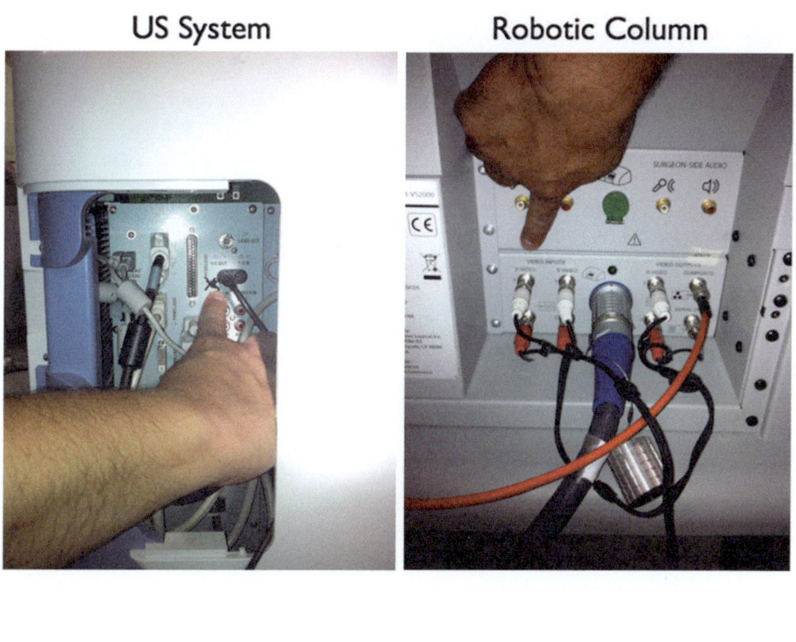

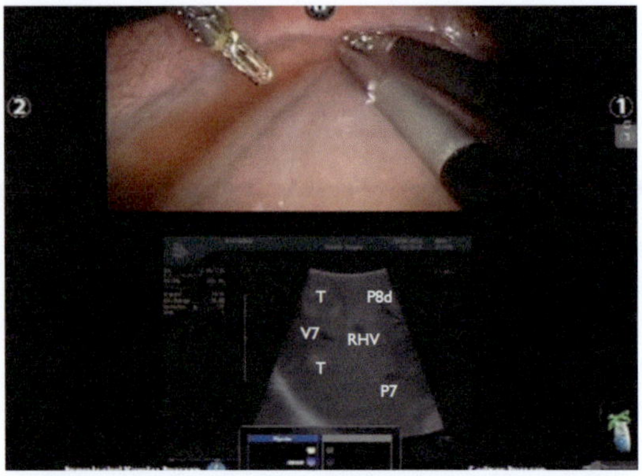

Fig. 14.3 Split-screen display mode using the BK transducer; tumor (*T*); portal branch for segment 8 dorsal (*P8d*); right hepatic vein (*RHV*); hepatic vein for segment 7 (*V7*); portal branch for segment 7 (*P7*)

toggled to present any two at a time to the console surgeon. Additionally, the data can be broadcasted to all monitors in the room so the assistants, nurses, and anesthesia teams can view the simulcast. The TilePro 'inbox' in the console view may be scaled depending on surgeon preference, with a 50 % display dimension having a resolution of 512 × 384 pixels. The sources of data are limitless; static images, graphical data, or even dynamic video, LIOUS, can all be input. The console surgeon with one click of the camera footswitch may perform changes or removal of the information [7]. The second issue of this technology pertains the US probe. With standard laparoscopic probes IOUS relies on the on-tale surgeon and, if not trained in ultrasound, on the console surgeon moving from the console to the table with a consequent time wasting and loss of information. Two different solutions have been proposed.

BK Medical has recently placed on the market an ultrasonograph equipped with a laparoscopic probe that can be manipulated by the robotic graspers (ProGrasp Forceps, Intuitive Surgical Inc., Sunnyvale, CA) (Fig. 14.3). The ProART Robotic Transducer Type 8826 is used together with a Flex Focus 800 Ultrasound system, which can be operated by wireless remote control UA1237 for use with the da Vinci Surgical System. The probe has a fin on its back that can be caught with ProGrasp forceps and manipulated by the console surgeon. The Flex Focus 800 is connected to the da Vinci Si console with a DVI cable for integration of picture-in-picture images with TilePro and can be remotely adjusted by the console surgeon. A similar system has been provided by Hitachi Aloka . A second solution has been tested in the preclinical setting. A prototype of a new robotic device for LIOUS has been developed by collaboration between the Johns Hopkins University and Intuitive. The device is composed by a linear transducer installed on an articulated probe controlled from the master tool manipulators of the surgical console [8]. In preclinical trials the probe was used with dedicated open-source software enabling to display the US images in different ways. The "split screen" display mode in which the surgeon sees the endoscopic and US views side-by-side. The "picture-in-picture" display mode that insets the US image into the endoscopic view and finally the "flashlight" display mode in which the US image is overlaid onto a 3D representation of the imaging plane in the stereo view of the console. The effect of this mode is to display the US image in the plane in which it is physically acquired by the transducer. Image magnification and camera filtering are other evolutions of the robotic view system with interesting future clinical applications. The key factor of this evolution is that the digital image at the console can be easily manipulated and the camera can be adapted to be sensible to different frequencies of light. Intuitive has recently cleared to the European market new system components including a surgical endoscope capable of visible light and near-infrared imaging. The 3D HD stereoscopic camera provides visible light and near-infrared illumination through the surgical endoscope via a flexible light guide. The system allows surgeons to view high-resolution near-infrared images of blood flow in vessels and microvessels, tissue and organ perfusion, and biliary excretion in real time during minimally invasive surgical procedures. The da Vinci robotic system with this new camera has been just adopted in clinical studies to replace intraoperative cholangiography using indocyanine green dye in order to delineate biliary anatomy and to detect bile leaks on the resection surface [9].

14.4 Operating Room Setup, Patient, and Trocar Position

Robot docking and patient position are of paramount importance to easily approach all the different liver segments for two motivations. Actually, the cart is heavy and once the robotic arms are connected to the trocars, changing position and operating field is relatively challenging. Second, a proper patient position is necessary to take advantage of gravity and the weight of the liver to improve exposure. Therefore, position of all the devices in the operating room, trocars, and patient has to be individualized according to the tumor location. When approaching anterior segments and segment 1 (Spiegel lobe) a reversed Trendelemburg supine patient position is optimal. The on-table surgeon stands between the legs and the scrub nurse and instruments are positioned lateral to the left leg (Fig. 14.4). The trocars are generally positioned along a bowl-shaped line passing through the umbilicus (Fig. 14.5).

For lesions located in the right posterolateral sector (upper segment 6 and segment 7) the patient is rotated on the left flank in order to facilitate liver mobilization and inferior vena cava dissection, when necessary. The camera port and the left-sided trocars should be placed as close as possible to the right costal margin, whereas the right trocar can be inserted in the intercostal space between the 10th and 11th rib close to the scapular line. At this level, the risk to accidental injury of the lung is very low and direct access to the posterolateral segments is

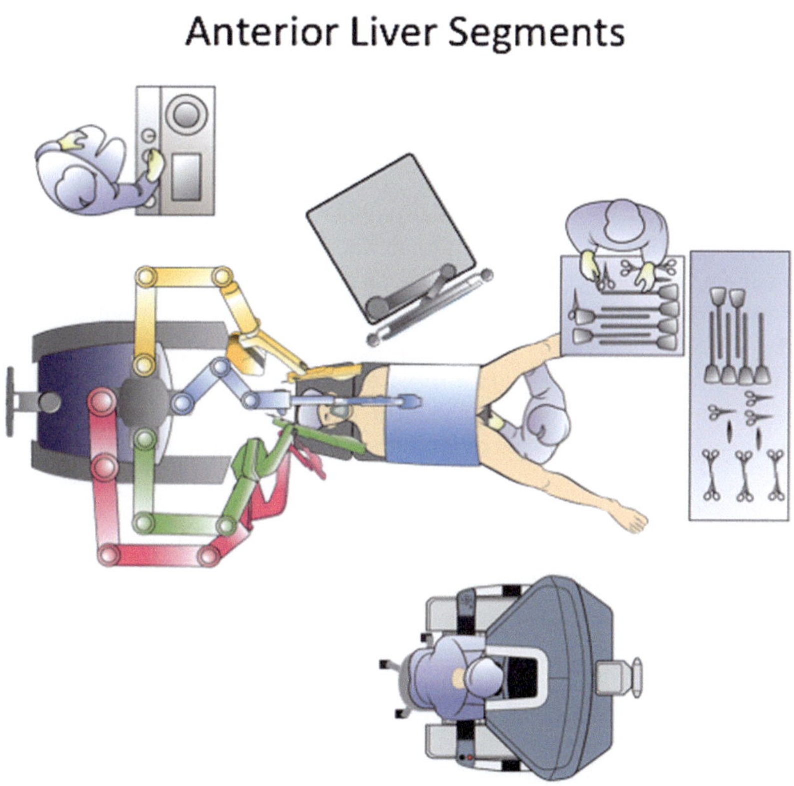

Fig. 14.4 Operating room setup for liver resections in the anterior segments

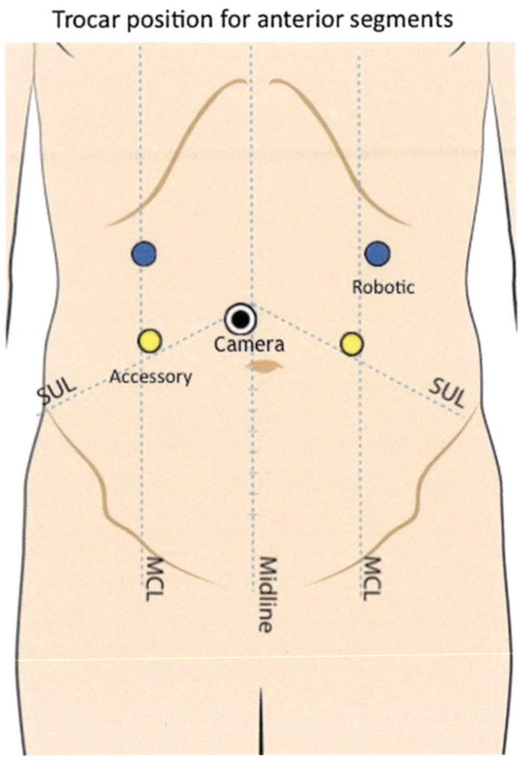

Fig. 14.5 Trocar position for liver resections in the anterior segments

provided (Figs. 14.6, 14.7, 14.8) [10]. For bilobar liver metastases with involvement of both anterior segments and S7-8 two options are equally effective; redocking the robot and changing patient position according to the tumor location; and using a semi-left lateral patient position with the robot over the patient's head (Fig. 14.9). The latter is preferred in our institution since it does not require robot redocking and changes during surgery of patient position with possible contamination of the surgical field.

14.5 Ultrasound Exploration

Ultrasound exploration follows the same general rules of traditional laparoscopic liver surgery. The typical frequency range adopted for LIOUS is 5–10 MHz. Access for the US probe to the peritoneal cavity is achieved through 10-or 11-mm ports which are usually the same ports used by the on-table surgeon for suction/irrigation and retraction (Figs. 14.5, 14.7). The supramesocolic space is instilled with saline solution until the space between the liver dome and the right diaphragm is completely filled in order to better explore the bare area of S7-8 and the hepatocaval confluence. A first ultrasound exploration of the liver is performed before the robot is docked and any other maneuver on the liver has been performed to avoid artifacts. This first exploration is intended to allow the surgical staff acquiring a clear 3D picture of liver vascular anatomy and lesion location. The examination is usually performed by contact scanning using the liquid film on the glissonian surface as a coupling agent. The hepatocaval confluence is usually visualized with the probe introduced through a right port and placed on S4a. Moving the probe between the diaphragm and the liver dome, the right hepatic vein is then identified. Portal bifurcation and right hepatic pedicles are visualized positioning the transducer on S4b and moving it to the right side. Left portal pedicles and left hepatic vein are better identified from the left upper quadrant. Using the linear probe, exploration of the diaphragmatic margins of S7-8 is carried out placing the probe on the water surface created in the right subdiaphragmatic area (Figs. 14.10, 14.11). Finally, the transection plane is outlined on the liver capsule with monopolar diathermy. When the robot is docked and resection begins, a continuous and meticulous ultrasound assessment of transection margin is imperative due to the lack of tactile feedback. Using a traditional laparoscopic US probe, the on-table surgeon checks the direction of the transection plane while the console surgeon can view on the screen the real-time ultrasonography and suggest to the on-table surgeon modifications of the probe position. Otherwise, the console surgeon has to move to the table to do it by him/herself. With the more sophisticated methods described above, the console surgeon can manipulate both the probe and US system during all the time of parenchymal transection. Concerning US-oriented anatomical resections for HCC, the two techniques described to identify

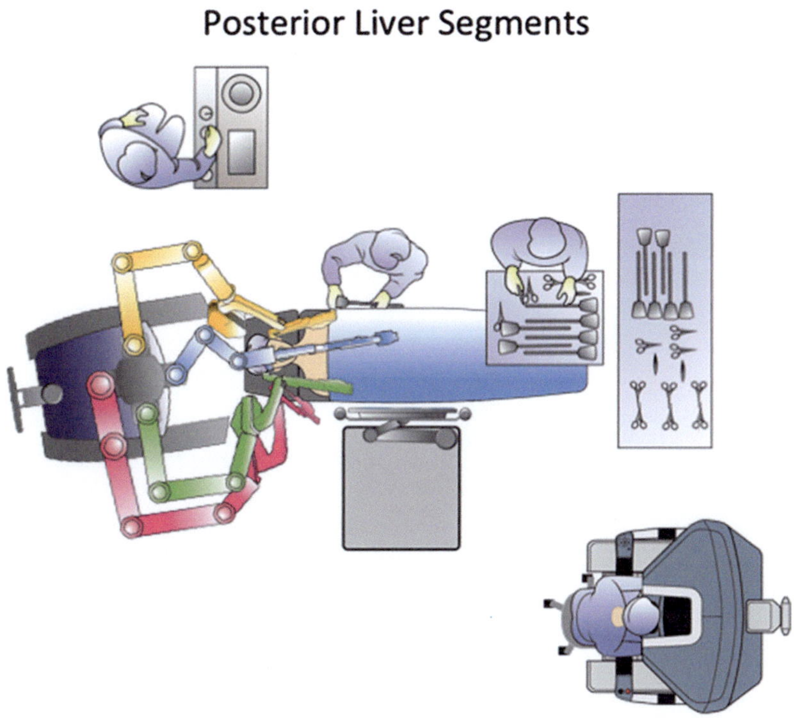

Fig. 14.6 Operating room setup for liver resections in the posterior segments

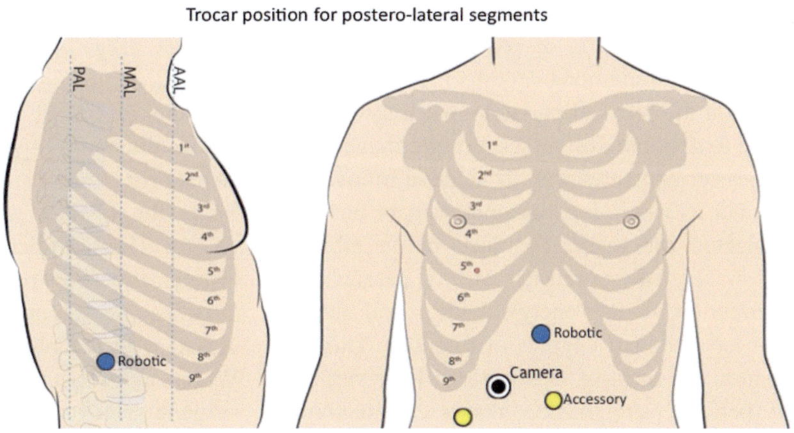

Fig. 14.7 Trocar position for liver resections in the posterior segments

the boundaries of liver segments were reproduced in minimally invasive surgery only in selected cases. The new generation laparoscopic US transducers—including those for robotic surgery—have a groove for needle guidance that allows performing the Makuuchi puncture technique. The "finger compression" described by Torzilli is more challenging to reproduce. The linear shape of the laparoscopic transducers, the scarce pressure applicable with the laparoscopic tools, thickness and stiffness of the liver are all factors that hamper laparoscopic compression of intrahepatic portal branches. Our personal experience is limited to segments 4b and 6 but current technological deficiency does not rule out the possible evolution of new devices to reproduce this technique in minimally invasive surgery (Fig. 14.12).

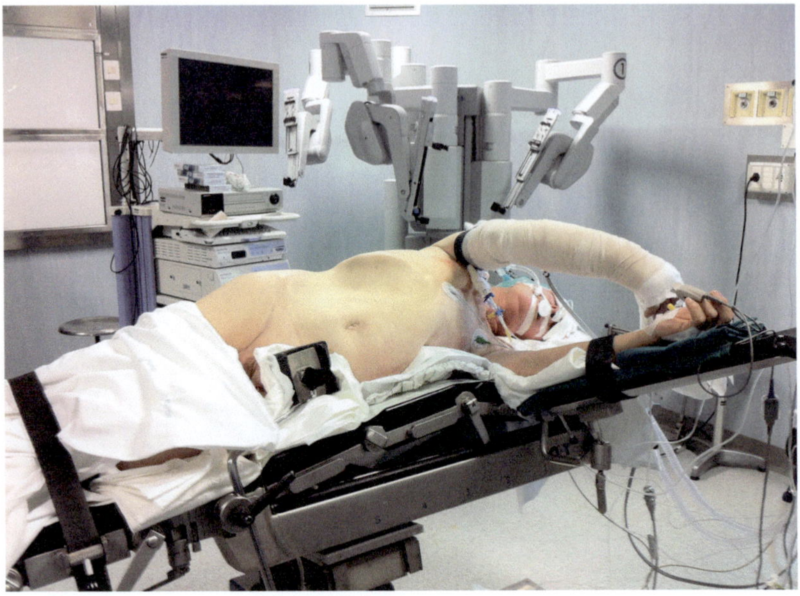

Fig. 14.8 Left lateral position for lesions in upper S6 and S7

14.6 Inflow Control

The availability of a system for intermittent inflow occlusion is of paramount importance when performing nonanatomical liver resections or when the planned parenchymal transection is close to a main liver vessel. Pringle maneuver is the easier and safer way to achieve inflow control but its use in laparoscopic surgery has been neglected for years. The lack of an effective inflow control favored the use for parenchymal transection of high-energy devices and staplers that have limited degrees of freedom. This has, in turn, led most of laparoscopic liver surgeons to perform straight-line major hepatectomies even for isolated PS lesions. A liberal use of Pringle maneuver in minimally invasive surgery is therefore imperative to safely perform echo-guided resections even for deeply located lesions or to handle large intraparenchymal vessels. An ideal system for laparoscopic Pringle maneuver should be cost effective and user friendly so as to permit intermittent inflow occlusion during parenchymal transection and guarantee a fast vascular control in case of bleeding. The device for inflow occlusion set in our institution is composed of a 20-Fr chest tube, an umbilical tape, and a plug used for occlusion of the Foley catheter (Fig. 14.13) [11]. The chest tube is inserted in the right upper abdominal quadrant and the umbilical tape is passed around the hepato-duodenal ligament with the use of an EndoWrist Cadiere forceps (Intuitive Surgical Inc., Sunnyvale, CA) (Figs. 14.14, 14.15, 14.16). The umbilical tape is then exteriorized through the chest tube with the use of a 5-mm laparoscopic forceps. The chest tube is finally closed with the plug in order to avoid air loss. When inflow occlusion is needed, the on-table surgeon removes the plug and pulls the umbilical tape. When the desired tape tension is achieved the chest tube is closed with the plug. With this technique the console surgeon can proceed in parenchyma transection while the on-table surgeon performs the intermittent pedicle clamping. The technique resulted to be safe when compared to the open counterpart in terms of postoperative bilirubin and liver enzymes blood levels [6].

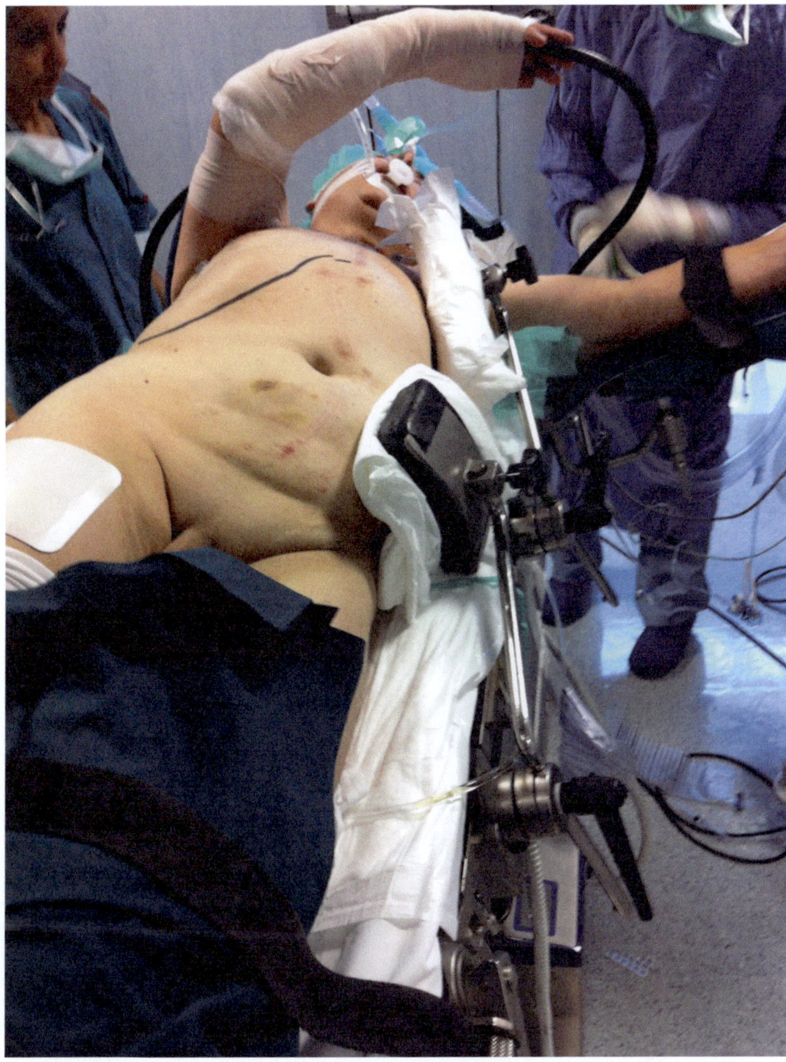

Fig. 14.9 Semi-left lateral patient position for bilobar lesions

14.7 Parenchymal Transection

With the attempt to perform RUGLR, a flexible and cost-effective device for parenchymal transection is required. The Kelly crush-clamp technique combined with intermittent Pringle maneuver is considered the safer and more accurate method of parenchymal transection in open liver surgery [12]. The major advantages of the Kelly crush-clamp technique are the low costs and the ability to fragment the parenchyma preserving the vascular structures that can be ligated and divided or preserved according to the resection plan. This economic and ingenious technique is not performed laparoscopically on a routine basis due to the inherent difficulties to perform the Pringle maneuver and the lack of dedicated instruments. Actually, robotics has renewed the interest for this technique. Using the EndoWrist bipolar precise forceps (Intuitive Surgical Systems, Sunnyvale, CA, USA) the parenchyma can be easily fragmented exposing the inner vessels as in open surgery (Fig. 14.17). The on-table surgeon uses it to perform the intermittent inflow occlusion, thereby allowing the console surgeon to focus his/her attention only on the

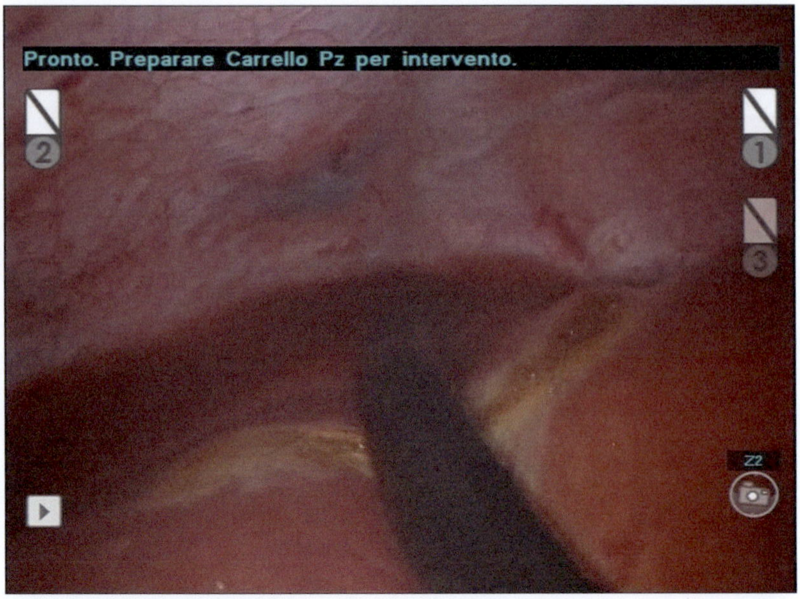

Fig. 14.10 LIOUS exploration of S7 before liver mobilization

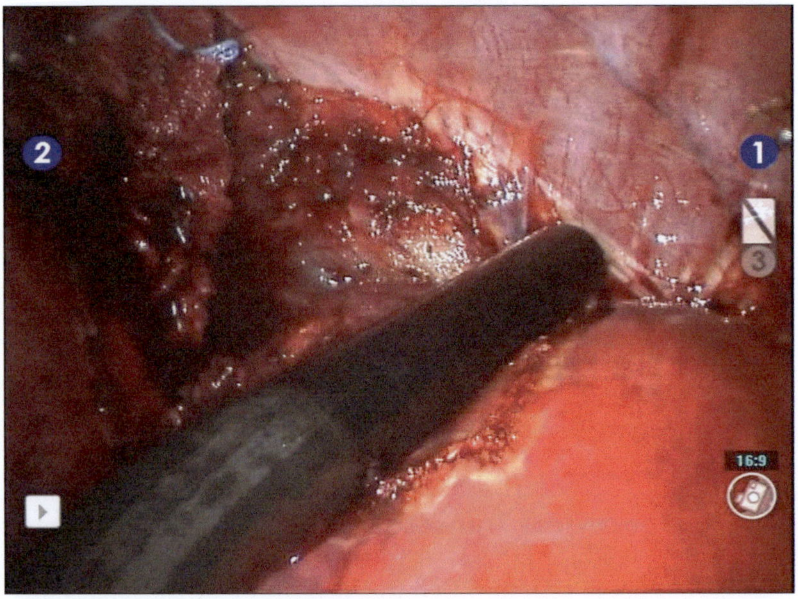

Fig. 14.11 LIOUS exploration after liver mobilization (same patient)

transection line. The wristed instruments gave back to the laparoscopic surgeon the option of performing curved and angled resections in all the liver segments, an ability lost with the rigid laparoscopic tools. Therefore, the robotic crush-clamp technique allows parenchymal preservation even for deeply located lesions, widening the indications for a minimally invasive approach even to lesions in the PS segments and located close to major liver vessels (Fig. 14.18). Hemostasis of small vessels is obtained with monopolar or bipolar cautery. To secure larger vessels on the transection line, we use Hem-o-lock® clips or ligatures with Vicryl® and Prolene®. The hepatic veins are usually divided with the laparoscopic linear

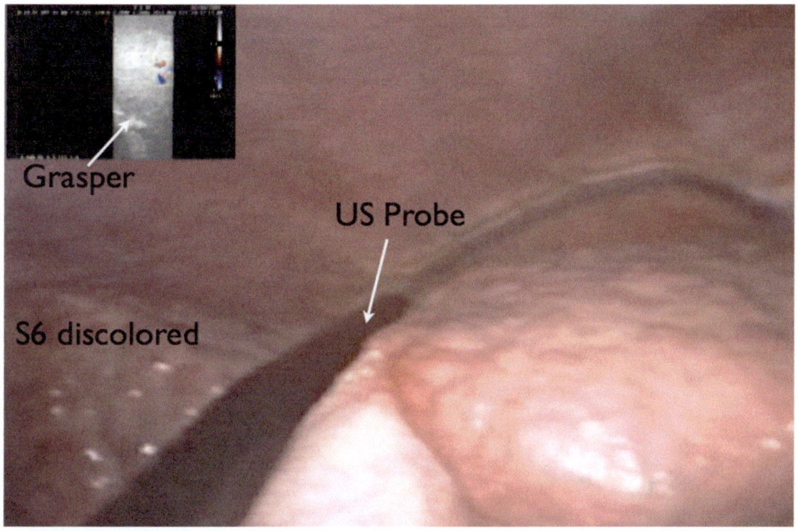

Fig. 14.12 Laparoscopic "finger compression technique"

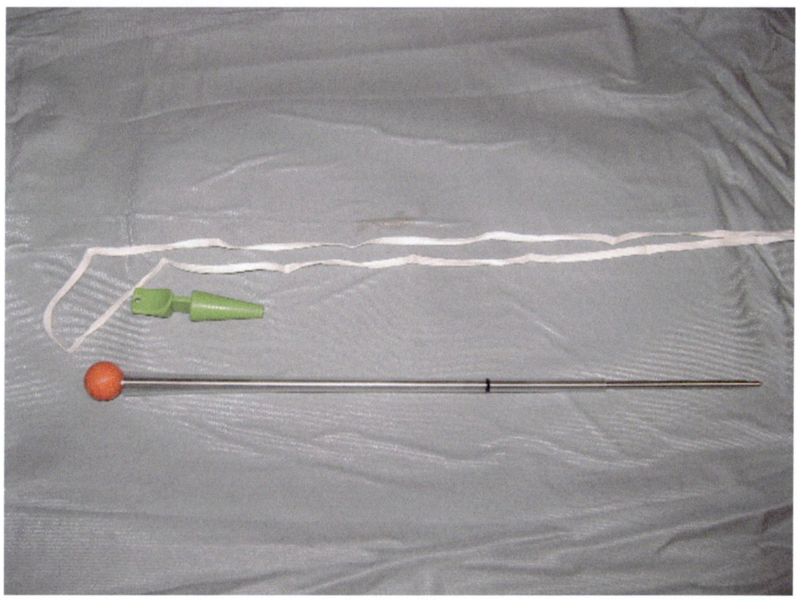

Fig. 14.13 Device for Pringle maneuver

stapler or sutured with Prolene®. Biliostasis is assessed by observation and the bile leaks controlled with sutures as in open surgery.

14.8 Liver Retraction

Retraction and tension have a great role in all aspects of surgery including liver resections. Once the proper resection plane has been identified with intraoperative ultrasound, in open surgery it is retraction of the specimen with the left surgeon hand to drive parenchymal transection. In minimally invasive surgery this simple act is reproduced with different tricks. For resections on anterior segments, left lateral sectionectomy included, some stay sutures can be useful to retract the specimen using the fourth robotic arm or the assistant grasper (Fig. 14.19). A vessel-loop held by the fourth arm around the left lobe can be used to stretch the parenchyma along the

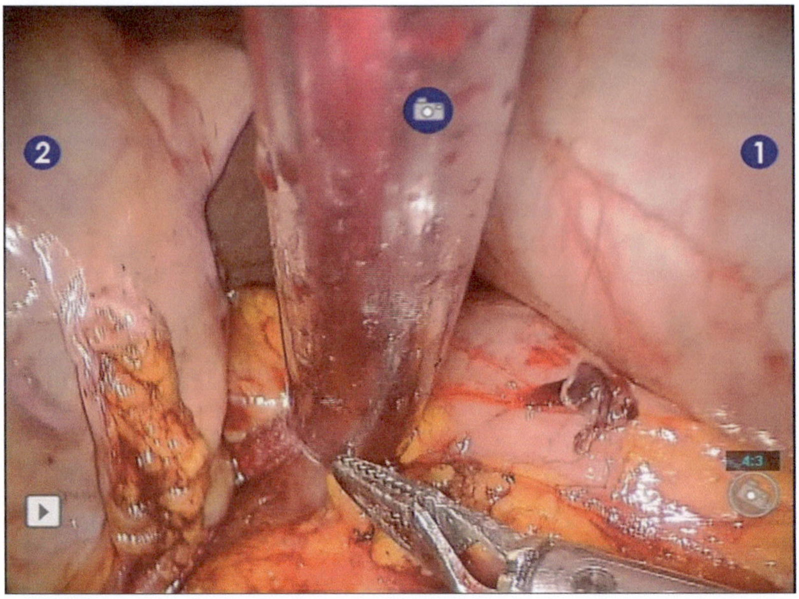

Fig. 14.14 Intraoperative view of the device for Pringle maneuver

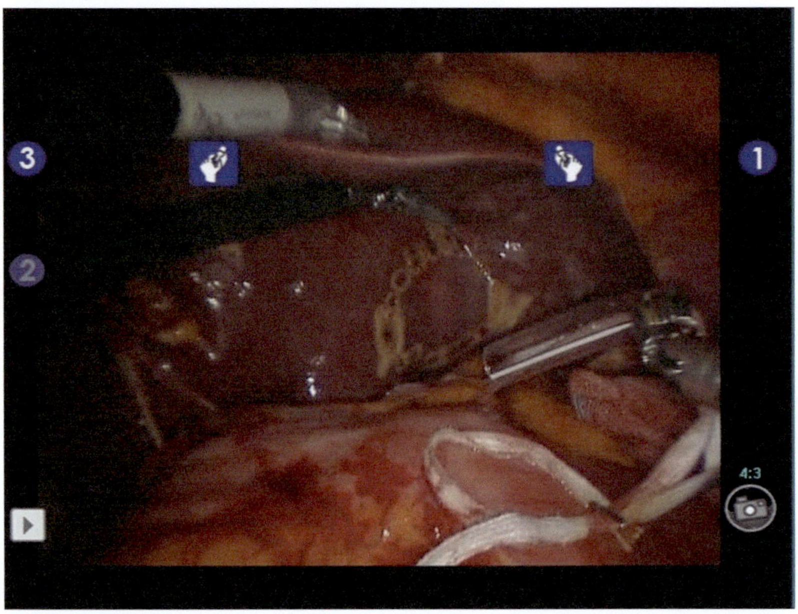

Fig. 14.15 Inflow control at the level of the liver pedicle and left hepatic artery arising from the left gastric artery

transection plane facilitating the effect of the Kelly crush-clamp technique (Fig. 14.20). For deeply located lesions or when the tumor is close to a major vessel the "corkscrew technique" can be reproduced (Fig. 14.21). After identification of the lesion by inspection and intraoperative ultrasound, Glisson's capsule is marked by electrocautery 1–2 cm away from the tumor margin. According to location of the tumor, the marked area is anchored by stitches with caution in order to prevent the needle from entering the tumor. The suture is held together by clips and upward traction is performed, facilitating the transection of the parenchyma and correct

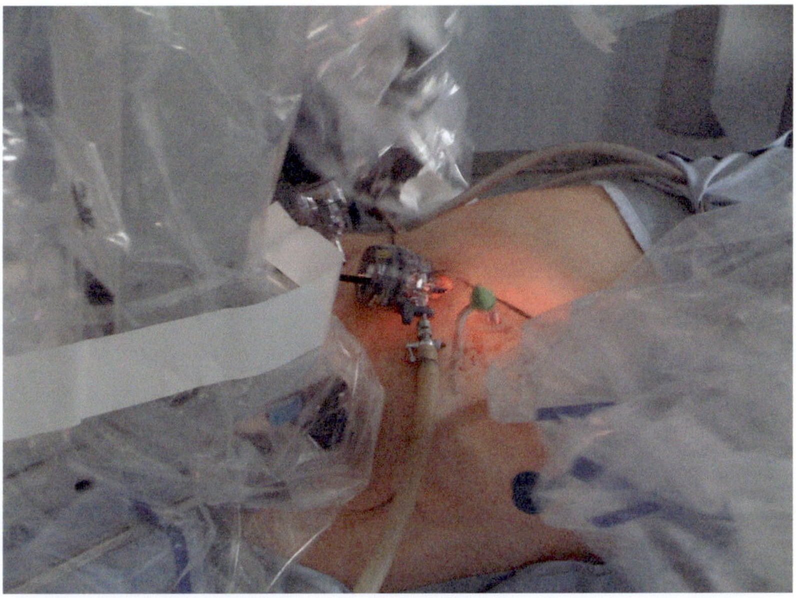

Fig. 14.16 External view of the device for Pringle maneuver

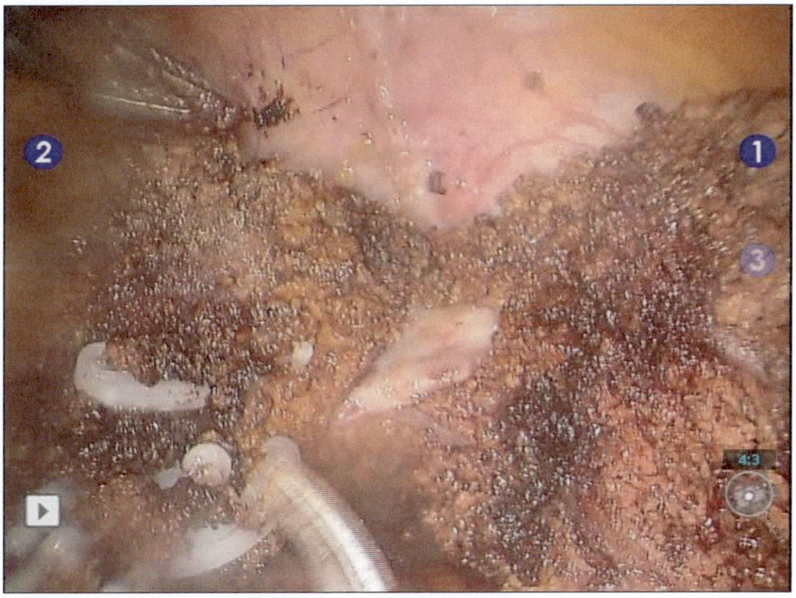

Fig. 14.17 Dissection of the left hepatic vein during a left lateral sectionectomy

identification of vascular and biliary structures. Parenchymal transection is performed with the monopolar shears for the first liver layer (1 cm from the Glisson capsule) and then with the Kelly crush-clamp technique. For steady exposure of the parenchymal transection plane in major hepatectomies, the "rubber band technique" can be used. Two sterile rubber bands are introduced into the abdominal cavity. One end of each rubber band is anchored with stay sutures at the right and left resection margins. The other end is pulled outside and fixed with appropriate tension [13].

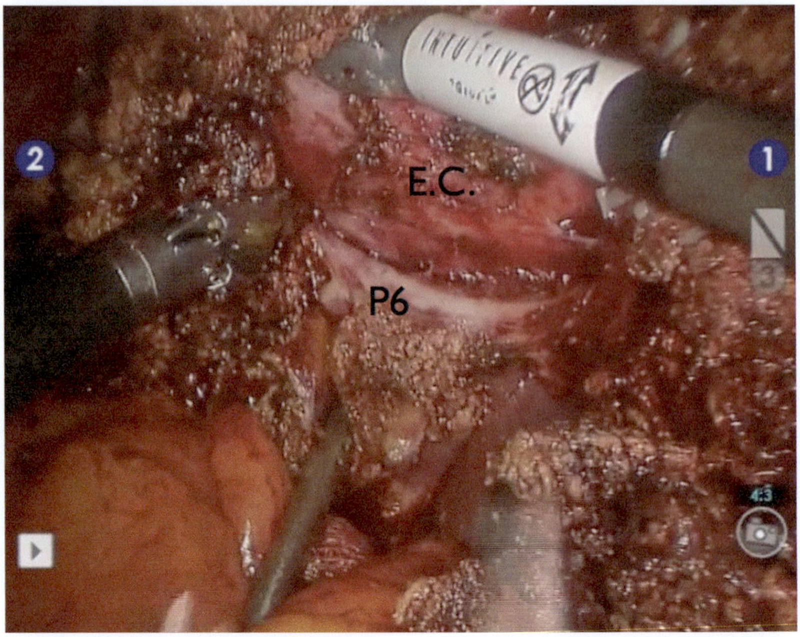

Fig. 14.18 Preservation of P6 during a pericystectomy for echinococcosis hydatid cyst

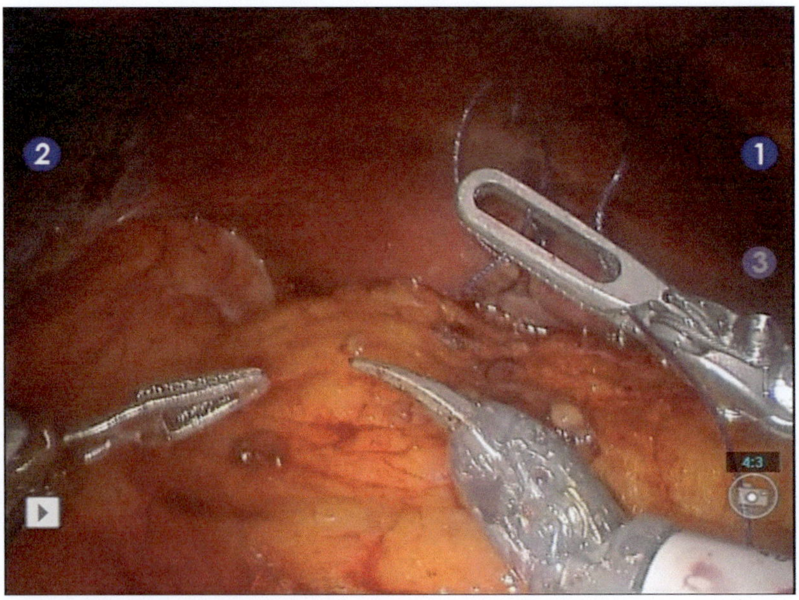

Fig. 14.19 Stay suture on the left lobe for retraction

14.9 Results of Robotic Liver Surgery

Interest in robotic liver resections dates back to 2008 when Choi et al. published their first series of four liver left lobectomies [14]. After this report, several series have been published investigating different aspects of robotic liver surgery [15–19]. The first study comparing laparoscopic and robotic liver resections was conducted by Berber et al. [20] who prospectively compared 9 patients that underwent robotic resection of peripherally located malignant

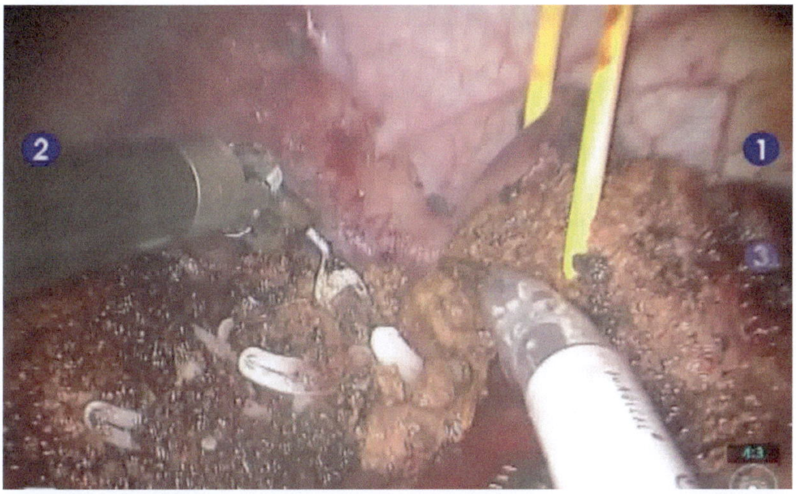

Fig. 14.20 A vessel-loop is used to hang the left lobe

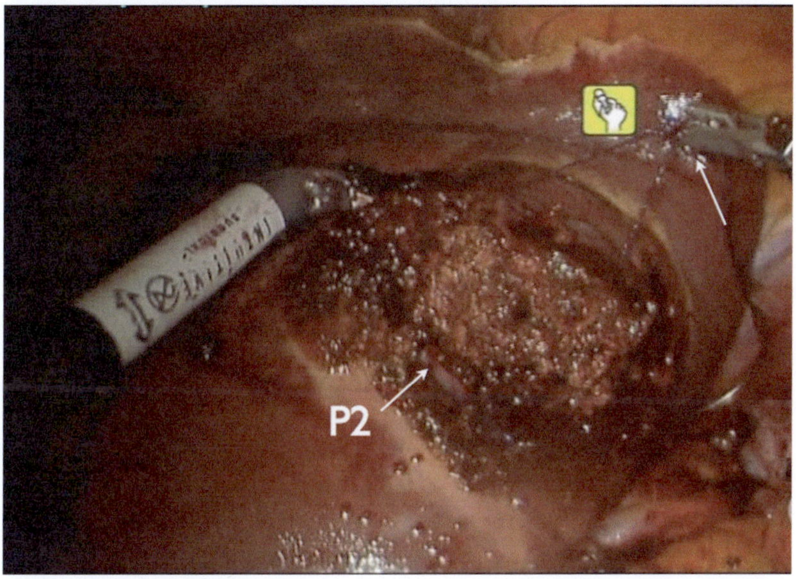

Fig. 14.21 The corkscrew technique at the level of S2

lesions with 23 matched patients that underwent laparoscopic resection at the same institution. The authors did not find significant differences between the two techniques even though robotic resection appeared to be more precise and bloodless [20].

A conceivable explanation to these results can be linked to the selection of patients with a tumor in the peripherally located liver segments. For easily accessible lesions or where there is no vascular involvement, laparoscopy and robotics seem to be equivalent. On the contrary, potential benefits of robotics in laparoscopic liver resections are highlighted approaching lesions located in the PS segments or involving vascular structures and when a complex reconstructive phase is required. Actually, two lines of research can be drawn in the current literature. The first aims to investigate the possibilities of robotics to perform major hepatectomies, even with biliary reconstruction. The other tries to delineate the technical aspects to carry out a robot-assisted parenchyma-sparing surgery. Casciola et al. [10] demonstrated that robotics allows an easy access to the PS segments to carry out parenchymal-saving resections instead of a major hepatectomy even when the tumor is in close contact with a great liver vessel. The use of EndoWrist instruments for parenchymal transection was the main technical trick evidenced in this study. Reproducing a traditional Kelly crush-clamp technique for curved resection planes, made possible to perform liver resections with a maximal parenchymal preservation even for lesions deeply located and in contact with the main liver vessels. Giulianotti et al. recently described the application of robotics in major liver surgery [17, 21]. A total of 24 right hepatectomies were carried out with zero mortality and with a low conversion rate (4.2 %). Postoperative morbidity was acceptable (25 %) with low blood loss. After a mean followup of 34 months, no port-site metastases were described among the oncologic cases. In the same center the da Vinci robotic system was used to complete complex biliary reconstructions with curative and palliative intent [16]. Asian surgeons achieved same results reporting series with a high rate of major hepatectomies [13, 18, 19]. Finally, possible advantages of robotics in hepatobiliary surgery are going to be delineated but prospective controlled studies involving a large number of patients are required for definitive results.

References

1. Torzilli G, Montorsi M, Del Fabbro D et al (2006) Ultrasonographically guided surgical approach to liver tumours involving the hepatic veins close to the caval confluence. Br J Surg 93(10):1238–1246
2. Torzilli G, Montorsi M, Donadon M et al (2005) Radical but conservative is the main goal for ultrasonography-guided liver resection: prospective validation of this approach. J Am Coll Surg 201(4):517–528
3. Torzilli G, Procopio F, Cimino M et al (2010) Anatomical segmental and subsegmental resection of the liver for hepatocellular carcinoma: a new approach by means of ultrasound-guided vessel compression. Ann Surg 251(2):229–235
4. Gold JS, Are C, Kornprat P et al (2008) Increased use of parenchymal-sparing surgery for bilateral liver metastases from colorectal cancer is associated with improved mortality without change in oncologic outcome: trends in treatment over time in 440 patients. Ann Surg 247(1):109–117
5. Cho JY, Han HS, Yoon YS, Shin SH (2009) Outcomes of laparoscopic liver resection for lesions located in the right side of the liver. Arch Surg 144(1):25–29
6. Patriti A, Ceribelli C, Ceccarelli G et al (2012) Noncirrhotic liver tolerance to intermittent inflow occlusion during laparoscopic liver resection. Updates Surg 64(2):87–93
7. Volonte F, Pugin F, Bucher P et al (2011) Augmented reality and image overlay navigation with OsiriX in laparoscopic and robotic surgery: not only a matter of fashion. J Hepatobiliary Pan 18(4):506–509
8. Schneider CM, Peng PD, Taylor RH et al (2012) Robotassisted laparoscopic ultrasonography for hepatic surgery. Surgery 151(5):756–762
9. Brouwer OR, Buckle T, Bunschoten A et al (2012) Image navigation as a means to expand the boundaries of fluorescence-guided surgery. Phys Med Biol 57(10):3123–3136
10. Casciola L, Patriti A, Ceccarelli G et al (2011) Robot-assisted parenchymal-sparing liver surgery including lesions located in the posterosuperior segments. Surg Endosc 25(12):3815–3824
11. Patriti A, Ceccarelli G, Bartoli A, Casciola L (2011) Extracorporeal pringle maneuver in robot-assisted liver surgery. Surg Laparo Endo Per 21(5): e242–e244
12. Gurusamy KS, Pamecha V, Sharma D, Davidson BR (2009) Techniques for liver parenchymal transection in liver resection. Cochrane Database Syst Rev (1):CD006880. doi:10.1002/14651858.CD006880.pub2
13. Choi GH, Choi SH, Kim SH et al (2012) Robotic liver resection: technique and results of 30 consecutive procedures. Surg Endosc 26(8):2247–2258
14. Choi SB, Park JS, Kim JK et al (2008) Early experiences of robotic-assisted laparoscopic liver resection. Yonsei Med J 49(4):632–638
15. Patriti A, Ceccarelli G, Bartoli A et al (2009) Laparoscopic and robot-assisted one-stage resection of colorectal cancer with synchronous liver metastases: a pilot study. J Hepatobiliary Pan 16(4):450–457
16. Giulianotti PC, Sbrana F, Bianco FM, Addeo P (2010) Robot-assisted laparoscopic extended right hepatectomy with biliary reconstruction. J Laparoendosc Adv S 20(2):159–163

17. Giulianotti PC, Coratti A, Sbrana F et al (2011) Robotic liver surgery: results for 70 resections. Surgery 149(1):29–39
18. Ji WB, Wang HG, Zhao ZM et al (2011) Robotic-assisted laparoscopic anatomic hepatectomy in China: initial experience. Ann Surg 253(2):342–348
19. Wakabayashi G, Sasaki A, Nishizuka S et al (2011) Our initial experience with robotic hepato-biliary-pancreatic surgery. J Hepatobiliary Pan 18(4): 481–487a
20. Berber E, Akyildiz HY, Aucejo F et al (2010) Robotic versus laparoscopic resection of liver tumours. HPB (Oxford) 12(8):583–586
21. Giulianotti PC, Sbrana F, Coratti A et al (2011) Totally robotic right hepatectomy: surgical technique and outcomes. Arch Surg 146(7):844–850

Trends and Future Prospects in the Use of Ultrasound in Liver Surgery 15

Guido Torzilli, Matteo Donadon, and Matteo Cimino

IOUS is the current method of choice for staging hepatic tumors, and improvements in sensitivity and specificity are expected by adding CEIOUS. Through IOUS, the surgeon can adequately understand the anatomy of the liver and the relations between tumors and intrahepatic vessels: crucial information for planning the resection. In this sense, the biggest strength of IOUS is in its guiding of the surgeon's hands in real time during liver parenchyma dissection. Further efforts to spread its use by means of education may help to more widely establish the different variants of this technique, as elaborated throughout this book, and to develop new applications.

15.1 Diagnosis and Staging

Contrast agents will most likely contribute in maintaining IOUS as reference standards for the purpose of tumor staging (as elaborated in Chaps. 5 and 6), irrespective of progress made in preoperative imaging. Further advances in unenhanced flow analysis may lead to the point of no longer requiring the injection of contrast agent (Fig. 15.1).

In the short term, one can expect the further spread of a combination of IOUS with such new technologies as fluorescent imaging, providing more crucial information for disease staging. Also, elastography has attracted the interest of many physicians for its potential in differentiating lesions based on their stiffness (Fig. 15.2a, b).

15.2 Surgical Strategy and Resection Guidance

Elastography may become beneficial not only for lesion differentiation but also may provide real-time information to help in defining the surgical strategy in terms of entity of parenchymal removal. It can be applied to evaluate liver stiffness intraoperatively, as the relation between the latter and the hepatic functional reserve are relevant in predicting the surgical risk [1, 2]. Preoperative evaluation together with elastography can add further information in defining the surgical strategy, allowing a more conservative operation in case the stiffness was preoperatively underestimated.

Further technical developments and dissemination of the navigation systems are also to be expected. However, they currently remain costly and feature a complex "plug and play", which limits their wide-spread use and, accordingly, their clinical relevance. New ultrasound

G. Torzilli (✉) · M. Donadon · M. Cimino
Department of Hepatobiliary Surgery,
University of Milan-School of Medicine,
Humanitas Research Hospital-IRCCS,
Via A. Manzoni 56, 20089 Rozzano, MI, Italy
e-mail: guido.torzilli@humanitas.it;
guido.torzilli@unimi.it

G. Torzilli (ed.), *Ultrasound-Guided Liver Surgery*,
DOI: 10.1007/978-88-470-5510-0_15, © Springer-Verlag Italia 2014

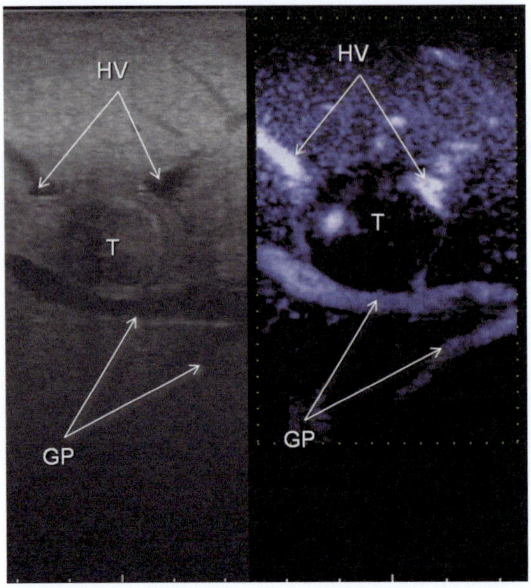

Fig. 15.1 Progress in flow ultrasound imaging may soon provide a contrast enhancement effect (*on the right*) without using any injected contrast agent; tumor (*T*); glissonian pedicle (*GP*); hepatic vein (*HV*)

systems, which can match in real time the preoperative imaging of CT and MRI with IOUS will improve intraoperative navigation modalities providing more simple and low-cost solutions than those currently proposed (Fig. 15.3a, b). They facilitate the interpretation of ultrasound images and thus the planning of the surgical strategy. Navigation with matched preoperative imaging will help to improve the detection of lesions otherwise not well visible by IOUS, as isoechoic lesions (Fig. 15.4). Similarly, navigation with matched imaging done prior to medical treatment will probably guide removal of those CLMs having disappeared after chemotherapy.

Such potential advancement can improve the role of IOUS guidance during liver resection. As described in this monograph, the aim is to guarantee, wherever possible, both anatomical and limited resection with a radical intent: this is relevant both for the effectiveness of the surgical treatment as for its safety. Without IOUS guidance, operations may involve useless major resections or inversely could result in incomplete tumor removal. The techniques of liver resection based on ultrasound guidance as herein extensively described show that for selected patients it is possible to closely approach the tumor burden without increasing the risk of incomplete removal or local recurrence [3]. Therefore, new oncological concepts are introduced. For HCC, tumor exposure on the cut surface does not contradict a full anatomical resection with respect to the oncological requirements for this kind of tumor [4], and this has been confirmed through several cases [5–7]. For CLM, getting closer to the tumor burden under IOUS guidance, even exposing it, is not in contradiction with a concept of radical surgery, at least not in cases that are not amenable by other approaches. Indeed, there is no increase in the risk of local recurrence and similar survival rates are observed [8–12].

An additional point of view in surgical practice introduced by IOUS consists in a new management concept of carriers of tumors that are at risk of compromised liver outflow. CFIOUS enables the disclosure of anatomical features otherwise not recognizable, such as the communicating veins [13], and has opened up new technical solutions allowing the introduction of new operation procedures [14–16]. This allows a more conservative approach to conditions that previously required major resections, complex and at-risk vascular reconstructions, or were even unsuitable for surgery. Further improvement of CFIOUS technology and the combination of IOUS with such new tools as fluorescent imaging can improve the information level. Also, the relation between degree of congestion and liver function based on fluorescence imaging during liver transplantions may allow new scenarios by having available additional criteria for

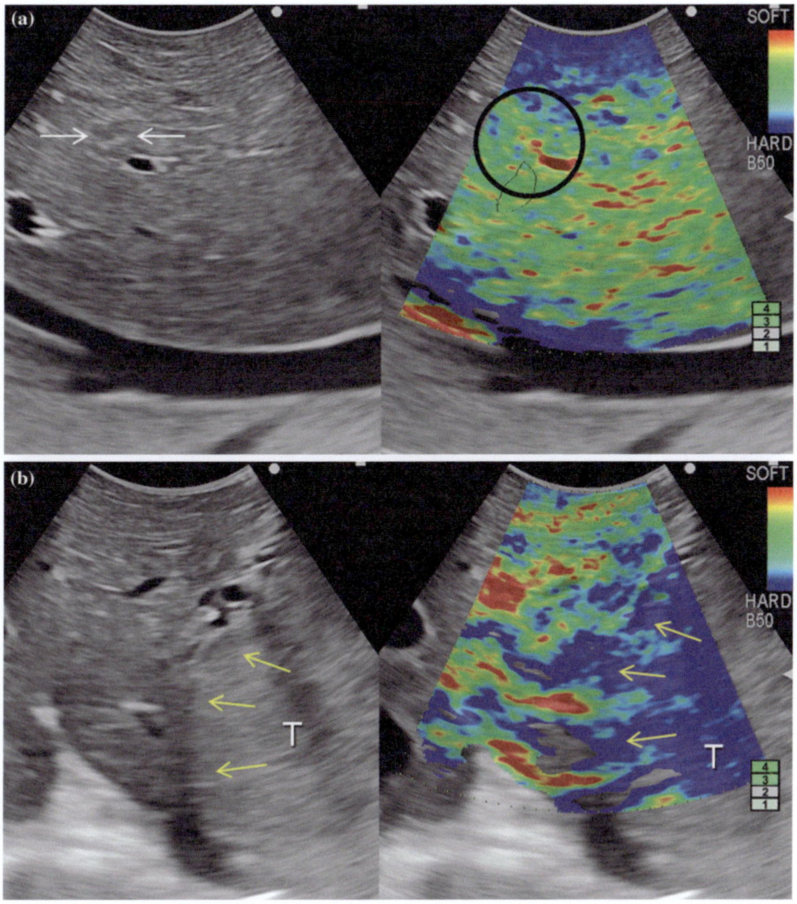

Fig. 15.2 **a** Based on the color scale on the upper right of the picture (soft is *red* and hard is *blue*) a hemangioma (*arrows*) as already seen in Chap. 4 almost remains invisible compared to the surrounding parenchyma (*black circle*) once elastography is activated; **b** inversely, the margins of a hepatocellular carcinoma (*yellow arrows*) grossly correspond with the blue area at elastography, meaning an increased stiffness compared to the surrounding parenchyma; tumor (*T*)

establishing whether intraoperatively detected communicating veins are sufficiently functional to decide whether to vicariate the hepatic vein to be resected or not.

This means that, with IOUS guidance it is possible to perform conservative but radical hepatectomies, and then to expand the surgical indications. With this approach the rate of major hepatectomies has been limited to 8 % in patients with tumors involving one or more hepatic veins close to their caval confluence, without performing any related vascular reconstruction [17], and to 4 % in patients with mutiple bilobar CLM with removal of up to 49 lesions at once [9]. Limitation of major hepatectomy has also been applied to advanced HCC, with less than 1 % mortality and improved long-term outcome [5]. Because this approach reduces the rate of major hepatectomies, the need for interventions such as preoperative PVE, adopted to prevent liver failure after major removal of liver parenchyma could be drastically reduced [18].

Therefore, in spite of the need for large exposure of the organ, IOUS-guided liver surgery should be considered a minimal invasive procedure having as main target just the sparing of the liver parenchyma, and its absolute safety is paradigmatic of what has been just affirmed: organ-targeted minimal invasion. Mostly because of that, surgery is still considered the treatment of choice for the majority of liver tumors in spite of the development and progress in other local

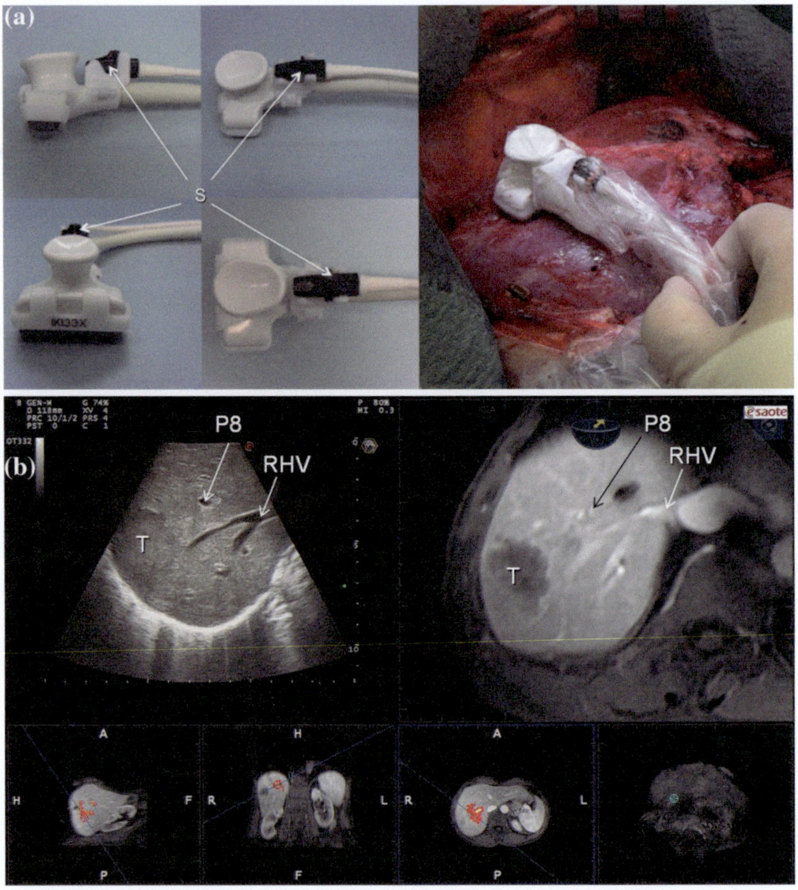

Fig. 15.3 **a** Ultrasound navigation using dedicated sensors (*S*) to read the movement of the probe; **b** combination of the ultrasound image with those of the computed tomography (*CT*) or the magnetic resonance (*MRI*) which are elaborated to reproduce exactly the ultrasound scan: this may facilitate the reading of the IOUS image while exploring the liver; portal branch to segment 8 (*P8*); right hepatic vein (*RHV*); tumor (*T*)

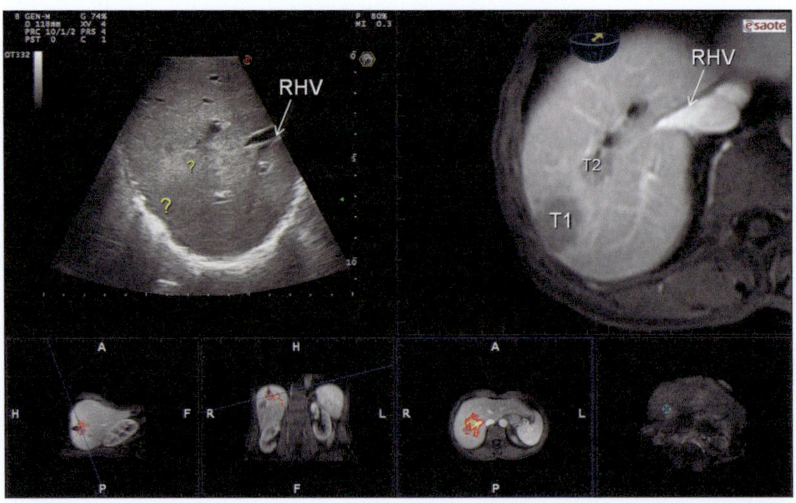

treatments such as ablation therapies and intravascular procedures. Furthermore, the of IOUS for expanding the indications for tumor removal, paradoxically, is in opposite trend with the introduction of ultrasound itself for guiding intraoperative tumor ablation. As a matter of fact, stressing the use of IOUS for guidance, it is possible to expand the surgical indications for HCC and CLM without recurring in any case to ablation treatment [5, 9]; the latter being certainly less radical than tumor removal [19, 20].

15.2.1 Laparoscopic Approach

Liver resections as discussed in the preceding chapters allow the combination of broad indications with a high level of safety, while they do demand large incisions with extensive mobilization and complex dissection plans. These requirements are opposite to the background motivating the anterior approach with or without a hanging maneuver [21, 22], promoted for reducing the need for mobilization, and even to that of laparoscopic hepatic surgery, introduced for reducing the length of the abdominal incisions. On the other hand, the complex IOUS-guided maneuvers herein described, and the complex dissection plans herein shown seem to be difficult to be transferred, at least at the highest levels of precision and safety, laparoscopically. However, perhaps for less complex presentations, the radical but conservative philosophy behind the advanced use of IOUS in open liver surgery, may find in the near future further acceptance in minimal access surgery. In this sense, our initial experience with a LUS-guided, radical, but conservative approach has shown some potential in reducing the sacrifice of parenchyma in conditions of tumor-vessel contact, which otherwise would have demanded, especially by minimal access, more extensive tissue removal (Fig. 15.5a–g). As hinted in this monograph, establishing this approach in laparoscopic or robotic minimal access liver surgery will be a challenge for hepatic surgeons once they have learned to appreciate the merits of using IOUS in liver surgery.

15.3 Educational

Education and training are of paramount importance for improving surgical outcomes. Postgraduate courses in IOUS and technologies devoted to interpreting ultrasound semiology have been introduced and their further implementation is expected. The educational introduction of navigation technology matching preoperative imaging and IOUS will hopefully help to improve the learning curve of surgeons in interpreting ultrasound images by having available the comparison in real time with CT and MRI scans (Fig. 15.6a, b): at the point where the system will be able to recognize matching processes as the modifications induced to the organ by the operating surgeon during handling, which is now still the weak point (Fig. 15.6c), this modality will become strongly established in clinical practice.

Surely, the complex 3D ultrasound images are difficult to interpret (Fig. 15.7a, b) even by expert surgeons, adding further complexity for the trainees. On the other hand, as repeatedly mentioned, most of the skill in transferring the ultrasound findings into surgical maneuvers comes from the capability of the surgeon to assemble in his mind a 3D picture of what the IOUS images show and what his hands are feeling. Thus, some experts perceive 3D IOUS as not really needed.

The future challenge should be to adequately educate and train young surgeons in ultrasound, particularly in the hepatic practice. Acceptance can be fostered by making available new ultrasound systems that are small and Wi-Fi connected to the probes for easier handling,

◀ **Fig. 15.4** Ultrasound navigation can be useful in disclosing lesions which are not well visible by IOUS, such as those that disappear after chemotherapy (combining the imaging done before chemotherapy) or that are isoechoic at intraoperative exploration (?) but well visible in preoperative imaging (*T1, T2*), for which the margin disclosure is helpful for defining the surgical strategy; right hepatic vein (*RHV*)

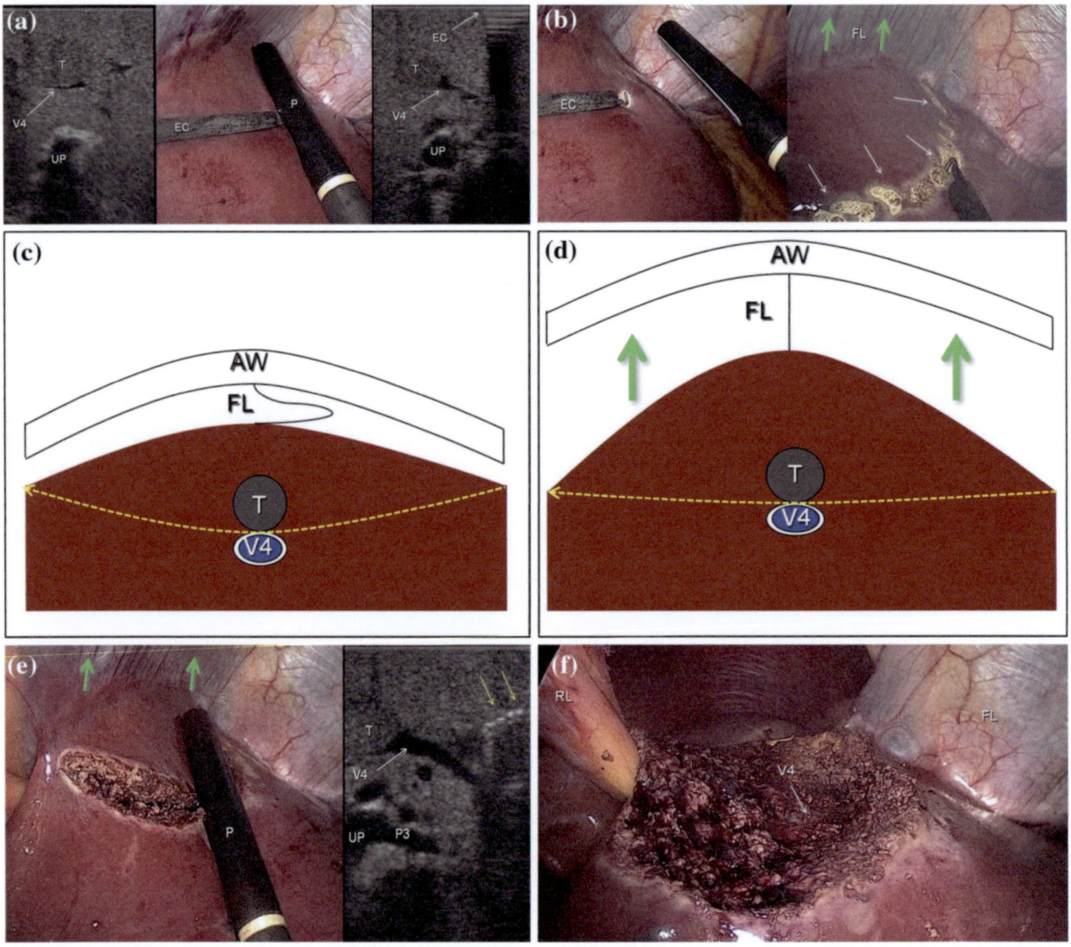

Fig. 15.5 A radical but conservative approach may be suitable also during laparoscopic surgery (at least for less complex conditions) introducing a maneuver that is thought useful for this purpose: then, an isoechoic tumor (*T*) in contact with the scissural vein (*V4*) at the edge between segments 2–3 and segment 4, and above the umbilical portion (*UP*), is selectively removed. **a** The edge of the resection area is marked under LUS guidance; **b** this is achieved by taking advantage of the lifted liver (*green arrows*) provided by the preserved falciform ligament (*FL*); **c–d** schematically the falciform ligament is under tension by the pneumoperitoneum and lifts the liver modifying slightly its profile and in fact straightening the virtual dissection plane (*dashed yellow arrow*); **e** therefore dissection (*yellow arrows*) proceeds easily under LUS guidance just passing in between the lesion and the hepatic vein; **f** resection is then carried out conservatively; abdominal wall (*AW*); electrocautery (*EC*); portal branch to segment 3 (*P3*); round ligament (*RL*)

providing real-time educational options such as direct web transmission, and by combining various imaging methods and elaborating images in a more readable format. For now, we hope to have at least succeeded in convincing the reader of the usefulness of these techniques and have encouraged surgeons in becoming more confident with their use in the clinical practice.

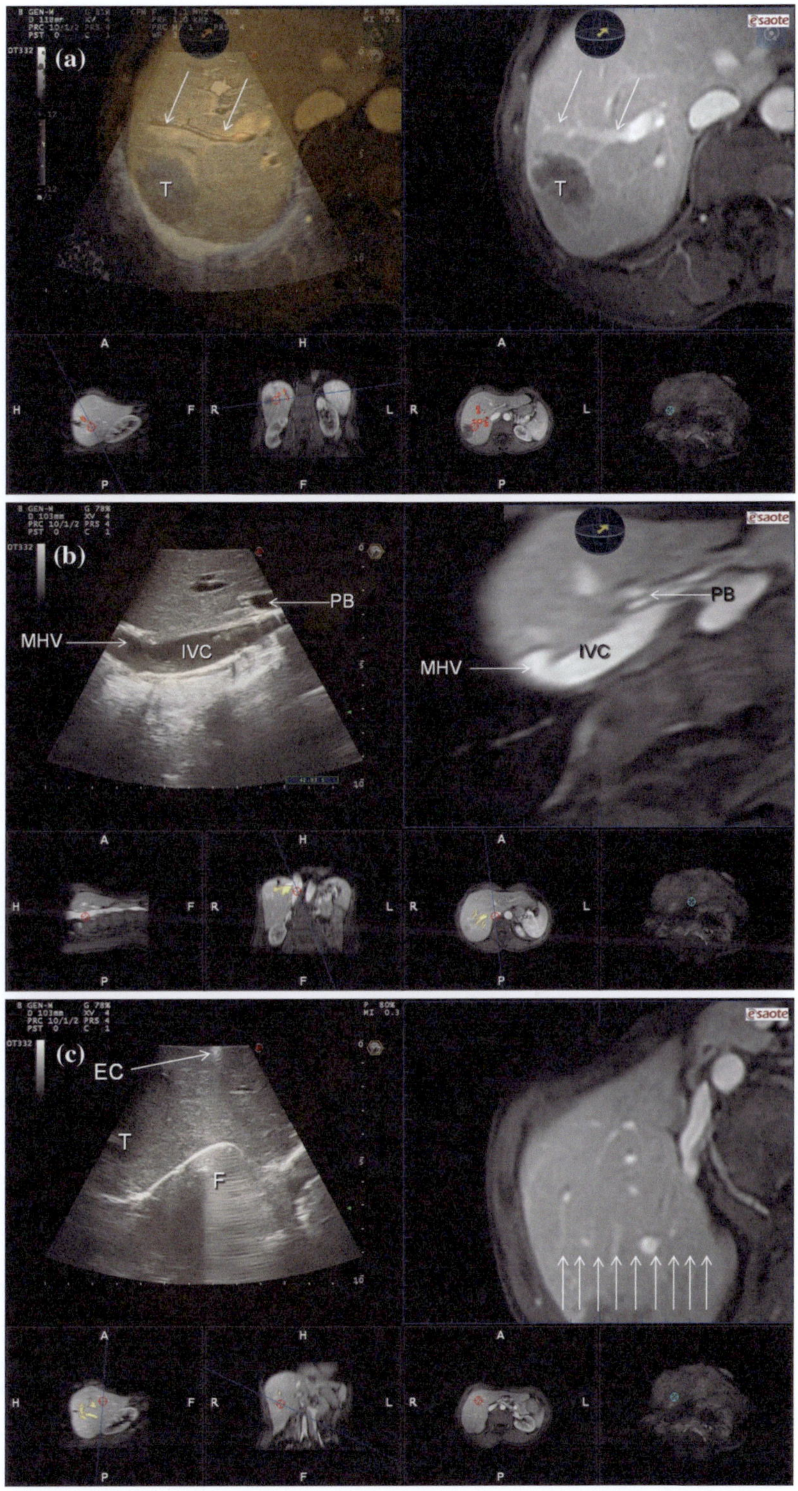

Fig. 15.6 **a** Matching IOUS and preoperative imaging is accurate and can be confirmed overlapping the images provided by both tools (*on the left*), and confirming the structure visualized simultaneously as a branch of the right hepatic vein in the example herein shown (*arrows*); **b** moreover, scans unfeasible with normal imaging can follow those provided by IOUS; **c** the future challenge for the systems will be to read the modification in the shape of the organ induced by the surgeon handling the liver, which nowadays are not taken: the *arrows on the right* indicate the missed repositioning of the MRI image of the liver; electrocautery (*EC*); fingertip (*F*); inferior vena cava (*IVC*); middle hepatic vein (*MHV*); portal bifurcation (*PB*); tumor (*T*)

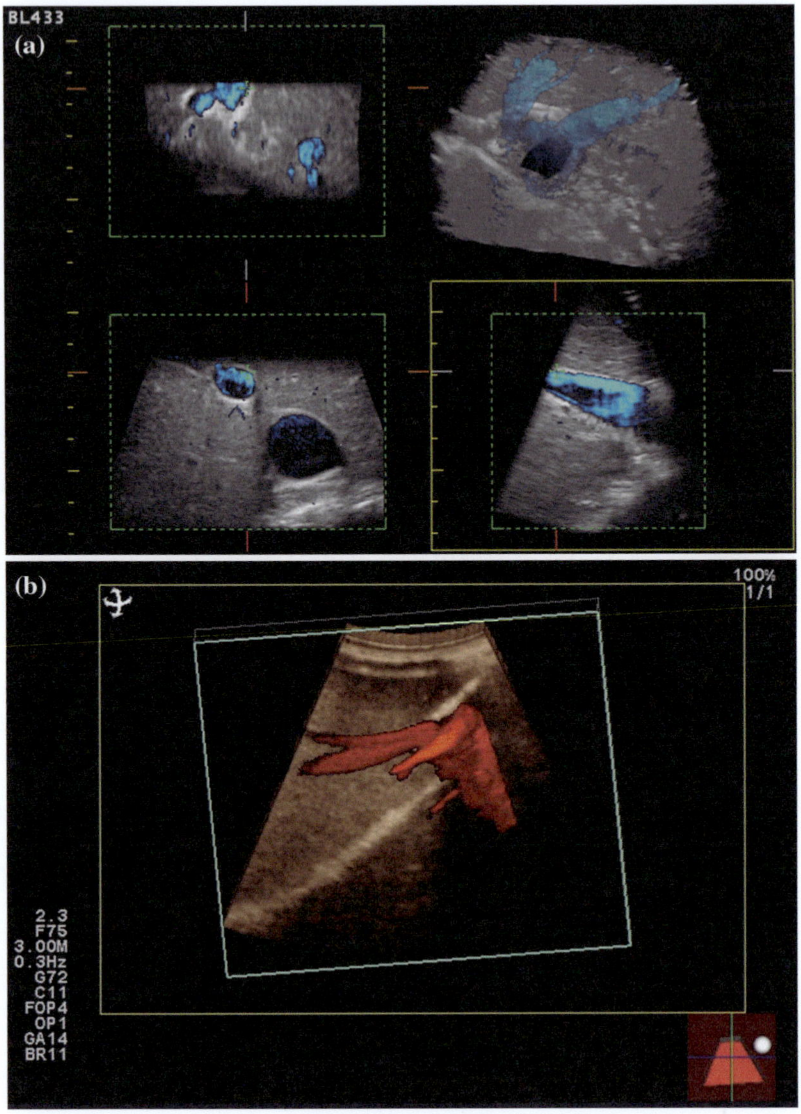

Fig. 15.7 3D ultrasound with all planes disclosed (**a**) and its reconstruction (**b**); the images are hard to interpret and thus of limited usefulness, where they actually should be able to facilitate the comprehension of the anatomical features

References

1. Kusaka K, Harihara Y, Torzilli G et al (2000) Objective evaluation of liver consistency to estimate hepatic fibrosis and functional reserve for hepatectomy. J Am Coll Surg 191(1):47–53
2. Cescon M, Colecchia A, Cucchetti A et al (2012) Value of transient elastography measured with FibroScan in predicting the outcome of hepatic resection for hepatocellular carcinoma. Ann Surg 256(5):706–712
3. Torzilli G, Montorsi M, Donadon M et al (2005) Radical but conservative is the main goal for ultrasonography-guided liver resection: prospective validation of this approach. J Am Coll Surg 201:517–528
4. Torzilli G, Donadon M, Montorsi M (2007) The surgical margin in liver resection for hepatocellular carcinoma: a real problem or not? Ann Surg 246(4):690–691
5. Torzilli G, Donadon M, Marconi M et al (2008) Hepatectomy for stage B and stage C hepatocellular carcinoma in the Barcelona clinic liver cancer classification: results of a prospective analysis. Arch Surg 143:1082–1090
6. Matsui Y, Terakawa N, Satoi S et al (2007) Postoperative outcomes in patients with hepatocellular carcinomas resected with exposure of the tumor surface: clinical role of the no-margin resection. Arch Surg 142:596–602

7. Ochiai T, Takayama T, Inoue K et al (1999) Hepatic resection with and without surgical margins for hepatocellular carcinoma in patients with impaired liver function. Hepatogastroenterology 46:1885–1889
8. Minagawa M, Makuuchi M, Torzilli G et al (2000) Extension of the frontiers of surgical indications in the treatment of liver metastases from colorectal cancer: long-term results. Ann Surg 231:487–499
9. Torzilli G, Procopio F, Botea F et al (2009) One-stage ultrasonographically guided hepatectomy for multiple bilobar colorectal metastases: a feasible and effective alternative to the 2-stage approach. Surgery 146:60–71
10. Pawlik TM, Scoggins CR, Zorzi D et al (2005) Effect of surgical margin status on survival and site of recurrence after hepatic resection for colorectal metastases. Ann Surg 241:715–722
11. Kokudo N, Miki Y, Sugai S et al (2002) Genetic and histological assessment of surgical margins in resected liver metastases from colorectal carcinoma: minimum surgical margins for successful resection. Arch Surg 137:833–840
12. de Haas RJ, Wicherts DA, Flores E et al (2008) R1 resection by necessity for colorectal liver metastases: is it still a contraindication to surgery? Ann Surg 248:626–637
13. Torzilli G, Garancini M, Donadon M et al (2010) Intraoperative ultrasonographic detection of communicating veins between adjacent hepatic veins during hepatectomy for tumours at the hepatocaval confluence. Br J Surg 97:1867–1873
14. Torzilli G, Donadon M, Marconi M et al (2008) Systematic extended right posterior sectionectomy: a safe and effective alternative to right hepatectomy. Ann Surg 247:603–611
15. Torzilli G, Palmisano A, Procopio F et al (2010) A new systematic small for size resection for liver tumors invading the middle hepatic vein at its caval confluence: mini-mesohepatectomy. Ann Surg 251:33–39
16. Torzilli G, Procopio F, Donadon M et al (2012) Upper transversal hepatectomy. Ann Surg Oncol 19(11):3566
17. Torzilli G, Montorsi M, Del Fabbro D et al (2006) Ultrasonographically guided surgical approach to liver tumours involving the hepatic veins close to the caval confluence. Br J Surg 93:1238–1246
18. Torzilli G, Donadon M, Palmisano A et al (2009) Ultrasound guided liver resection: does this approach limit the need for portal vein embolization? Hepatogastroenterology 56:1483–1490
19. Abdalla EK, Vauthey JN, Ellis LM et al (2004) Recurrence and outcomes following hepatic resection, radiofrequency ablation, and combined resection/ablation for colorectal liver metastases. Ann Surg 239:818–825
20. N'Kontchou G, Mahamoudi A, Aout M et al (2009) Radiofrequency ablation of hepatocellular carcinoma: long-term results and prognostic factors in 235 Western patients with cirrhosis. Hepatology 50:1475–1483
21. Liu CL, Fan ST, Cheung ST et al (2006) Anterior approach versus conventional approach right hepatic resection for large hepatocellular carcinoma: a prospective randomized controlled study. Ann Surg 244:194–203
22. Ogata S, Belghiti J, Varma D et al (2007) Two hundred liver hanging maneuvers for major hepatectomy: a single-center experience. Ann Surg 245:31–35

Index

A
Abdominal incision, 117
Abdominal surgery, 164
Aberrant duct, 33
Ablation, 51, 141
Ablation therapies, 271
About staging laparoscopies, 217
Accessory duct, 33
Accessory hepatic veins, 80
Accuracy, 222
Adhesions, 15, 51, 125
Agreement between the two procedures, 222
Air bubbles, 129
Anatomical resection, 268
Anatomic structure, 219
Anechoic, 43
Anesthesiologist, 56
Anterior approach, 150, 271
Arantius ligament, 125
Arterial elements, 25
Arterial phase, 57
Artifacts, 28

B
Background liver, 125
Balloon catheter, 141
Barcelona Clinic Liver Cancer (BCLC), 231
Bare area, 122
Bile duct, 18, 33, 219
Bile duct dilation, 77
Bile duct drainage, 169
Bile duct resection, 169
Bile ducts are dilatated, 219
Bile leak, 203, 253
Biliary, 169
Biliary complications, 169, 203
Biliary elements, 25
Bilobar liver metastases, 254
Biopsy, 45
Black-hole effect, 60
Bright liver, 62
Brisbane terminology, 17, 25

C
Calcified pattern, 49
Camera system, 250
Cantlie's line, 143
Capsulated HCC, 77
Carbon dioxide, 55
Caudate lobe, 130
Caval confluence, 16, 269
Characterization, 218
Chemotherapy, 48, 62
Cirrhotic appearance, 55
Cirrhotic liver, 15, 51, 128
Clamping, 80
Clots, 148
Color flow modes (CFIOUS), 10, 87, 268
Color-Doppler, 9
Colorectal liver metastases (CLM), 45, 55, 79, 126, 249, 268
Communicating veins (CV), 79
Compression maneuvers, 10
Computed tomography (CT), 158, 268
Condoms, 52
Congestion, 268
Contrast agent, 9, 267
Contrast-enhanced IOUS (CEIOUS), 4, 45, 267
Contrast-enhanced laparoscopic ultrasound, 244
Contrast enhancement, 43
Convex, 5
Cooling technique, 232
Corkscrew technique, 260
Coronary ligament, 125

G. Torzilli (ed.), *Ultrasound-Guided Liver Surgery*,
DOI: 10.1007/978-88-470-5510-0, © Springer-Verlag Italia 2014

Counterstaining technique, 130
Cut surfaces, 148
Cystic lesions, 62

D
Da Vinci Si platform, 251
Detection, 43
Detection of known lesions, 218
Diastolic flow, 185
Differentiation, 43
Disclosure of additional nodules, 218
Dissection plane, 63
Dissection plans, 271
Domino transplantation, 197
3D screen, 251
Ducts, 33
Dysplastic nodules, 57

E
Early HCC, 59
Echoes, 3
Echogenic line, 148
Echogenicity, 59
Echoprobes, 4
Elastography, 45, 267
Electrocautery, 131
Electromagnetic sensor, 164
Endoscopic column, 250
EndoWrist bipolar precise forceps, 257
EndoWrist instruments, 250
Expert surgeons, 121
Exposure, 117
Extranodular growth, 127

F
Falciform ligament, 15, 28, 141
Finger compressing, 80
Finger compression, 125
Flashlight display, 252
Flex Focus 800 Ultrasound system, 252
Flexible tip, 8
Fluorescent imaging, 52, 267
Focus level, 43
Free-hand technique, 128

G
Gain, 43
Galactose shell, 55
Gauze, 148
Glisson's capsule, 17
Glissonian pedicle, 77
Glissonian skeleton, 25
Gloves, 52
Gray scale, 43
Guidance to surgical procedures, 217

H
HA stenosis, 189
Hanging, 117
Hanging maneuver, 271
Head-and-neck surgery, 164
Hemangioma, 45
Hepatic artery, 130
Hepatic artery complications, 185
Hepatic hilum, 125
Hepatic vein, 15, 25, 78, 269
Hepatic veins confluence, 222
Hepatocaval confluence, 25, 254
Hepatocellular Carcinoma (HCC), 45, 55, 76, 126, 231, 249, 268
Hepatofugal blood flow, 80
Hepatopetal, 80
Hepatospecific, 12, 55
High-frequency probe, 16
Hilar dissection, 143
Hitachi Aloka, 252
Hooking, 130
Hooking technique, 141
HV stenosis or thrombosis, 197
Hyperechoic shadow, 43
Hypoechoic, 43, 55

I
Indigo carmine dye, 128
Indocyanine green dye, 253
Indocyanine green (ICG), 52
Indocyanine green (ICG) fluorescence imaging, 174
Inferior right hepatic vein (IRHV), 25, 80
Inferior vena cava (IVC), 88, 123, 222
Inflow, 16, 75
Infrared-based optical line, 158
Infrared camera, 175
Inspection, 15
Intercostal space, 253
Interdigital, 5
Intermittent inflow occlusion, 256
Intermittent Pringle maneuver, 257
Interstitial treatments, 226
Interventional procedure, 231
Intrahepatic biliary tree, 31
Intrahepatic vascular occlusion, 241
Intraoperative cholangiography (IOC), 169
Intraoperative planning of the operation, 222
Intraoperative ultrasonography, 250
Intraoperative ultrasound (IOUS), 3
Intravascular contrast agents, 55
Intravascular procedures, 271
Isoechogenicity, 60

Isoechoic, 48, 55
IVC stenosis or thrombosis, 197

J
J-shaped laparotomy, 121
J-shaped thoracophrenolaparotomy, 121
J-shaped thoracophrenolapatotomic, 90

K
Kelly crush-clamp technique, 257, 264
Keyboard, 10, 15
Kupffer cells, 55

L
Laparoscopic cholecystectomy, 174
Laparoscopic liver resection, 251
Laparoscopic liver surgery, 217
Laparoscopic port, 8
Laparoscopic surgery, 249
Laparoscopic transducers, 8
Laparoscopic ultrasonography, 217
Laparoscopic ultrasound (LUS), 9, 231
Large incisions, 271
Late phase, 57
LCD monitors, 251
Left bile duct, 169
Left hand, 117
Left hemiliver, 131
Left hepatectomy, 33, 47
Left hepatic vein (LHV), 25, 87
The left lateral sectionectomy, 222
Left portal pedicles, 254
Left portal vein (LPV), 143
Left-sided hepatectomies, 169
Linear, 5
Liver anatomy, 222
Liver exposure, 75
Liver function, 268
Liver metastases, 232
Liver mobilization, 117
Liver outflow, 268
Liver stiffness, 267
Liver surgery, 232
Liver tunnel, 78
Liver vascular skeleton, 75
Lower inferior hepatectomy, 78

M
Main portal bifurcation, 28
Magnetic resonance (MRI), 158, 268
Major hepatectomy, 75, 169, 249, 269
Major liver surgery, 264
Median incision, 121
Medical robotics, 250
Mesenteric vein, 141
Microbubbles, 11, 55
Microconvex, 5
Microwave (MWA), 231
Mid-low-frequency probe, 16
middle hepatic vein, 226
Middle hepatic vein (MHV), 87, 155, 266
Middle inferior right hepatic vein (MIRHV), 25
Minimal invasive procedure, 269
Minimally invasive surgery, 250
Mirror effect, 43
Mobilization, 75, 271
Mortality, 269
Mosaic, 45
Multinodularity, 60
Mutiple bilobar CLM, 269

N
Navigation systems, 267
2nd order portal branch, 28
Near-infrared imaging, 252
Neo-vascularity, 59
New detected lesions, 218
New nodules, 217, 222
Nonanatomical resection, 225

O
Operative decision making, 59, 75
Optical, 158
Outflow, 17, 75

P
P5-8, 88
Palpation, 15, 75
Paracaval portion, 117
Parachute technique, 146
Parenchymal sparing resections, 75
The parenchymal transection, 222
Patient-side Cart, 250
Percutaneous contrast-enhanced ultrasound (CE-US), 57
Perfluorobutane, 12
Picture-in-picture display, 252
Piezoelectric crystals, 3
P4inf, 88
Planning the liver resection, 224
Plug and play, 267
Portal bifurcation, 254
Portal branch, 15, 29, 80, 222
Portal elements, 25
Portal vein complications, 190
Portal vein (PV), 192
Power-Doppler, 9
Pringle maneuver, 256
ProART Robotic Transducer Type 8826, 252
Probes, 117
Pseudoaneurysms, 189
PVE, 269

R
Radiation risk, 174
Radical but conservative, 271
Radiofrequency (RFA), 231
3rd order portal branch, 28
Regenerative nodules, 57
Relationships between lesions and vasculo-biliary structures, 218
Relationships with vascular and biliary structur, 218
Reliability, 221
Remote control UA1237, 252
Resection area, 63
Resection guidance, 63, 75
Reversal flow, 88
Right anterior glissonean sheat, 82
Right anterior, 76
Right hepatectomies, 264
Right hepatectomy, 47
Right hepatic pedicles, 254
Right hepatic vein (RHV), 29, 155
Right inferior phrenic vein, 123
Right portal branch (RPV), 143
The right posterior, 82
Right posterior section, 86
Right posterior sectional bile duct (B6-7), 33
Right posterolateral sector, 253
Robot-assisted parenchyma-sparing surgery, 263
Robotic liver resections, 262
Robotic liver surgery, 9, 262
Round, 15
Round ligament, 43
Rubber band technique, 261

S
Satellites, 127
Scars, 51
Screen, 10, 15
Second generation, 55
Second-order portal branches, 78
Section, 76
Sectionectomies, 122
Segment, 117
Segment 1, 253
Segmentectomies, 122
Sensitivity, 221
Serpiginous path, 18
Short hepatic vein, 123
Silicon gauze, 148
Simple hepatic cysts, 43
Skip-areas, 43
Small-for-size grafts, 192
Software, 158
Sonazoid, 12
SonoVue, 11, 56
Specificity, 57, 221
Split screen display, 251, 252
Staging of liver diseases, 217
Stained area, 128
Steatotic appearance, 55
Stenosis, 194
1st order portal branch, 28
Stiffness, 45
Stitch, 150
Subsegmentectomies, 122
Sulfur hexafluoride, 11, 56
Surgeon Console, 250
Surgical risk, 267
Surgical strategy, 16, 63
Surgical theater, 165
Systematic segmentectomy, 128

T
Three-dimensional reconstruction, 75
Thrombosis, 185, 192
TilePro software, 251
To mark the planes, 225
Tourniquet, 141
Tracking systems, 158
Tract anatomy, 169
Transducer, 3
Transection plane, 225
Transient ischemia, 131
Trapezoid scanning window, 5
Trendelemburg supine patient, 253
Triangular ligament, 123
T-shaped, 5
Tumor burden, 63
Tumor thrombus, 77, 79, 219
Tumor vascularity, 57
Tumor-vessel relationship, 63, 75

U
Ultrasound color-Doppler, 226
Ultrasound semiology, 271
Ultrasound system, 9, 15, 117
Umbilical portion, 29, 43
Unpaired arteries, 57

V
Vascular reconstruction, 88, 268
Vasculobiliary anomalies, 222
Vein encirclement, 125
Vessel wall, 76
Visual plane, 121

W
Water bath, 165
Wi-Fi, 271
Wound hernias, 122

X
Xiphoid process, 117

MIX
Papier aus verantwortungsvollen Quellen
Paper from responsible sources
FSC® C105338

If you have any concerns about our products,
you can contact us on
ProductSafety@springernature.com

In case Publisher is established outside the EU,
the EU authorized representative is:
Springer Nature Customer Service Center GmbH
Europaplatz 3, 69115 Heidelberg, Germany

Printed by Libri Plureos GmbH
in Hamburg, Germany